Contemporary Pediatric and Adolescent Sports Medicine

Series editor

Lyle J. Micheli, Boston, MA, USA

More information about this series at http://www.springer.com/series/11729

Ruth Solomon · John Solomon
Lyle J. Micheli
Editors

Prevention of Injuries in the Young Dancer

Springer

Editors
Ruth Solomon
University of California
Santa Cruz, CA
USA

John Solomon
Santa Cruz, CA
USA

Lyle J. Micheli
Division of Sports Medicine
Boston Children's Hospital
Boston, MA
USA

ISSN 2198-266X ISSN 2198-2678 (electronic)
Contemporary Pediatric and Adolescent Sports Medicine
ISBN 978-3-319-85553-0 ISBN 978-3-319-55047-3 (eBook)
DOI 10.1007/978-3-319-55047-3

Softcover reprint of the hardcover 1st edition 2017

Printed on acid-free paper

This Springer imprint is published by Springer Nature
The registered company is Springer International Publishing AG
The registered company address is: Gewerbestrasse 11, 6330 Cham, Switzerland

The Micheli Center for Sports Injury Prevention

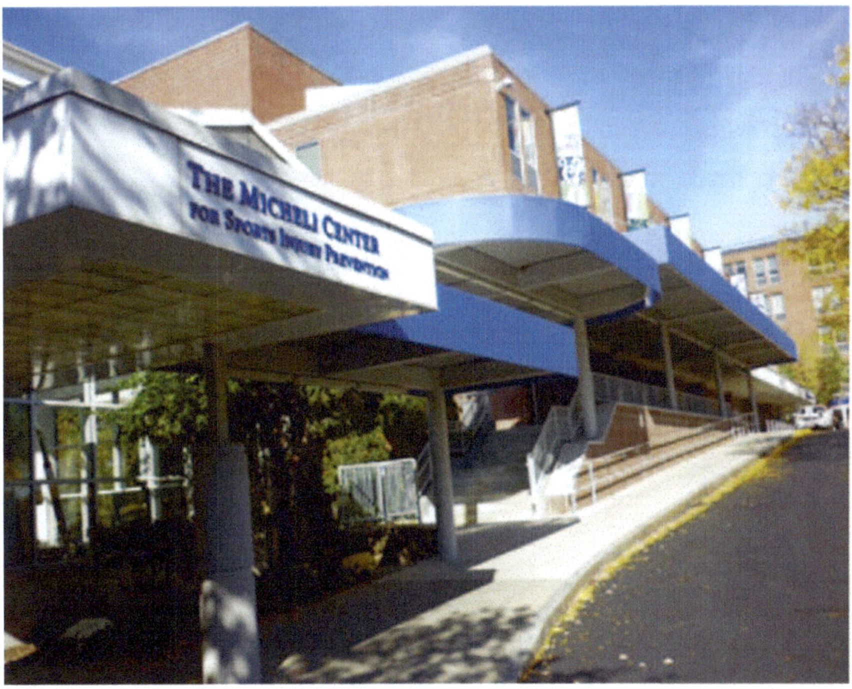

The mission of the Micheli Center for Sports Injury Prevention is at the heart of the *Contemporary Pediatric & Adolescent Sports Medicine series*.

The Micheli Center uses the most up-to-date medical and scientific information to develop practical strategies that help young athletes reduce their risk of injury as they prepare for a healthier future. The clinicians, scientists, activists, and technologists at the Micheli Center advance the field of sports medicine by revealing current injury patterns and risk factors while developing new methods, techniques, and technologies for preventing injuries.

The Micheli Center, named after Lyle J. Micheli, one of the world's pioneers in pediatric and adolescent sports medicine, had its official opening in April 2013. Thus far, The Micheli Center has served more than 2800 athletes and has published more than 100 studies. Dr. Micheli is the series editor of *Contemporary Pediatric & Adolescent Sports Medicine*.

Consistent with Dr. Micheli's professional focus over the past 40 years, The Micheli Center conducts world-class medical and scientific research focused on the prevention of sports injuries and the effects of exercise on health and wellness. In addition, the Micheli Center develops innovative methods of promoting exercise in children.

The Micheli Center opens its doors to anyone seeking a healthier lifestyle, including those with medical conditions or illnesses that may have previously limited their abilities. Fellow clinicians, researchers, and educators are invited to collaborate and discover new ways to prevent, assess, and treat sports injuries.

Series Editor Biography

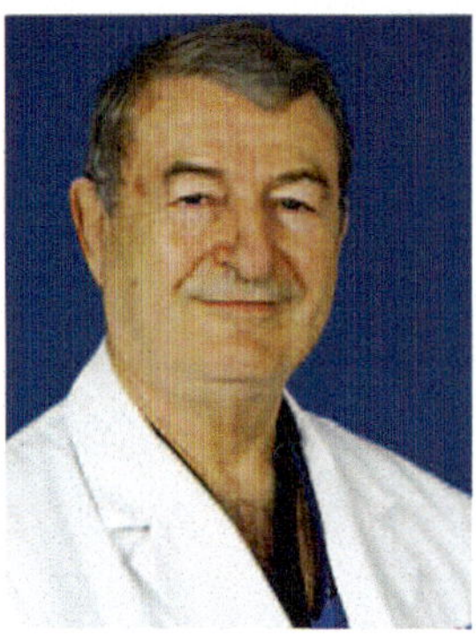

Dr. Lyle J. Micheli is the series editor of *Contemporary Pediatric & Adolescent Sports Medicine*. Dr. Micheli is regarded as one of the pioneers of pediatric and adolescent sports medicine, a field he has been working in since the early 1970s when he co-founded the USA's first sports medicine clinic for young athletes at Boston Children's Hospital.

Dr. Micheli is now director of the Division of Sports Medicine at Boston Children's Hospital, and Clinical Professor of Orthopaedic Surgery at Harvard Medical School. He is a past president of the American College of Sports Medicine and is currently the Secretary General for the International Federation of Sports Medicine. Dr. Micheli co-chaired the International Olympic Committee consensus on the health and fitness of young people through physical activity and sport.

In addition to many other honors, Dr. Micheli has served as Chairperson of the Massachusetts Governor's Committee on Physical Fitness and Sports, on the Board of Directors of the United States Rugby Football Foundation, as Chairman of the USA Rugby Medical and Risk Management Committee, and on the advisory board of the Bay State Games. He served as Attending Physician for the Boston Ballet from 1977–2016 and is Medical Consultant to the Boston Ballet School.

Dr. Micheli received his undergraduate degree from Harvard College in 1962 and his medical degree from Harvard Medical School in 1966. As an undergraduate student, Dr. Micheli was an avid athlete, competing in rugby, gridiron football, and boxing. Since graduating, Dr. Micheli has played prop for various Rugby clubs including, the Boston Rugby Football Club, the Cleveland Blues Rugby Football Club, Washington Rugby Club and Mystic Valley Rugby Club, where he also served as team coach.

Dr. Micheli has authored over 300 scientific articles and reviews related to sports injuries, particularly those sustained by children. His present research activities focus on the prevention of sports injuries in children. Dr. Micheli has edited and authored several major books and textbooks.

Preface

Dear Reader:

We would like to introduce you to this book by way of a brief word to and about the authors represented here. These are all MDs or PTs who have taken time out from their extremely busy practices to compose the chapters you will be reading, and for that we are eternally grateful. You should also know that the majority of them are affiliated with the newly opened Micheli Center for the Prevention of Sports Injuries, in Waltham, MA. This highlights two important points: First, that dance is finally in the process of being recognized, from the standpoint of both medical and dance personnel, as a form of athletic activity. What this means to the dance community is that it is increasingly enjoying access to the extensive resources of sports medicine. Hence, if you are a dancer, or the parent of a dancer, and should make your way to the Micheli Center, you might well find yourself in the hands of one of our authors and can be confident that he or she will be fully conversant with your needs.

Second, it is a highly significant development that with the emergence of the Micheli Center the prevention of injuries has been institutionalized for the use of the general public. In essence, the mission of the Center mirrors the screening procedures that are now being implemented in many colleges, universities, conservatories, and some professional dance companies (as described in two chapters of this book), but the majority of dance students still do not have access to programs of that sort. To the best of our knowledge, the Center remains unique as of this date, but its early popularity provides reason to believe that it will soon be replicated elsewhere.

Finally, a cautionary note about the text you are about to encounter. A few of the chapters are laced with medical terminology that may be unfamiliar to you. This is the result of two factors: (1) the need to appeal to both dance and medical readers, who we have assumed would mutually comprise the book's readership, and (2) the fact that the way medical personnel conceive of prevention involves an understanding of the potential injuries that could result from a given activity (like dance), and that kind of understanding can only be communicated in the language of medicine. Each chapter begins with definitions of its key terms, but if this remains an issue for you, our advice is to just stay with it, as brushing up against these terms here can come in handy when faced with an injury.

We salute your interest in keeping young dancers healthy so that they can realize their full potential. As we all know, "prevention is the better part of cure."

Cordially,

Ruth Solomon
John Solomon
Santa Cruz, CA, USA

Contents

Contributors

Derrick D. Brown, MSc Institute of Sport Science/Dance Science, University Bern, Bern, Switzerland; National Centre Performing Arts Onderlangs 9, Arnhem, The Netherlands

Maribeth Crupi, PT Maribeth Crupi Physical Therapy LLC, Wilmington, MA, USA; Physical Therapy LLC, Wilmington, MA, USA

Pierre d'Hemecourt, MD Division of Sports Medicine, Department of Orthopedics, Boston Children's Hospital, Boston, MA, USA

Avery D. Faigenbaum, EdD Department of Health and Exercise Science, The College of New Jersey, Ewing, NJ, USA

Joana L. Fraser, MBChB, BSc Division of Sports Medicine, Department of Orthopedics, Boston Children's Hospital, Boston, MA, USA

Marina G. Gearhart, BA Division of Sports Medicine, Boston Children's Hospital, Boston, MA, USA

Peter G. Gerbino, MD Department of Orthopedic Surgery, Community Hospital of the Monterey Peninsula, Monterey, CA, USA

Sarah Jackson, MD, CSCS Division of Sports Medicine, Department of Orthopedics, Boston Children's Hospital, Boston, MA, USA

Nancy J. Kadel, MD Seattle Dance and Performing Arts Medicine (SeaPAM), Seattle, Washington, USA

Mininder S. Kocher, MD, MPH Division of Sports Medicine, Department of Orthopaedic Surgery, Boston Children's Hospital, Boston, MA, USA

Gregory D. Myer, PhD, FACSM, CSCS*D The Micheli Center for Sports Injury Prevention, Waltham, MA, USA; Division of Sports Medicine, The SPORT Center, Cincinnati Children's Hospital Medical Center, Cincinnati, OH, USA; Departments of Pediatrics and Orthopaedic Surgery, University of Cincinnati, Cincinnati, OH,

USA; Department of Orthopaedics, University of Pennsylvania, Philadelphia, PA, USA

Emily Niu, MD Division of Sports Medicine, Boston Children's Hospital, Boston, MA, USA

Lindsay N. Ramey, MD Physical Medicine and Rehabilitation, Rehabilitation Institute of Chicago, Chicago, IL, USA

Miriam R. Rowan, MS PGSP-Stanford Psy.D. Consortium, Palo Alto, CA, USA

Itzhak Siev-Ner, MD Department of Orthopedic Rehabilitation, Sheba Medical Center, Tel-HaShomer, Tel Aviv, Israel

Ruth Solomon Professor Emerita, Department of Theater Arts, University of California, Santa Cruz, CA, USA

Heather Southwick, PT, MSPT Boston Ballet, Boston, MA, USA

Nili Steinberg, PhD The Wingate College of Physical Education and Sports Sciences, Wingate College, Wingate Institute, Netanya, Israel

Andrea Stracciolini, MD, FAAP, FACSM The Micheli Center for Sports Injury Prevention, Waltham, MA, USA; Division of Sports Medicine, Department of Orthopedics, Boston Children's Hospital, Boston, MA, USA; Division of Emergency Medicine, Department of Medicine, Boston Children's Hospital, Boston, MA, USA

Katherine L. Wilson, MSW Boston Ballet School, Boston, MA, USA

Amy X. Yin, MD Department of Orthopedics, Podiatry, and Sports Medicine, Kaiser Permanente San Leandro Medical Center, San Leandro, CA, USA

Abbreviations

ACL	Anterior cruciate ligament
ACT	Acceptance and commitment therapy
AIIS	Anterior inferior iliac spine
AIS	Adolescent idiopathic scoliosis
AMDQ	Athletic Milieu Direct Questionnaire
AN	Anorexia nervosa
ATFL	Anterior talofibular ligament
BMAD	Bone mineral apparent density
BMC	Bone mineral content
BMD	Bone mineral density
BMI	Body mass index
BN	Bulimia
CFL	Calcaneofibular ligament
DAFT	Dance-specific aerobic fitness test
DJD	Degenerative joint disease
DXA	Dual energy X-ray absorptiometry
ED	Eating disorder
FABER	Flexion-abduction-external rotation
FAI	Femoroacetabular impingement
FAST	Female Athlete Screening Tool
FDL	Flexor digitorum longus
FHL	Flexor hallucis longus
GH	Growth hormone
HCTD	Heritable connective tissue disorders
HR	Heart rate
IP	Interphalangeal
ISIJ	Inferior sacroiliac joint
IT	Iliotibial
ITB	Iliotibial band
KPR Test	Kasch Pulse Recovery Test

LCL	Lateral collateral ligament
LEAF-Q	Low Energy Availability in Females Questionnaire
MCL	Medial collateral ligament
MDD	Major depressive disorder
MPFL	Medial patellofemoral ligament
MTP	Metatarsal phalangeal
NSAIDs	Non-steroidal anti-inflammatory drugs
OSS	Osgood-Schlatter syndrome
PCL	Posterior cruciate ligament
PFPS	Patellofemoral pain syndrome
PRP	Platelet-rich plasma
PSIS	Posterior superior iliac spine
PST	Physiological Screening Test
ROM	Range of motion
SI	Sacroiliac
SIJ	Sacroiliac joint
SLJS	Sinding-Larsen-Johansson syndrome
SLR	Straight leg raise
TLSO	Thoraco-lumbo-sacral orthosis
VMO	Vastus medialus obliquus

Chapter 1
Epidemiology of Injury in the Young Dancer

Lindsay N. Ramey, MD and Amy X. Yin, MD

Pertinent Definitions

Pediatric: The term pediatric is used to describe pre-pubertal (skeletally immature) and pubertal (approaching skeletal maturity) dancers. Studies referenced in this chapter include patients aged 3–20 years. In this chapter the term "child" typically refers to the pre-pubertal group, while the term "adolescent" typically refers to the peri-pubertal or pubertal group.
Airplane test: A functional test for pointe readiness. The trunk is pitched forward and the non-supporting leg is raised straight in extension, bringing the trunk and non-supporting leg into a line parallel to the floor with the pelvis square to the ground. The dancer passes if he/she performs 4 of 5 pliés with arms moving from second position to the floor while maintaining lower extremity alignment.
Sauté test: A functional test for pointe readiness. The dancer passes if he/she performs at least 8 of 16 consecutive single-leg sauté jumps while maintaining neutral pelvis and lower extremity alignment, stable trunk, toe-heel landing, and fully extended knee with pointed foot in the air.

L.N. Ramey, MD
Physical Medicine and Rehabilitation, Rehabilitation Institute of Chicago,
345 E. Superior Street, Chicago, IL 60611, USA
e-mail: lnr8t@virginia.edu; lramey@ric.org

A.X. Yin, MD (✉)
Department of Orthopedics, Podiatry, and Sports Medicine,
Kaiser Permanente San Leandro Medical Center, 2500 Merced Street,
San Leandro, CA 94577, USA
e-mail: amy.x.yin@kp.org

R. Solomon et al. (eds.), *Prevention of Injuries in the Young Dancer*,
Contemporary Pediatric and Adolescent Sports Medicine,
DOI 10.1007/978-3-319-55047-3_1

Topple test: A functional test for pointe readiness. The dancer passes if she performs a pirouette en dehors from fourth position with the gesture leg in full retiré and the support leg fully extended while maintaining a vertical trunk and demonstrating a controlled landing.
Soft tissue injury: Damage to muscles, tendons, or ligaments throughout the body.
Strain: An injury to muscles or tendons that causes fibers to be stretched and/or torn.
Sprain: An injury to one or more of the ligaments that support a joint.
Tendon injury: Includes tendinitis (acute inflammatory tendon injury), tendinosis (chronic tendon injury with cellular degeneration and no inflammation), and tendinopathy (chronic tendon injury of any etiology). Specific examples in this chapter include groin, ankle, and foot (pedis) tendon injury.
Jumper's knee: Patellar tendon injury resulting in pain at the anterior, inferior knee.
Bony injury: Injury to bone or cartilage.
Growth plate or physis: A hyaline cartilage plate in the metaphysis of long bones that is responsible for the longitudinal growth. Growth plates close as the child ages and are not present in mature, adult bone.
Physeal injury: Injury to the growth plate, or physis.
Apophysis: A secondary ossification center in bone that acts as an insertion site for a tendon.
Apophysitis: Injury, irritation, or inflammation of the apophysis.
Chondromalacia patella: Damage to the cartilage on the undersurface of the patella.
Patellofemoral pain: Anterior knee pain arising from the patella subchondral bone.
Spondylolysis: Bony defect or fracture within the pars interarticularis of the vertebral arch in the spinal column, typically lumbar.
Ankle impingement: Painful mechanical limitation of ankle range of motion due to osseous or soft tissue abnormality.

Introduction

Dancing requires a unique blend of artistry and athleticism. It is studied by individuals of all ages and comes in many forms. Given the variability of its participants and its demands, it can be associated with a broad profile of injuries. For young dancers, while some enjoy it as a form of recreation, others undergo intense and prolonged training starting at an early age with the hope of embarking on a professional career. Some researchers consider the intensity of dance second only to football [1]. Because of its high physical demand, the risk of injury can be significant. Furthermore, young dancers may be more vulnerable to such injuries due to the physiological growth process [1, 2]. Here, we highlight some important factors to be considered in assessing and managing injuries in this special population.

The Young Dancer Population

A substantial portion of American youth participate in dance. Approximately 3.5 million children receive dance instruction from dance specialists across 32,000 private dance schools in the USA [3]. A recent national survey of adolescents showed a 20% prevalence of dance participation, ranging from 8% for males to 38.4% for females [4].

Young Dancer Injury Statistics

The self-reported rate of injury among adolescent pre-professional dancers has been cited as high as 4.7 injuries per 1000 dance hours [5]. This injury rate is similar to that reported in other adolescent sports—comparable to youth indoor soccer (4.5 injuries/1000 h) [6] and higher than elite adolescent gymnastics (2.6 injuries/1000 h) [7] and figure skating (1.4/1000 h) [8]. In addition, dance injuries can be quite severe, and often require urgent evaluation. Between 1991 and 2007, 113,084 children and adolescents aged 3–19 years were reportedly treated in US emergency departments due to dance injuries [9].

Studies have shown that pre-professional dancers, aged 9–18 years, report higher rates of injury (0.77–4.71/100 h) [10–12] than adult professional ballet and modern dancers, aged 17–55 years (0.51–4.4/1000 h) [13–16]. Between 42.1 and 77% of ballet students aged 9–20 years have reported being injured at least once during their training [10–12]. For pre-professional dancers, these injuries can have significant effects throughout their dance careers.

Injuries do not plague only elite dancers; reported injury rates among recreational dancers are also high. A 2013 study of 569 injured recreational dancers, aged 8–16 years, found that 42.4% had reported a prior dance-related injury [17].

Given the high rate of dance participation, in conjunction with the high rate of injury among young dancers, it is critical to understand risk factors, injury patterns, and prevention and treatment strategies for dance injuries in the pediatric population.

Risk Factors for Dance Injuries

Risk factors for dance injury are commonly classified as intrinsic or extrinsic. Intrinsic factors are characteristics of the individual, while extrinsic factors are related to the environment or training.

Among the intrinsic risk factors, age is of particular interest, as the prevalence and type of injuries reported have been shown to vary by age [17]. Dance involves repetitive movements in non-physiologic positions and requires significant neuromuscular control and balance, which places heavy loads on the joints and their supporting structures [9, 14]. It has been theorized that pediatric dancers are vulnerable to such stressors due to maturing growth plates and the growth process itself [1, 2, 18]. There is evidence to suggest that young dancers may be at particular risk of injury during the peri-pubertal period and its associated growth spurt. While determination of pubertal onset for males can be difficult as there is no one defining characteristic, puberty typically occurs around age 12 in females, usually marked by the onset of menarche [19]. Recent research has shown that cartilage active throughout the pubertal growth spurt may be more susceptible to injury than immature or mature bone [1]. The loss of flexibility that occurs during this time period, as bones grow faster than ligaments and tendons, has also been theorized to increase injury risk [20, 21]. Overall, the intensive and specialized training required of dancers may create conditions that cause the growth process to predispose the adolescent dancer to injury. However, there is no clear consensus based on the current literature confirming the relationship between age, growth, and injury.

While other intrinsic risk factors have been studied extensively, few high-quality studies have emerged. A recent systematic review evaluated the current evidence regarding risk factors for musculoskeletal injury in pre-professional ballet and modern dancers, aged 18 years or younger, but, due to the lack of studies worthy of full consideration in the review, no definitive conclusions could be reached [22]. There was low-level evidence suggesting that previous injury, insufficient psychological coping skills, low body mass index, poor aerobic capacity, abnormal lower extremity alignment in turnout, and perfectionism may be associated with increased risk of injury in pre-professional young dancers [22]. Studies on additional intrinsic risk factors in young dancers have shown inconsistent results.

Extrinsic risk factors hypothesized as contributors to dance injury include poor technique, improper training, inappropriate scheduling to prevent fatigue, lack of strengthening to prevent muscular imbalances, and suboptimal equipment, including footwear and floor type [23]. These are areas of particular interest, as they are modifiable aspects of training. In the aforementioned systematic review, only jump landing technique and fatigue had low-level evidence to suggest an association with injuries in young dancers [22]. In a study by Liederbach et al., adult professional dancers were shown to have different landing kinetics/kinematics and increased resistance to fatigue-induced changes compared to other female athletes, who incur higher rates of ACL injuries. Prevention of fatigue and proper jump technique were therefore proposed as protective mechanisms against specific injuries, including ACL injuries [24, 25]. These results have been echoed in studies that have linked training intensity with increased injury incidence among adolescent dancers [21]. However, despite the vast quantity of studies examining extrinsic risk factors, insufficient high-quality data exist to make definitive conclusions regarding extrinsic risk factors for musculoskeletal injury in young dancers.

Injuries by Dancer Demographics

Age

For reasons previously described, age and growth have been hypothesized to be risk factors for dance injuries. Studies have shown that young dancers in the peri-pubertal period have a higher rate of injury than young dancers at other ages [10, 21, 26]. In a 2014 survey-based study of 806 young dancers, 11–12 year olds were found to have a higher rate of injury (1.55/1000 h) than 13–18 year olds (1.17–1.24/1000 h) [21]. This was consistent with prior studies showing that dancers ≤ 10 years or 14–16 years of age had lower injury rates than dancers aged 11–13 years [10, 26].

Injury location has been shown to differ among age groups. The lower extremity has consistently been identified as the most common site of injury in pediatric dancers of all ages and all dance styles [17, 20, 21, 26]. However, younger dancers, aged 8–11 years, have shown high rates of injury to the foot and ankle [17, 20, 26], while older dancers, aged 12–18 years, have shown increased rates of injury to the knee and hip [17, 20, 21, 26]. Results regarding the distribution of injury at the spine and upper extremities among age ranges are conflicting [17, 20, 21, 26].

The type of tissue injured has also been shown to differ among age groups [17, 20, 21, 26]. A recent study of young dancers of any discipline showed that pediatric dancers, aged 8–11 years, more commonly injured bony structures, while adolescent dancers, aged 12–18 years, had similar rates of bony and soft tissue injuries, suggesting that soft tissue injuries increase in frequency as the young dancer grows [20]. Similarly, Steinberg et al. [17] found that ligament and tendon injuries increased in frequency with increasing age (from 4% in 8–10-year olds to 13.7% in 16–18-year olds) among young dancers of all disciplines.

Gender

Gender-specific research is limited in young dancers. The majority of dance research has been performed in ballet and has largely focused on females, likely due to their increased participation compared to males [4]. In a 2002 prospective study of 39 adolescent dancers of various disciplines, aged 14–18 years, males reported injuries twice as frequently as females (8.4 vs. 4.1 injuries/1000 dance hours) [5]. However, in a recent study of 266 pre-professional ballet dancers, aged 15–19 years, no significant difference in the rate of injury was found between sexes [12]. Likewise, in a recent systematic review, the rate of injury in adolescent male ballet dancers (1.08 injuries/1000 dance hours) was similar to that of adolescent female ballet dancers (0.99 injuries/1000 dance hours). These findings suggest that adolescent male ballet dancers have equivalent injury rates to females, while male dancers of other disciplines may have an increased risk for injury compared to females. Further research for causation and replicability is needed. Of note, these results somewhat contrast with the literature in adults, which suggests that professional male ballet dancers have a higher rate of injury than their female counterparts [16, 27].

No consistent gender differences have been found in the types of injuries reported among adolescent dancers. In 2011, Leanderson et al. [10] found that young ballet dancers reported a similar breakdown of overuse (77%) and traumatic (23%) injuries, regardless of sex. In 2014, Steinberg et al. [21] found no significant gender differences in injury type or location among adolescent dancers of various disciplines. Again, this contrasts with the literature published for professional adult ballet dancers, which suggests males more commonly suffer from acute injuries [14, 28, 29] and injuries to the upper extremity when compared to females [14]. The conflicting data between adolescent and adult male dancers may reflect the unique demands of the older male dancer, which include increased partnering work (especially lifts), particularly in ballet.

Injuries by Dance Discipline

Ballet

The vast majority of dance research has been conducted in ballet, at either the professional or pre-professional level. A few studies have evaluated musculoskeletal injuries in ballet dancers aged 21 years or younger. A recent systematic review encompassing four retrospective studies of 1147 amateur ballet dancers, mean age 16.2 years, reported a rate of ballet-related injuries of 0.97 injuries/1000 dance hours [29]. This is lower than the 4.7 injuries/1000 dance hours reported by Luke et al. for dancers of all disciplines [5]. While this may truly reflect a decreased injury rate among adolescent ballet dancers compared to adolescent dancers of other disciplines, it should be noted that different reporting methods were used in these studies (i.e., retrospective review vs. self-reporting), which may also contribute to this discrepancy. Limited data are available comparing the rate of injury among adolescent ballet dancers to other dancers. A 1996 study noted that new lower extremity injuries were less common in ballet students than modern students by about half; however, this was not the primary purpose of the study, and data presentation makes confirmation and/or other comparisons unavailable [30].

In the aforementioned review, overuse injuries were reported to account for approximately 75% of injuries in amateur ballet dancers, ranging from 72 to 82.9% [10–12, 31], which was slightly higher than that reported in adult professional ballet dancers (66%) [29]. No data were available for comparison to other dance styles.

Among young ballet dancers, the lower extremity is the most commonly affected body region [10–12, 32]. Within the lower extremity, injuries have been reported most commonly at the foot and ankle region [10–12, 32]. In a 2008 study by

Gamboa et al., the majority of injuries among elite American ballet students aged 9–20 years were found to occur at the foot/ankle (53%), followed by the hip (21.6%), knee (16.1%), and back (9.4%) [11]. In 2011, Leanderson et al. found a similar breakdown during a retrospective review of 476 elite Swedish ballet students, aged 10–21 years, with 76% of injuries occurring in the lower extremity and 51.6% of those at the foot/lower leg [10]. More recently, Ekegren et al. performed a one-year prospective study of 266 elite British ballet students, aged 15–19, and, similarly, found that the majority of injuries (77%) occurred in the lower extremity, with 33% in the ankle, 22% in the lower leg, 20% in the foot, 13% in the knee, and 10% in the hip/groin [12]. This study also assessed the type of tissue injured and found that injuries to the joints and their supporting ligaments, particularly at the ankle, were most common. A similar distribution of injuries has been reported in adult ballet dancers. In a 5-year study of 98 professional Swedish ballet dancers, 75% of injuries were reported in the lower extremities, with the ankle and foot region being most commonly affected [14]. Details on specific diagnoses are discussed further in the "Injury Diagnosis" section below.

Though less common than lower extremity injuries, spine and trunk injuries have also been reported among young ballet dancers. In a recent review by Caine et al., spine and trunk injuries accounted for 9.8 to 24% of injuries in young ballet dancers [32]. The majority of these injuries involved soft tissues, including low back strain [32]. While bony injuries have been less reported, stress fractures of the lumbar spine are worthy of particular mention, as they have been found to account for 10% of all stress fractures affecting pre-professional ballet dancers aged 15–19 years [33].

While different styles of ballet exist and have been studied in the adult population, this has not been done in young dancers. Of particular interest is the effect of en pointe dancing on injury patterns in the developing dancer. Limited data exist regarding the appropriate time to introduce pointe in the young dancer. There is some evidence to suggest that functional tests, such as the Airplane, Sauté, and Topple tests, may be more useful for gauging pointe readiness than chronological age, though this has not been shown to affect injury rates [34]. It has also been suggested that dancers who use demi-pointe shoes prior to transitioning to pointe may have a lower risk of injury to the foot and ankle [35]. The relationship between the intensity of pointe training and injury has also been brought into question. A 2013 study found that young dancers, aged 8–16 years, who spent more than 60 min/week en pointe had a higher rate of back injuries and foot and ankle tendinopathy compared to dancers who did not [17], though these results have not been consistently reproduced. A detailed discussion of pointe readiness and pointe training intensity is beyond the scope of this chapter.

Irish Dance

In recent years, Irish dance has grown in popularity. As more children are participating in competitive Irish dancing, more injuries are being reported. While research is limited, a few studies have evaluated patterns of youth dance injury in this genre. A chart review of 255 patients attending Irish dance schools requiring evaluation at a sports medicine or orthopedic clinic noted that almost all injuries (95%) occurred in the pediatric population [36]. Like most other dance styles, the majority of injuries were overuse (80%) and occurred in the lower extremities (95.9%), specifically at the foot (33.2%), ankle (22.7%), knee (19.7%), and hip (14.4%). Specific diagnoses included tendon injury (13.3%), apophysitis (11.4%), patellofemoral pain (10.8%), and stress injury (10.1%), all of which are commonly seen in other dance styles [36]. A more recent survey-based study of 36 competitive Irish dance students, aged 12 years or older, attending an accredited dance school in Calgary, supported the finding that Irish dance injuries most commonly occur at the foot and ankle (67%). However, in this study the majority of injuries were recorded in elite-level dancers and dancers over 18 years of age [37]. Both studies are small, but mutually suggest that Irish dancers most often suffer from foot and ankle injuries. However, it is unclear which age groups are most vulnerable; further study may reveal more consistent injury trends.

Other

Limited data are available regarding other dance styles, and nearly all studies have focused on adult populations. As noted above, one study comparing 107 ballet and 41 modern pre-professional dancers attending the North Carolina School of the Arts found that modern dancers had a higher rate of lower extremity injury [31]. No other studies focused on adolescent modern dancers were identified.

Studies evaluating injuries associated with other styles of dance, including Broadway, hip-hop, tap, jazz, ballroom, ethnic, and breakdance, have focused on adult populations or included mixed age groups. Therefore, no conclusions can be reached about injuries associated with these dance styles among pediatric dancers.

Injuries by Characteristics

Injury Location

The distribution of injury by anatomical location among dance students has been assessed in multiple studies, though most have focused on ballet students and are discussed in the ballet section above.

A few studies have been conducted in young dancers participating in any dance discipline and have, similarly, shown a high rate of injury in the lower extremities. The knee has been shown to be most commonly involved in all dancers, followed closely by the foot and ankle [17, 21, 38]. In a 2013 epidemiological study of 569 injured female recreational dancers from the Israel Performing Arts Medicine Center, aged 8–16 years, the lower extremity was the most commonly injured area of the body. Knee injuries were most common (40.4%), followed by "other injuries" (23.4%), back injuries (19.2%), and ankle and foot tendinopathy (17.0%) [17]. This high rate of knee injury was reproduced by Yin et al. in a 2015 retrospective cross-sectional epidemiological study of 181 injured pediatric dancers, aged 5–17 years. Injuries most commonly occurred in the lower extremity, with the majority affecting the knee (28%), ankle (21.2%), foot/toe (16.7%), hip (13.1%), and spine (11.7%). Similar results were found in a 2014 study assessing the injury profile of 806 young dancers, aged 10–18 years, attending UK Centres for Advanced Training, in which "other lower extremity" injuries (including the knee) accounted for the majority of injuries (21.8%), followed closely by foot and ankle injuries (19.3%) [21].

Of note, the use of different classification systems of body regions and the use of unspecified "other" categories make comparing results across studies difficult and likely contributes to the discrepancies seen among studies. A standardized system to specify body regions of dance-related injuries is needed.

Injury Etiology

The etiology of injury is commonly classified as either traumatic (acute) or overuse (chronic). The majority of research on the etiology of injury among young dancers has focused on ballet students, and has shown that most injuries in this population are overuse in nature [10–12, 32], as discussed above.

Injury Type

In recent research, dance injuries have been classified by the type of tissue involved; common groupings including bone, joint, soft tissue (tendons and/or muscles), and, rarely, physeal injuries. As this type of reporting has only been included in more recent studies of pediatric dancers, literature in this area is limited. Among ballet dancers, only one study was identified that assessed injury type based on tissue. In the aforementioned study by Ekegren et al., injuries most commonly involved joint structures or their supporting ligaments (46%), followed by muscles and tendons (30%), bones (19%), and "other" (5%) [13]. While other studies have not focused on tissue type specifically, the most common diagnoses have involved tendons, ligaments, or other joint structures [6, 11], supporting the hypothesis that these are frequently affected tissue types among young ballet dancers.

A few studies of dancers in other styles have assessed tissue type involved in injury. Their results have been conflicting. In the Steinberg et al. study of young British dancers, muscle injuries were most common among all ages, though ligament and tendon injuries increased with age [22]. However, in the Yin et al. study of young American dancers, joints injuries (42%) were most common among all ages, followed closely by soft tissue injuries (including muscles; 31%). Injuries less often involved bones (20%) and growth plates (7%) [39]. Of note, this was the first study that included physeal injuries as a tissue category among pediatric dancers. Further research is needed in this area, as physeal injuries, which are unique to the skeletally immature, can result in long-term growth abnormalities.

As shown above, different grouping systems have been used in each study, making direct comparisons between studies difficult. Despite this limitation, it seems that young dancers of all disciplines commonly injure joints and supporting soft tissue structures.

Injury Diagnosis

Numerous studies have assessed the most common dance-related injuries that occur in the pediatric population [2, 5, 10–12, 17, 20, 21, 26, 29, 32, 38]. Again, a majority of these have evaluated ballet dancers. Studies have reported high rates of tendinopathy, ligament sprains, and muscle strains, and low rates of fractures or bony stress reactions [5, 10]. Leanderson et al. found that the most common diagnoses were tendinosis pedis (12.8%) and ankle sprain (11.4%). These were followed closely by low back pain (10.3%), groin tendinosis (9.4%), jumper's knee (7.1%), and chondromalacia patellae (5.7%). Few fractures were seen (2.7%); of those that occurred, the metatarsals (67%) were the most common site [10]. Similarly, Luke et al. reported Achilles tendinopathy to be the most common foot/ankle injury among adolescent ballet dancers [5]. In contrast, Ekegran et al. found the most common diagnosis to be "lower leg overuse injury" (10.3%), with shin splints being the most common type of overuse injury (8.7%). This was followed closely by ankle synovitis/impingement/bursitis (8.7%) and ankle tendon injury (7.1%). Similar to Leanderson et al., foot and tibial stress reactions/fractures were found to account for only a small portion of injuries (4.0 and 1.3%, respectively), though these injuries accounted for the longest time out of dance [12]. Studies among adult professional ballet dancers have shown similar results, with the most common injuries being ankle sprains and tendinosis, most frequently to flexor hallucis longus, the Achilles, or the peroneals [14].

In addition to the above diagnoses, dancers involved in other disciplines commonly suffer from knee injuries, specifically patellofemoral pain [21, 38]. Of the 181 dancers in the Yin et al. study, 25 suffered from tendinopathy (11.3%) and 23 from patellofemoral pain (10.4%) [38]. In contrast to ballet dancers, patellofemoral pain was seen almost as frequently as tendinopathy. Other common diagnoses included apophysitis (6.3%), ankle impingement (6.3%), hip labral tear (5.9%), joint instability (5.0%), sprain (5.0%), strain (4.5%), pars stress reaction/spondylolysis (4.5%), and other stress reaction/fractures (4.1%) [38]. While no other studies were identified that clearly described injury diagnosis among pediatric dancers, a higher incidence of injury at the knee has been described and is discussed in detail above in the Injury Location section [17].

Interpretation of data from these studies is limited due to inconsistent categorization of diagnoses, inadequate definitions of each injury, and lack of specificity of all diagnoses (e.g., include only the most common injuries).

Conclusion

While by no means comprehensive, this chapter provides an overview of the current literature on musculoskeletal injuries in young dancers. Hopefully, as we better understand the patterns of injury in these dancers, focus can turn to prevention strategies. Given the diversity of movement requirements, a unified protocol of injury prevention may be difficult to develop. However, some key concepts and themes have emerged from the available studies that may already be applied. First, given the role of fatigue as a potentially modifiable extrinsic risk factor, periodization in dancer training may be a way not only to improve performance, as demonstrated in other sports, but also to reduce injury rates [39]. Also, individualized conditioning programs using injury history and functional movement screen have been demonstrated to be effective in reducing injuries in adult professional ballet dancers [40]. Ultimately, a personalized program involving an interdisciplinary team, including parents, dance teachers, and healthcare providers, who work together to evaluate growth, technique, and training intensity may be the best way to ensure the health of young dancers.

References

1. Flachsmann R, Broom ND, Hardy AE, Moltschaniwskyj G. Why is the adolescent joint particularly susceptible to osteochondral shear fracture? Clin Orthop Relat Res. 2000;381:212–21.
2. Micheli L. Overuse injuries in children's sports: the growth factor. Orthop Clin North Am. 1983;14(2):337–60.
3. Statistics: General US Education and Dance Education. National Dance Education Organization. 2014. Available from: http://www.ndeo.org/content.aspx?page_id.22&club_id.893257&module_id.55774.
4. O'Neill JR, Pate RR, Liese AD. Descriptive epidemiology of dance participation in adolescents. Res Q Exerc Sport. 2011;82(3):373–80.
5. Luke AC, Kinney SA, D'Hemecourt PA, Baum J, Owen M, Micheli LJ. Determinants of injuries in young dancers. Med Probl Perform Art. 2002;17(3):105–12.

6. Emery CA, Meeuwisse WH. Risk factors for injury in indoor compared with outdoor adolescent soccer. Am J Sports Med. 2006;34(10):1636–42.
7. Kolt G, Kirby R. Epidemiology of injury in elite and subelite female gymnasts: a comparison of retrospective and prospective findings. Br J Sports Med. 1999;33(3):312–8.
8. Kjaer M, Larsson B. Physiological profile and incidence of injuries among elite figure skaters. J Sports Sci. 1992;10(1):29–36.
9. Roberts KJ, Nelson NG, McKenzie L. Dance-related injuries in children and adolescents treated in US emergency departments in 1991–2007. J Phys Act Health. 2013;10(2):143–50.
10. Leanderson C, Leanderson J, Wykman A, Strender LE, Johansson SE, Sundquist K. Musculoskeletal injuries in young ballet dancers. Knee Surg Sports Traumatol Arthrosc. 2011;19(9):1531–5.
11. Gamboa JM, Roberts LA, Maring J, Fergus A. Injury patterns in elite preprofessional ballet dancers and the utility of screening programs to identify risk characteristics. J Orthop Sports Phys Ther. 2008;38(3):126–36.
12. Ekegren CL, Quested R, Brodrick A. Injuries in pre-professional ballet dancers: incidence, characteristics and consequences. J Sci Med sport. 2014;17(3):271–5.
13. Shah S, Weiss DS, Burchette RJ. Injuries in professional modern dancers: incidence, risk factors, and management. J Dance Med Sci. 2012;16(1):17–25.
14. Nilsson C, Leanderson J, Wykman A, Strender LE. The injury panorama in a Swedish professional ballet company. Knee Surg Sports Traumatol Arthrosc. 2001;9(4):242–6.
15. Bronner S, Ojofeitimi S, Rose D. Injuries in a modern dance company: effect of comprehensive management on injury incidence and time loss. Am J Sports Med. 2003;31 (3):365–73.
16. Allen N, Nevill A, Brooks J, Koutedakis Y, Wyon M. Ballet injuries: injury incidence and severity over 1 year. J Orthop Sports Phys Ther. 2012;42(9):781–90.
17. Steinberg N, Siev-Ner I, Peleg S, Dar G, Masharawi Y, Zeev A, et al. Injuries in female dancers aged 8–16 years. J Athl Train. 2013;48(1):118–23.
18. Poggini L, Losasso S, Iannone S. Injuries during the dancer's growth spurt: etiology, prevention, and treatment. J Dance Med Sci. 1999;3(2):73–9.
19. Malina R, Bouchard C, Bar-Or O. Growth, maturation and physical activity. 2nd ed. Champaign, IL: Human Kinetics Press; 2004. p. 50–100.
20. Stracciolini A, Yin AX, Sugimoto D. Etiology and body area of injuries in young female dancers presenting to sports medicine clinic: a comparison by age group. Phys Sportsmed. 2015;43(4):342–7.
21. Steinberg N, Aujla I, Zeev A, Redding E. Injuries among talented young dancers: findings from the U.K. Centres for advanced Training. Int J Sports Med. 2014;35(3):238–44.
22. Kenny SJ, Whittaker JL, Emery CA. Risk factors for musculoskeletal injury in preprofessional dancers: a systematic review. Br J Sports Med. 2016;50(16):997–1003.
23. Russell JA. Preventing dance injuries: current perspectives. Open Access J Sports Med. 2013;4:199–210.
24. Orishimo KF, Liederbach M, Kremenic IJ, Hagins M, Pappas E. Comparison of landing biomechanics between male and female dancers and athletes, part 1: influence of sex on risk of anterior cruciate ligament injury. Am J Sports Med. 2014;42(5):1082–8.
25. Liederbach M, Kremenic IJ, Orishimo KF, Pappas E, Hagins M. Comparison of landing biomechanics between male and female dancers and athletes, part 2: influence of fatigue and implications for anterior cruciate ligament injury. Am J Sports Med. 2014;42(5):1089–95.
26. Steinberg N, Siev-Ner I, Peleg S, Dar G, Masharawi Y, Zeev A, et al. Injury patterns in young, non-professional dancers. J Sports Sci. 2011;29(1):47–54.
27. Wanke EM, Arendt M, Helmgard M, Groneberg DA. Occupational accidents in professional dance with focus on gender differences. J Occup Med Toxicol. 2013;8:35.
28. Klemp P, Learmonth ID. Hypermobility and injuries in a professional ballet company. Br J Sports Med. 1984;18(3):143–8.

29. Smith PJ, Gerrie BJ, Varner KE, McCulloch PC, Lintner DM, Harris JD. Incidence and prevalence of musculoskeletal injury in ballet: a systematic review. Orthop J Sports Med. 2015;3(7):2325967115592621.
30. Wiesler ER, Hunter DM, Martin DF, Curl WW, Hoen H. Ankle flexibility and injury patterns in dancers. Am J Sports Med. 1996;24(6):754–7.
31. Negus V, Hopper D, Briffa NK. Associations between turnout and lower extremity injuries in classical ballet dancers. J Orthop Sports Phys Ther. 2015;35(5):307–18.
32. Caine D, Goodwin BJ, Caine CG, Bergeron G. Epidemiological review of injury in pre-professional ballet dancers. J Dance Med Sci. 2015;19(4):140–8.
33. Lunden K, Melcher L, Bray K. Stress fractures in ballet: a twenty five year review. J Dance Med Sci. 1999;3(3):101–7.
34. Richardson M, Liederbach M, Sandow E. Functional criteria for assessing pointe-readiness. J Dance Med Sci. 2010;14(3):82–8.
35. Pearson SJ, Whitaker AF. Footwear in classical ballet: a study of pressure distribution and related foot injury in the adolescent dancer. J Dance Med Sci. 2012;16(2):51–6.
36. Stein CJ, Tyson KD, Johnson VM, Popoli DM, d'Hemecourt PA, Micheli LJ. Injuries in Irish dance. J Dance Med Sci. 2013;17(4):159–64.
37. Eustergerling M, Emery C. Risk factors for injuries in competitive Irish dancers enrolled in dance schools in calgary. Canada Med Probl Perform Art. 2015;30(1):26–9.
38. Yin AX, Sugimoto D, Martin DJ, Stracciolini A. Pediatric dance injuries: a cross-sectional epidemiological study. PM R. 2016;8(4):348–55.
39. Wyon M. Preparing to perform: periodization and dance. J Dance Med Sci. 2010;14(2):67–72.
40. Allen N, Nevill AM, Brooks JH, Koutedakis Y, Wyon MA. The effect of a comprehensive injury audit program on injury incidence in ballet: a 3-year prospective study. Clin J Sport Med. 2013;23(5):373–8.

Chapter 2
Screening the Young Dancer: Summarizing Thirty Years of Screening

Nili Steinberg, PhD and Itzhak Siev-Ner, MD

Pertinent Definitions

Screening: The process of applying tools that measure functional capacities in individual dancers such as range of motion (ROM), body alignment, and relevant anatomic deviations. The goal is to help prevent injuries by providing guidance for training adaptations and skill acquisition.
Joint range of motion (ROM): Refers to the number of degrees of motion that are present in a joint, as commonly assessed by use of a goniometer.
Turnout: The ability of a dancer to stand and move with the legs externally rotated at the hip so that the toes are directed diagonally away from the midline of the body.
Joint hypermobility: Joint hypermobility is characterized by increased joint flexibility, where the joints move beyond the "normal" limits. The primary cause of hypermobility is attributed to changes in the collagen fiber structure, which is inherent and determined by the fibrous protein genes. This characteristic is often assessed by use of the Beighton scale.
Anatomical alignment: The arrangement of body segments as seen in various postural positions. The ideal or standard alignment involves a minimal amount of stress and strain and is conducive to maximal efficiency of the body.
Incorrect dance technique: Bad habits or patterns of movement, frequently involving lack of sufficient ROM in a specific joint that is compensated for at other joints, causing excessive shear forces that may result in a breakdown of tissue.

N. Steinberg, PhD (✉)
The Wingate College of Physical Education and Sports Sciences,
Wingate College, Wingate Institute, Netanya, Israel
e-mail: knopp@wincol.ac.il

I. Siev-Ner, MD
Department of Orthopedic Rehabilitation, Sheba Medical Center,
109 Rothschild Blvd., Tel-HaShomer, Tel Aviv, Israel
e-mail: zivner@netvision.net.il

R. Solomon et al. (eds.), *Prevention of Injuries in the Young Dancer*,
Contemporary Pediatric and Adolescent Sports Medicine,
DOI 10.1007/978-3-319-55047-3_2

Introduction

As most dance injuries are caused by overuse or misuse, many dance medicine researchers have been occupied with finding a means to prevent these injuries. In general, this research aims to ascertain whether the injury in question was the result of one or more of the following:

- A structural flaw (i.e., are some anatomical characteristics particularly conducive to injury?);
- A specific dance style (ballet, modern, jazz, etc.);
- Faulty technique that exposes the tissues to excessively high loads;
- Intensity (i.e., the tolerance of load is related to the scale of training);
- Age (growth and development);
- Hormonal factors;
- Environment (floor, shoes, studio temperature, etc.); and
- Inadequate nutrition.

It has become obvious that the risks involved are multifactorial, and that in order to draw meaningful and significant conclusions a Sisyphean task is required. These authors set out to develop and implement a screening instrument that could be used with groups of dancers to analyze each individual's potential for overuse injury. The larger, more defined, and uniform the studied groups were, we believed, the more accurate the conclusions drawn would be. The challenge we faced was to know what parameters to examine, record, and compare. At the start we took a decision to collect as many parameters as possible, bearing in mind that some would prove to be insignificant—yet this could not be known until we tested and verified the usefulness of each one. The interpretation of the studies enabled us to understand what is important to ask, collect, and measure. Thus, we now may be able to suggest a target-oriented screening process that is reproducible and can focus on the issues that matter most to the dancers.

Such an effort is worthwhile if the conclusions reached can be implemented and make a difference—e.g., reduce the rate of injuries; prevent unrealistic expectations of young dancers, their parents, and teachers; offer better health and functioning, and longer-lasting careers.

Screening and profiling runs the risk of blocking opportunities to talented students who do not have the "ideal" body type. We should be very careful in establishing what the "best" profile is for a successful dancer. However, if we use the screening information wisely we may be able to anticipate injuries and focus on prevention through proper guidance and cautious teaching.

After a journey that has lasted several decades, screened over 3000 dancers, and involved many skilled scientists, medical personnel, and teachers, we now better understand the risks for injuries, and some of that knowledge is presented in this chapter. The best proof of the value of this information is that the rate of some typical injuries has diminished in the dancers we have screened. Dancers now have a better chance of completing a long career, despite the increasing demands and expectations of such a dynamic and competitive occupation, where the bar keeps moving higher and higher.

Background

The desire to create the "ideal" dancer should not distract us from selecting what are regarded as the best characteristics for a professional dancer. Possessing certain anatomical structures may facilitate achieving the high demands of dance technique, yet much more has to do with talent, artistic qualities, etc. The role of the medical team is not to judge who is going to become a good dancer; our responsibility is to enable each student to do the best they can with their innate qualities, and to promote proper technique and use of their body. As such, the medical team acts as an **advisor** to teachers, dancers, and choreographers; it does not replace them.

Aims of Screening the Young Dancer

The individual student dancer, as well as the teachers and medical team, benefit from the outcomes of screening. The former will be informed of his/her risk factors and how to prevent personal injuries; the latter will better understand the risk factors and mechanisms of injury by deducing conclusions from the accumulated data and its analysis presented in scientific studies.

The art and responsibility of the teachers and medical team is to determine what to assess and what conclusions can be drawn. Thus, the goals are:

1. To detect risk factors at an early stage in order to prevent injuries.
2. To learn the body characteristics of the individual dancer so that they can be used as a baseline for comparison when injuries occur.
3. To collect data for research in order to be able to distinguish between "normal" and any deviation (i.e., to build an ideal profile of the dancer by defining what is "normal").

Collect the Maximum Data

1. Record previous and current impacting factors, such as years of training, age at which female students started pointe work, current hours dancing per day/week, dance style.
2. Measure anatomical and morphological characteristics, such as height and weight, leg length, joint ROM, alignment, and anatomical variations.

3. Obtain information regarding factors that may affect performance (e.g., dance technique), as well as more holistic factors (nutrition, emotional and psychological, etc.).
4. Assess any current injury; record previous medical problems and resulting deficits; identify unrecognized injury.

Timing

Dance students should be screened at the earliest opportunity, preferably prior to, or immediately after, joining a high-level dance class. A full screening should be performed initially, followed by modified screening usually performed at the commencement of each school year.

There may be some specific concerns about the screening protocol during the growth and developmental stages of the young dancer, bearing in mind the different individual (hormonal) maturation rates.

Pre-pubertal Dancers (Age 6–10 Years)

Youngsters may start dance lessons as early as 4 or 5 years old. There are mainly two considerations with the pre-pubertal age group:

1. The manifestation of previously unrecognized congenital deviations;
2. At this age students usually do not sustain high impact injuries; they take one to three classes a week and the classes are short in duration. Yet, during this period they may acquire "imprinting," i.e., faulty movement habits that may follow them for years and eventually become injurious. Hence, the screening staff should make every effort to determine whether the student is being exposed to good instruction.

The medical staff can exert a great deal of influence on the dancer's education, because habits are just being established and brain plasticity is still quite malleable. After the correct methods of dance technique are explained a high degree of compliance can be expected.

Pubertal Dancers (Age 11–14 Years)

Most dancers at this age are involved in a considerable number of practice hours per week (h/week), and the effect of time and highly demanding exercises on their maturation should be addressed. During the pubertal period dancers are undergoing rapid growth and developmental changes, accompanied by risk factors related to the "growth spurt". Bones normally grow faster than ligaments and tendons (which become "shorter" relative to bone length), and dancers who force their soft tissues into larger ROM expose themselves to a higher incidence of injury [1, 2]. Students who sense that their ROM is decreasing may force the joints beyond their limit, creating mini tendon and muscle tears that will scar the soft tissues and further limit the joints' range, thus initiating a vicious cycle. Simple explanations by a teacher or screener may avert these consequences.

Excessive repetitive movements such as working en pointe and demi-pointe may create high load and strain on muscles and ligaments and have been found to increase the prevalence of injuries during the pubertal period [3, 4]. Most dance educators and healthcare practitioners would agree that dancers need a minimum of 3–4 years of ballet training and the attainment of the chronological age of 12 years before they can acquire the technical skill and motor control necessary to begin en pointe work [5, 6].

Adolescent Dancers (Age 15–18 Years)

This group includes students who usually have had some years of practice, yet there may also be some beginners. At this age the intensity as well as the total number of training h/week increases significantly, sometimes reaching a "semi-professional" level and load. These dancers are at the highest exposure to risk. Their motivation and ambition might exacerbate the risk, as this is also the time they will elect or be selected to devote themselves to becoming professional dancers.

Insights from the Screening

Age

Young (age 6–18 years) dancers are a unique group. As previously stated, they are in the phase of growth and development. Their dance intensity and hours of practice can place a great physical load on their growing musculoskeletal system. Certain dance techniques (such as dancing en pointe) may exceed the young dancer's ability to cope with the high demands during this period.

The results from screening 1336 young dancers demonstrated an increased prevalence of injuries in the age group of 8–16; whereas at 8 years old one out of 10 girls experienced an injury, by the age of 16 every third girl had suffered an injury [7]. On the other hand, another study of 806 young dancers attending Centres for Advanced Training (UK) demonstrated no difference in the rate of injuries with increasing age (11–18 years) [8]. Most dancers trained from 6 to 11 years before their first injury occurred [7]. A high rate of dancers with recurrent injury (27.7%) is already noted in dancers of a very young age (9 years), a rate that rises to 46% at the age of 16 years [7]. The average time elapsed between the first and second injury is age-dependent; the older the dancer, the smaller the time gap between the first and second injury [7].

Dance History

Obtaining the students' dance history reveals information regarding the number of years they were exposed to dancing and its possible accumulative impact on their bodies. Specific screening questions should refer to the age that they started the following:

- Dance classes,
- Ballet dancing,
- Modern dancing,
- Other types of dancing,
- Dancing more than 10 h per week, and
- Dancing en pointe.

Impact of the Current Training Program

Specific questions concerning the current impact of dance training should include the following:

- Total hours of practice per week in each technique,
- Number of days per week that the dancer practices more than 4 h/day, and
- Total h/week of en pointe work.

Screening of 1336 young dancers showed no statistically significant association between total h/week of dance training and injuries, although the injured girls tended to dance more h/week than the non-injured dancers. A significant association between dance practice in a specific position (en pointe) and injury was observed ($p < 0.001$): 43% of the dancers who trained en pointe more than 60 min per week had an injury compared with just 29% of the dancers who practiced this position for less than 60 min per week [9]. Among the 806 UK dancers mentioned earlier the young injured dancers practiced more h/week than the non-injured dancers of the same age cohort. The percentage of injured dancers who practiced more than 2 h/week in modern dance style was higher than the percentage of injured dancers who practiced between 1 and 2 h/week of modern dance. No differences were found between dancers who practiced >3 h/week of ballet and dancers who practiced <3 h/week of ballet [8].

Age at Onset of Menarche

The screening should address:

- Age at onset of menarche,
- Frequency of menarche (regular/irregular), and
- Dysmenorrhea (yes/no).

Extensive involvement in sport may delay physical development and menstrual function [10], unless the activity is reduced [11]. Young female dancers showed delayed age at menarche and higher frequency of delayed menarche compared with age-matched controls [12–14].

Dancers who began training before menarche have been shown to experience a later menarche and had an increased incidence of menstrual dysfunction when compared to girls who began training after menarche [12–14]. Dancers with delayed menarche have manifested lower body weight, lower bone mass, and higher frequency of stress fractures at the transitional stages of puberty than dancers with normal age onset of menarche [15, 16]. As a certain percentage of body fat (>17%) is necessary for regular ovulatory cycles, it is understandable that nutritional shortcomings, low body fat, and a high ratio of lean mass to body weight in young dancers will delay the adolescent growth spurt, retard the onset of menarche, and cause menstrual disturbance [2, 17]. Comparing age at menarche of injured and non-injured dancers showed no significant difference. Injured dancers had more occasions when their menarche stopped for ≥ 3 months compared to non-injured dancers [8]. Screening a large group of young non-professional dancers demonstrated no association between the age of onset of menarche and injuries, manifestation of scoliosis, joint hypermobility, or hallux valgus [4, 18–20].

Anthropometric Measures

Data concerning weight, height, and BMI are essential for understanding the anthropometric characteristics of the young dancer. Young dancers are significantly leaner and have lower BMI compared to age-matched non-dancer controls [21–23]. The low body weight found in young ballet dancers is most likely associated with a light skeletal frame and below average amount of muscle tissue [23].

Other anthropometric data, such as leg length (Fig. 2.1) and foot length discrepancies, are important mainly for identifying any deviations from the normal posture. Segmental discrepancies should be noted as they might be predisposing factors for posture mal-alignments such as scoliosis, some common compensatory mechanisms during certain dance movements, and overuse syndromes commonly found among dancers [24, 25].

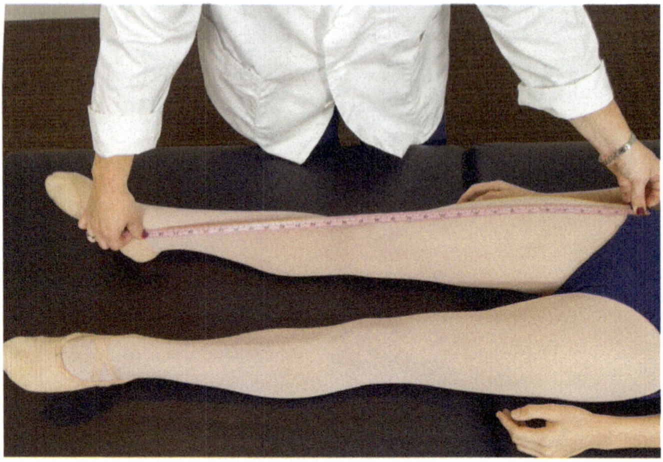

Fig. 2.1 Leg length measurement. Photograph courtesy of James Koepfler

Joint Hypermobility Syndrome

Joint hypermobility is a condition in which most of the synovial joints move beyond the "normal" limits. It is recognized as a feature of heritable disorders of the connective tissue (changes in the collagen fiber structure regulated by the fibrous protein genes) and is generally identified by use of the Beighton scale [26]. Among dancers hypermobility refers to weak joint stability. It is the result of long and loose ligaments and certain structural deviations such as shallow joint surfaces, making dancers with hypermobility more vulnerable to musculoskeletal injury and to prolonged periods of post-injury recovery [27–30].

Hypermobility characteristics are considered by dancers to be of great aesthetic benefit, with general agreement that they confer advantages in career advancement [31, 32]. From a medical point of view, hypermobility is a genetic phenomenon [33, 34], yet some authorities claim that it is related to years of incorrect technical execution of dance exercises, which is capable of exacerbating the condition [35].

Among young dancers (aged 8–16 years) joint hypermobility was found to be very common and showed an increased prevalence with increasing age [20]. This is likely due in part to some self-selection of body type, with dancers who could not match what is perceived to be the "perfect" dance movements performed by their hypermobile counterparts dropping out [2, 36, 37]. Teachers frequently promote this process by favoring those dancers who exemplify the aesthetically "correct body shape" to become professionals [2, 36, 37].

Hypermobility should be addressed in young dancers, as pubertal hypermobile female dancers are at high risk for suffering from chronic musculoskeletal pain and arthralgia [2, 36, 37]. It has been frequently observed that young female dancers with hypermobility and resulting pain have lower motivation, higher prevalence of dropout from their ballet career, and greater risk for injuries compared to their peers [32, 35, 36, 38].

Knee Laxity

Screening examination should include:

- Laxity around the knee joint: medial/lateral laxity of the knee (Fig. 2.2);
- Lachman test and drawer test;
- Medial/lateral mobility of patella in extended knee; and
- Medial/lateral mobility of patella in 30° of knee flexion.

In one study adolescent dancers (12–14 years old) with patellofemoral pain syndrome were found to have greater prevalence of patellar laxity in the extended knee and in 30° flexion of the knee compared to non-injured dancers [39]. It was suggested that excessive lateral tracking of the patella increased the forces and stresses between the patellar articular surface and the femur throughout knee ROM [39]. Although another study showed that patellar mobility was not associated with the development of patellofemoral pain syndrome [39], knee instability should be screened as it might predispose the dancer to overuse injuries [40].

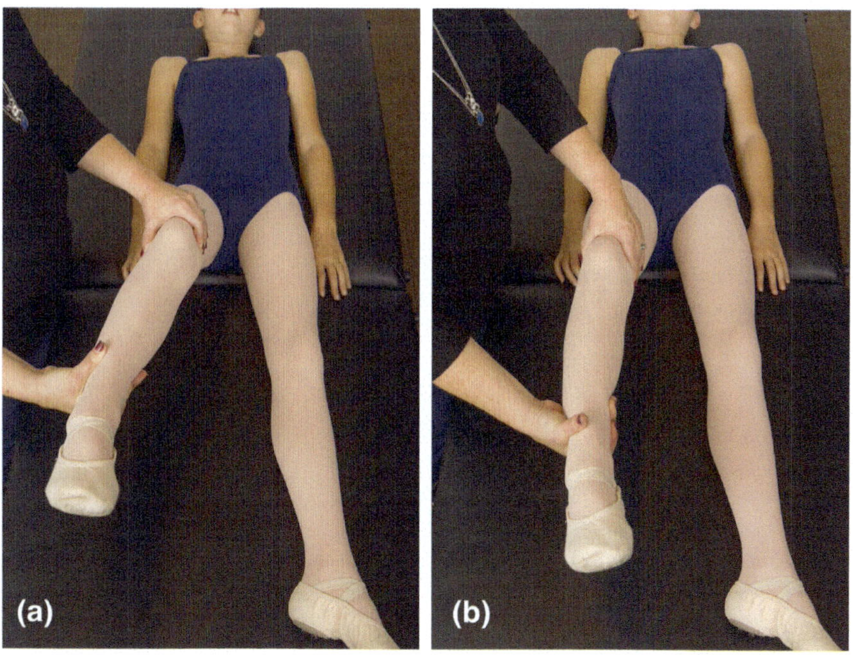

Fig. 2.2 Knee lateral (**a**) and medial (**b**) laxity assessments. Photographs courtesy of James Koepfler

Passive Joint ROM

Dancers should be screened for the most important joints' ROM (Fig. 2.3):

- Hip (flexion, extension, abduction, external rotation, internal rotation);
- Knee (flexion, extension);
- Ankle (dorsiflexion, plantar flexion);
- Foot (en pointe); and
- Combined joints' ROM (lower back and hamstring).

The ROM measurement procedure was described previously by a number of experts in dance medicine who determined the norms and movements essential in dance-related screening [41, 42] (Table 2.1).

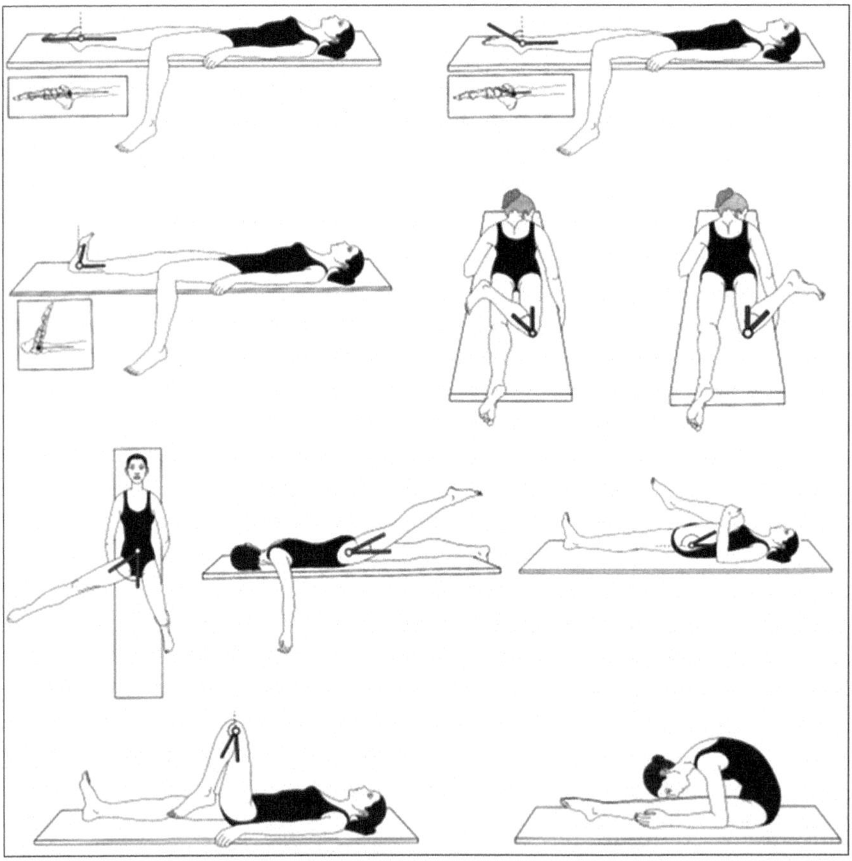

Fig. 2.3 From *left to right*: *Upper row*, combined passive ankle and foot plantar flexion (pointe); passive plantar flexion of the ankle joint. *Second row*, passive dorsiflexion of the ankle joint; passive external rotation of the hip joint; passive internal rotation of the hip joint. *Third row*, passive abduction of the hip joint; active extension of the hip joint; passive flexion of the hip joint. *Bottom row*, passive flexion of the knee joint; lower back and hamstring flexibility. Reprinted with permission from Steinberg et al. [43]

Table 2.1 Passive joint ROM: physician observations and classifications into 3 groups: hypo ROM (> −1 S.D. of mean), average ROM (±1 S.D. of mean), and hyper ROM (> +1 S.D. of mean), based on ROM distribution for each joint obtained from 1314 dancers aged 8–16 years [43]

Joint	Passive movement	Physician observations	Classifications
Foot and ankle	Dorsiflexion	The angle between the long axis of the medial border of the tibia and the long axis of the medial aspect of the foot	Limited ROM ≤ 5° Average ROM 6–15° Hyper ROM ≥ 16°
	Plantar flexion	The angle between the long axis of the medial border of the tibia and the manually palpated navicular	Limited ROM ≤ 45° Average ROM 46–64° Hyper ROM ≥ 65°
	En pointe	The angle between the long axis of the medial border of the tibia and the manually palpated distal head of the first metatarsal	Limited ROM ≤ 75° Average ROM 76–90° Hyper ROM ≥ 91°
Knee	Extension	In the extended knee, the angle between the long axis of the thigh and the long axis of the tibia	Average ROM 0° Hyper ROM ≥ 5°
	Flexion	In the flexed knee, the angle between the long axis of the thigh and the long axis of the tibia	Limited ROM ≤ 140° Average ROM 141–150° Hyper ROM ≥ 151°
Hip	Active extension	In the active extended hip, the angle between the midaxillary line (the axis on the greater trochanter) and the long axis of the thigh between the greater trochanter and the lateral epicondyle of the femur	Limited ROM ≤ 20° Average ROM 21–39° Hyper ROM ≥ 40°
	Flexion	In flexed hip, the angle between the midaxillary line (the axis on the greater trochanter) and the long axis of the thigh between the greater trochanter and the lateral epicondyle of the femur	Limited ROM ≤ 135° Average ROM 136–150° Hyper ROM ≥ 151°
	Abduction	Hip abducted in frontal plane in neutral rotation (of the hip) with the foot perpendicular to the floor. Range was measured between a line from the umbilicus and the symphysis pubis and the long axis of the abducted thigh (between the umbilicus and the patella)	Limited ROM ≤ 45° Average ROM 46–59° Hyper ROM ≥ 60°

(continued)

Table 2.1 (continued)

Joint	Passive movement	Physician observations	Classifications
	External rotation	In the flexed knee and externally rotated hip, the angle between the vertical axis and the anterior border of the tibia	Limited ROM $\leq$ 50° Average ROM 51–60° Hyper ROM $\geq$ 61°
	Internal rotation	In the flexed knee and internally rotated hip, the angle between the vertical axis and the anterior border of the tibia	Limited ROM $\leq$ 45° Average ROM 46–65° Hyper ROM $\geq$ 66°
Lower back and hamstrings	Flexion	In extended knees and planter-flexed ankles, the dancer leaned forward with the forehead toward her knees	Limited ROM $\leq$ 1 cm distance between forehead and knees. Hyper ROM $\geq$ forehead touching the knees

The term joint ROM is defined by the "musculotendinous unit length" and the "musculotendinous unit flexibility," and thus refers to the ROM available in a single joint [44, 45]. Several factors affect joint ROM in a particular joint, including the shape of the articulating surface, the shape of the articular capsule, ligamentous structures, the structure of the bony surfaces, muscle fat content, and muscle tension. All of these are genetically determined [46, 47]. There are clinical guidelines and norms for evaluating each specific joint (such as the hip, knee, and ankle joints) and each specific passive movement (such as flexion, extension, and rotation), which are normally measured with a goniometer [48, 49]. Increased joint ROM can create the illusion of perfect movements or positions, and has therefore been identified as a prerequisite for successful dancers [2, 50].

The classic question "Which came first, the chicken or the egg?" is relevant with regard to ROM. There are two schools of thought; for decades there was an argument in the literature as to whether joint ROM is solely dictated by genetics or if long periods and intensity of dance training may increase joint ROM. We should also question whether deviant joint ROM (insufficient or excessive) increases the risk of injury. With regard to the first question, in most studies dancers manifested greater joint ROM compared to non-dancers [43, 51]. A study of 1314 young female dancers found that ROM did not improve or diminish with age, but rather was preserved [43]. The ability of dancers to retain joint flexibility with age is probably due to regular training, as ROM in non-dancers tends to decrease with age [43]. Conversely, Hamilton et al. [2] explain that the desired dancer en pointe ROM (90°–100°) results from constant stretching and skeletal modeling while the bones are growing. It was suggested that improvement in hip external rotation ROM was attributable to structural changes in the femur (anteversion/retroversion of the femoral neck) as a result of the growth process controlled by hormonal changes during the spurt period, along with capsular stretching [2, 52].

Concerning the relationship between a deviated joint ROM and the risk of injury, insufficient or excessive joint ROM have been suggested as important intrinsic characteristics that may alter the biomechanics of dance movements and therefore be associated with dance injuries [2, 9, 50, 53, 54]. For example, insufficient ankle plantar flexion was found to be more common among injured dancers [53]; hyper (increased) joint ROM in the lower extremity was found to be associated with increased rate of ankle/foot paratendonitis [4]; and dancers who practice en pointe in "turnout" position with insufficient joint stability predispose themselves to injury [55].

Dancers with increased (hyper) joint ROM may exhibit excessive motion, inappropriate direction of forces, and failure of the muscles acting around the joints to keep the correct kinematic movement pattern, which can result in injuries to the affected tissues [56, 57]. Conversely, dancers who lack the required joint ROM for ideal positions tend to develop compensatory strategies [56, 58], which, in turn, may lead to an injury [28, 57]. Nevertheless, a study by Steinberg et al. [9] reported opposing results: dancers with decreased hip and ankle/foot joint ROM were found to be less prone to develop patellofemoral pain syndrome [54], and Wiesler et al. [59] reported no predictive relationship between ankle ROM measurements and injury in 148 elite adolescent pre-professional dancers.

The correct conclusion probably lies in the sample size and the cohort studied. Most compensatory movements probably contribute to pathologies. However, the large group studied [52] who underwent screening demonstrated that lack of "ideal" ROM does not necessarily cause injuries if ROM is not forced by compensations.

Unlike hypermobile (unstable) joints, which demand greater effort from the muscles around the joint to stabilize and control movement in order to prevent injuries, the mirror image of limited ROM needs "only" to avoid forcing a non-existing range, and hence prevent negative compensation and injuries.

Anatomical Alignment

Screening young dancers for joint malalignment and structural deviations may reduce the risk for related injuries (Table 2.2):

- Knee valgum/varum
- Forefoot adduction
- Hind-foot varum/valgum
- Longitudinal arch cavus/planus (splay foot)
- Hallux valgus
- Lordosis
- Scoliosis

Table 2.2 Anatomical anomalies

Joint	Anomalies	Physician observations (in an anatomical position)	Definition of a positive test[a]
Foot and ankle	Longitudinal arch planus (LAP)/ Longitudinal arch cavus (LAC)	Viewing the medial aspect of the foot, an increased height of the medial longitudinal arch indicates LAC, and reduced height of the medial longitudinal arch, with its margins touching the ground, indicates LAP.	Planus: Forefoot inversion, pes planus Cavus: Forefoot eversion
	Calcaneal valgus/varum	Viewed from behind, for varum the calcaneus is inverted when the subtalar joint is in a neutral position; for valgus the calcaneus is everted when the subtalar joint is in a neutral position	Varum: >5° inversion from calcaneal midline Valgus: <5° eversion from calcaneal midline
	Hallux valgus	Viewing the dorsal aspect of the foot, hallux valgus is present when the first metatarsal is lateromedially oriented and the proximal phalanx mediolaterally oriented. A callus is also present at the medial aspect of the head of the first metatarsal.	>15° at MTP
Knee	Valgus/varum	Viewing the anterior aspect of the lower extremities, with the knees fully extended: valgus is considered if the tibia has a valgus angulation in comparison to the femur (the dancer's knees touch and the ankles do not); varum is considered present if the tibia has a varum angulation in comparison to the femur (the dancer's ankles touch and her knees do not). The knees are in correct alignment when the hips are neutral in rotation and the patellae are facing directly forward.	Knee valgus: Q angle >22° in females, >18° in males with knees extended. Knee varum: Space between the right and left knee with feet together in stance
	Genu-recurvatum	Viewing the lateral aspect of the lower extremities with the knees fully extended, genu-recurvatum is considered present if the femur is fully extended and the legs have a posterior angulation	>10° Hyperextension

(continued)

Table 2.2 (continued)

Joint	Anomalies	Physician observations (in an anatomical position)	Definition of a positive test[a]
Back	Scoliosis	(A) Magee's "skyline" view: any deviation from the normal posture: the head is straight on the shoulders; the posture of the jaw is normal; the tip of the nose is in line with the sternum; the trapezius neck line is equal on both sides; the shoulders are level; the clavicles are level; there is no protrusion, depression, or lateralization of the sternum, ribs, or costocartilage; the waist angles are equal, and the arms are equidistant from the waist; the carrying angle at each angle is equal, the palms of both hands face the body in the relaxed standing position; the high points of the iliac crest are the same on both sides; the ASIS are level; the pubic bone is level; the knees are straight; the heads of fibula are level; the ankles are level; the arches of the feet are equal on both sides; the feet angle out equally; there is no bowing of bones. (B) The Adams forward-bend test: when the dancer flexes her spine forward from a standing position scoliosis is considered when any hump on one side and a hollow on the other is detected. A positive test means that a rib hump deformity is noted in the thoracic region, or that an angle of trunk rotation is evident in the thoracolumbar or lumbar region.	Adams forward-bend test: thoracic: no posterior rib hump at 30° Lumbar: no increased muscle bulk at 90° of forward flexion

[a]According to Karim et al. [60]

Limited data are available regarding an association between static postural alignment and injuries. One study found a correlation between scoliosis and injuries among dancers aged 8–16 years [9]. Most other studies measured the *dynamic* alignment of dancers during active dance movements, suggesting that poor *dynamic* lower extremity alignment increased the risk of injury among young dancers [53, 61].

Hallux Valgus

Hallux valgus is a common deformity in the female population as a whole, and among athletes and dancers in particular [19, 62]. Prevalence of hallux valgus among young dancers (age 8–16 years) is very high (40%), and increases from pre-pubertal age (8–10 years: 32.7%) to pubertal age (11–13 years: 45.6%) [19]. Hallux valgus in dancers may result from various factors, such as the genetic component; the increased lever arm of the long hallux acting on the MP joint through an extreme ROM; increased stress on the MP joint during demi-pointe work; forced turnout (leading to rolling in) in demi-plié that also leads to excessive internal rotation of the tibia; and excessive movements such as en pointe work [62–64]. It has been suggested that hyper-pronation ("rolling in") can result in abnormal pressure distribution throughout the foot, which can place the dancer at risk for developing hallux valgus [65]. To summarize, genetic predisposition together with faulty technique might be the inappropriate combination that explains the high rate of hallux valgus in dancers. The greater the deformity the higher the chance that it will adversely influence the dancing by causing pain, bursitis, and limited ROM—all of which negatively impact the performance of the dancer. As surgical correction of hallux valgus deformities in dancers may decrease the power or ROM at the first MP joint muscles and ligaments [66], the most common recommendation for dancers is to adhere to conservative measures and avoid corrective surgery, preserving the range of dorsiflexion at the joint, which is a necessity for dancers [62].

Hallux valgus was found to be associated with other spinal and lower extremity joint mal-alignments such as scoliosis and knee varum [19], but no correlation between h/week of ballet practice and hallux valgus or h/week of en pointe dancing and hallux valgus have been reported among dancers [19, 63]. Given the prevalence and severity of hallux valgus with increasing age, it is suggested that hallux valgus is mostly related to hereditary anatomical factors and to incorrect technical execution [63].

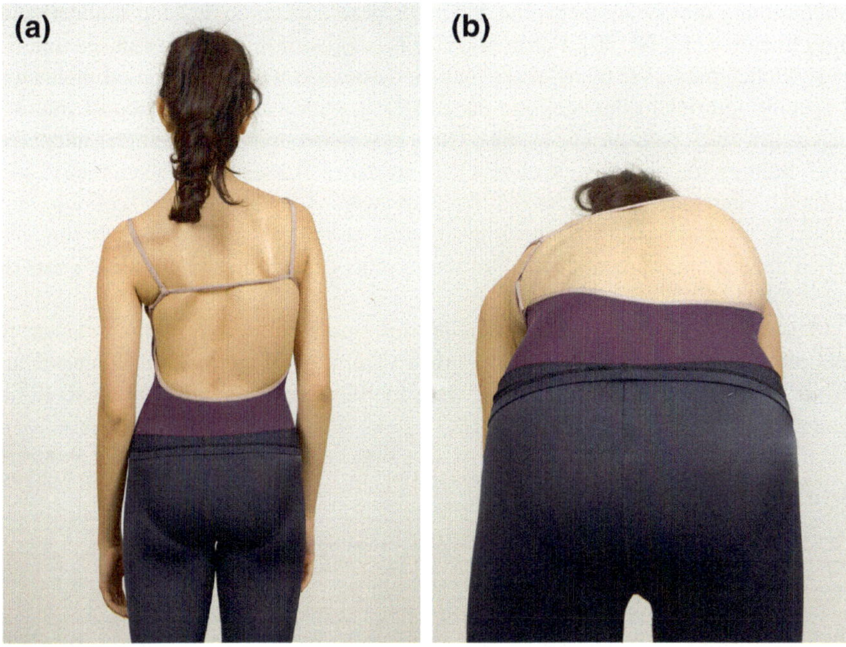

Fig. 2.4 Magee's "skyline" view (**a**) and the Adams forward-bend test (**b**). Photographs courtesy of James Koepfler

Scoliosis

There is a high incidence of scoliosis in athletic girls and dancers compared to their age-matched controls [67, 68]. In a screening examination performed by an orthopedic surgeon utilizing the Magee's "skyline" view (Fig. 2.4a) and the Adams forward-bend test (Fig. 2.4b), the prevalence of scoliosis was found to be 24–30% among recreational dancers, 30% among adolescent ballet dancers, and 24% in young professional dancers [15, 18, 69]. Scoliosis had already been noted in 22.6% of dancers at the age of 9, a prevalence that increased slightly to 26.3% at 16 years old [18].

The relationship between factors such as growth processes, intensive exercise, and scoliosis is not clear. A number of researchers have claimed that dance is a highly repetitive activity that imposes high stress on the immature spine, and that ballet training may delay menarche and predispose dancers to develop scoliosis and stress fractures [15, 68, 70]. Furthermore, it is suggested that the stresses exerted on the scoliotic spine over many years may be associated with an increased incidence of specific injuries to the scoliotic dancers [70], with a high incidence of injuries such as low back pain [9, 15, 18, 53]. Other researchers have claimed that intensive dance training may improve scoliosis [71], as dance classes involve symmetric and balanced exercises. Hence, no differences were found between scoliotic and non-scoliotic dancers in training impact parameters (mean age at which students started dance classes, mean h/week of dance practice, and mean number of years of practice) [18].

Identifying other anatomical anomalies during screening of a scoliotic dancer is important, as mal-alignments such as knee varum, genu-recurvatum, long-plantar planus, splay foot, and hallux valgus were found more frequently among scoliotic dancers than non-scoliotic dancers [18].

Physical Fitness (Muscle Strength Assessments)

Dance physical fitness depends on individuals' ability to work under aerobic and anaerobic conditions, and on their capacity to develop high levels of fitness parameters, such as muscle strength. Although no fitness measurement can predict success in dance, detection of muscle weakness is a powerful indicator of future injury [46].

Previous data have suggested that dance injuries are related mainly to the simultaneous presence of strong and weak muscles in the same limb [46]. Most injuries to the knee and lower leg occur due to diminished hip and knee muscle strength, which leads to faulty lower extremity alignment [52, 72]. Decreased strength may lead to faulty biomechanics of the lower extremity, particularly when the dancer tries to maintain neutral alignment during single leg landings [73]. Monitoring the strength of hip abductors, knee extensors, and ankle evertors is important, as during movement those muscles should control alignment of the lower extremities so that the patella remains in line with the second toe and the foot is placed in the correct position [74]. Thus, any muscle deficits or imbalance might predispose dancers to higher risk of injury [2]. Studies of young dancers showed that female dancers aged 8–11 years had weaker hip muscles than age-matched controls, except for hip abductor strength, which was similar. Yet, the dancers had the ability to improve their hip strength (in specific dance-related muscles) in a 12-month strengthening program, suggesting that hip strength can be trained at this young age [52, 58].

Dance Technique (Sickling in, Rolling in, and Hyperlordosis)

"Sickling in" refers to varus alignment of the foot, with increased stress on the lateral structures of the ankle [64, 66]. "Rolling in" refers to valgus heel with forefoot pronation [64, 75, 76] (Fig. 2.5). Hyperlordosis refers to anterior pelvic tilt or lumbar lordosis, which generates undue stress on the posterior elements of the spine [64] (Fig. 2.6; Table 2.3).

Screening young dancers for improper posture and technique is important, as using compensatory strategies is known to be a common phenomenon among ballet dancers and has been strongly linked to overuse injuries [9, 76–78]. Screening programs should address postural compensations in specific positions and should increase the dancers' self-awareness of their physical limitations, as well as the teachers' awareness.

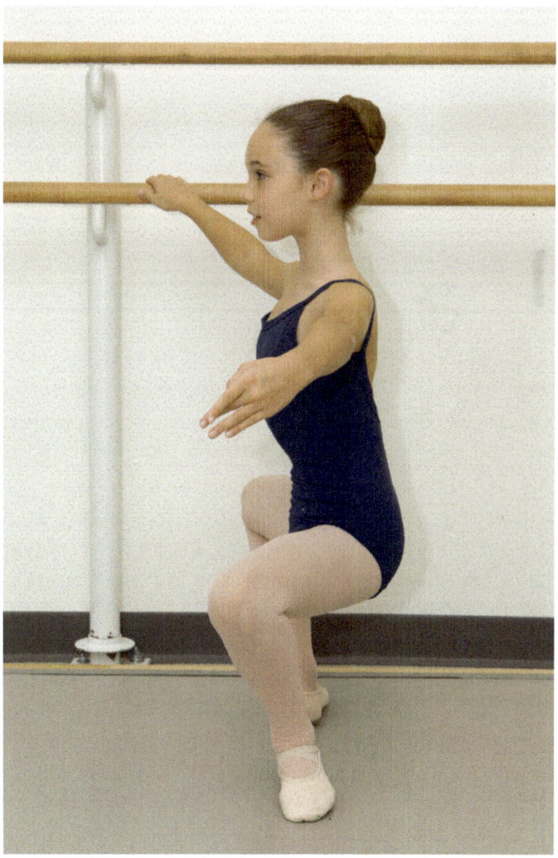

Fig. 2.5 "Rolling in" during turnout. Photograph courtesy of James Koepfler

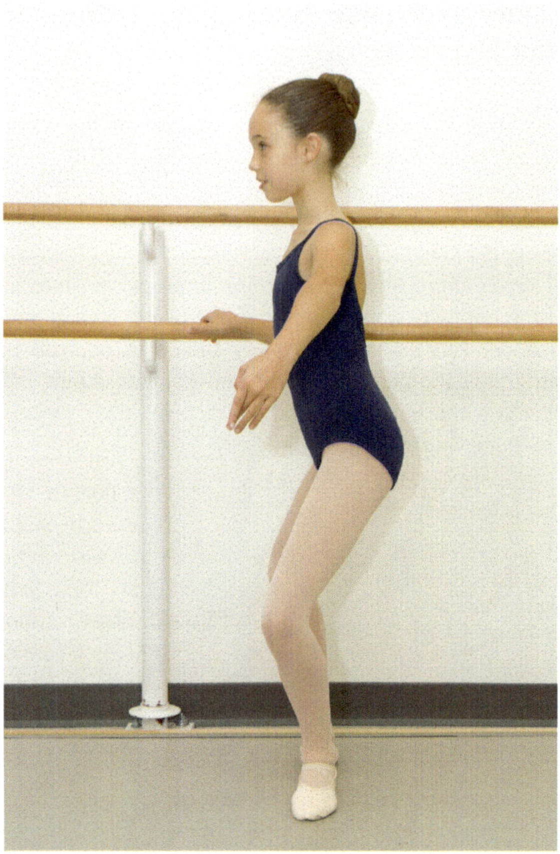

Fig. 2.6 Hyperlordosis during turnout. Photograph courtesy of James Koepfler

Considering the fact that limited joint ROM may trigger technique compensations that can lead to injury [2], education of dancers and teachers should emphasize correct dance positions and avoidance of compensation and stress, in accordance with the anatomic structure of each individual and based on his/her natural ROM [43, 76]. For example, dancers who try to achieve perfect "turnout" often compensate for insufficient hip motion by rotating at the knees, everting the heels, pronating the feet, and increasing the lordosis in their lumbar spine, which may be the origin of some of the spinal and lower extremity injuries seen in dancers [4, 77–80]. In addition, dancers with limited ankle plantar flexion compensate for this by using poor techniques that shift much of the load to their adjacent joints, including the knees [81]. Improving dance technique (e.g., correcting for neutral lower extremity alignment) may reduce the need for compensatory strategies, and therefore reduce the risk of injury [73].

Table 2.3 Dance technique

Technique	Physician observations	Comments
Sickling out/sickling in	The dancer was asked to perform a relevé: Correct technique is when the dancer rises up on the ball of the foot and the weight is in a straight line with the forefoot. Incorrect technique is when the dancer places weight onto the lateral (sickling out) or medial (sickling in) borders of her feet.	(1) The dancer is asked to demonstrate each technique 1–3 times at her usual speed, and 1–3 times as slowly as possible. (2) Technique movements were categorized as either correct or incorrect.
Hyperlordosis	The dancer was asked to perform a turnout position: correct technique is when the dancer externally rotates her hips, legs, and feet, without anterior pelvic tilt; incorrect technique is when the dancer tries to compensate for poor "turnout" by tilting the pelvis forward (hyperlordosis).	
Rolling in	The dancer was asked to perform a plié in first position: correct technique is when the patella is above the second toe; incorrect technique is when the patella is above or medial to the first toe (rolling in).	

Extrinsic Relevant Factors

Motivation and Adherence to Dance

The benefits of dancing include improvement in psychological well-being, increased self-esteem, and anxiety reduction. Thorough understanding on the part of teachers and screeners of the motivational stimulus of young dancers through readily available and reliable tools (such as the "Dance Motivation Inventory-DMI") is recommended [82, 83]. One should consider the high level of competition between students, the role model of the teacher, the body image confronting dancers in the mirror during classes, the emotional stress of adolescence, and stage fright.

Eating Habits

When a dancer is found to be at risk for disordered eating on the basis of screening measures (weight significantly lower than expected for age and height) a detailed assessment of eating habits and exploration of risk factors for disordered eating and poor self-image should be undertaken [84]. Validated screening tools exist for the detection of disordered eating behavior in athletes, including the Athletic Milieu Direct Questionnaire (AMDQ) [85], the Female Athlete Screening Tool (FAST) [86], the American Physiological Screening Test for eating disorders among Female College Athletes (PST) [87], the Low Energy Availability in Females Questionnaire (LEAF-Q) [88], and others designed to identify female athletes at risk for the "Triad" (a syndrome comprised of disordered eating, menstrual irregularity, and impaired bone health).

Musculoskeletal Injuries

The aim of musculoskeletal screening is to assess recovery from any previous injury and the presence of risk factors for future injury. The dancer should be asked about any previous or current injury/pain [7]. When a positive answer is obtained the dancer should be asked to describe the mechanism of injury—that is, the movements or exercises that precipitated the injury—and the extent to which the injury affects dancing and daily life activities. Dancers who report pain or dysfunction should be examined by a physician specializing in dance medicine. A clinical examination is required to reveal reproduction of pain or signs of injury (such as swelling, instability, reduced ROM.) [7, 9]. When additional confirmation is required, radiographs, ultrasound, computed tomography, or magnetic resonance imaging should be performed.

Injury Prevention

The medical screening process is an opportunity to identify potential risk factors and implement measures designed to reduce those risks. It is also an opportunity to ensure that medical equipment and assistive devices (such as scoliosis braces and proprioceptive insoles) are being used appropriately by injured dancers.

Summary

Screening provides an opportunity for the young dancer to be examined by experts in dance medicine—often for the first time in his/her life. The screening process may provide the dancers, their parents, their dance teachers, and the clinical team with useful information relevant to the future management of the dancer.

Most authors describe the majority of injuries in dancers as occurring in the lower leg and lumbar regions [5, 6, 89], with a different distribution of injuries between the youngest dancers (age 6–10 years) and adolescent dancers (age 14–18 years) [5, 6], and a different distribution between the two genders [89]. Injury incidence per 1000 h of practice indicated that the average for young dancers ranged from 0.8 to 8.4 [5, 6, 43, 90].

The data provided by methodological screenings and processing of accumulated knowledge from the literature enable teachers and medical staff to formulate solid conclusions that improve their care of the student dancer.

The task has not been completed; further intervention and longitudinal research will assist in determining associations between screening results and outcomes, with a better understanding of the relationship between various characteristics of the young dancer and risk factors for dance injuries.

Acknowledgements We gratefully acknowledge Prof. Israel Hershkovitz (the Department of Anatomy and Anthropology, Sackler Faculty of Medicine, Tel-Aviv University, Israel) for providing insight and expertise throughout the whole research and writing processes. For more than a decade prof. Hershkovitz supervised me and taught me (N.S.) how to adjust scientific tools from the field of anatomy and physical anthropology to the clinical field of dance medicine and science; Miss Aviva Zeev (Wintage College of Physical Education and Sports Sciences, Wingate Institute, Israel) for the statistical analysis; the Authority for Research and Development; and, Miss Anna Bechar (the Department of Anatomy and Anthropology, Sackler Faculty of Medicine, Tel-Aviv University, Israel) for the drawings.

References

1. Ivkovic A, Franic M, Bojanic I, Pecina M. Overuse injuries in female athletes. Croat Med J. 2007;48(6):767–78.
2. Hamilton WG, Hamilton LH, Marshall P, Molnar M. A profile of the musculoskeletal characteristics of elite professional ballet dancers. Am J Sports Med. 1992;20(3):267–73.
3. Nilsson C, Leanderson J, Wykman A, Strender LE. The injury panorama in a Swedish professional ballet company. Knee Surg Sports Traumatol Arthrosc. 2001;9(4):242–6.
4. Steinberg N, Hershkovitz I, Peleg S, Dar G, Masharawi Y, Siev-Ner I. Paratenonitis of the foot and ankle in young female dancers. Foot Ankle Int. 2011;32(12):1115–21.
5. Richardson M, Liederbach M, Sandow E. Functional criteria for assessing pointe-readiness. J Dance Med Sci. 2010;14(3):82–8.
6. Weiss DS, Rist RA, Grossman G. When can I start pointe work? Guidelines for initiating pointe training. J Dance Med Sci. 2009;13(3):90–2.
7. Steinberg N, Siev-Ner I, Peleg S, Dar G, Masharawi Y, Zeev A, et al. Injury patterns in young, non-professional dancers. J Sports Sci. 2011;29(1):47–54.
8. Steinberg N, Aujla I, Zeev A, Redding E. Injuries among talented young dancers: findings from the U.K. centres for advanced training. Int J Sports Med. 2014;35(3):238–44.
9. Steinberg N, Siev-Ner I, Peleg S, Dar G, Masharawi Y, Zeev A, et al. Extrinsic and intrinsic risk factors associated with injuries in young dancers aged 8–16 years. J Sports Sci. 2012;30(5):485–95.
10. Loucks AB. Effects of exercise training on the menstrual cycle: existence and mechanisms. Med Sci Sports Exerc. 1990;22(3):275–80.
11. Twitchett E, Brodrick A, Nevill AM, Koutedakis Y, Angioi M, Wyon M. Does physical fitness affect injury occurrence and time loss due to injury in elite vocational ballet students? J Dance Med Sci. 2010;14(1):26–31.

12. Malina RM. Menarche in athletes: a synthesis and hypothesis. Ann Hum Biol. 1983;10(1):1–24.
13. Steinberg N, Siev-Ner I, Peleg S, Dar G, Masharawi Y, Hershkovitz I. Growth and development of female dancers aged 8–16 years. Am J Hum Biol. 2008;20(3):299–307.
14. Steinberg N, Siev-Ner I, Peleg S, Dar G, Masharawi Y, Zeev A, et al. Injuries in female dancers aged 8 to 16 years. J Athl Train. 2013;48(1):118–23.
15. Warren MP, Brooks-Gunn J, Hamilton LH, Warren LF, Hamilton WG. Scoliosis and fractures in young ballet dancers. Relation to delayed menarche and secondary amenorrhea. N Engl J Med. 1986;314(21):1348–53.
16. Warren MP, Brooks-Gunn J, Fox RP, Holderness CC, Hyle EP, Hamilton WG. Osteopenia in exercise-associated amenorrhea using ballet dancers as a model: a longitudinal study. J Clin Endocrinol Metab. 2002;87(7):3162–8.
17. Abraham SF, Beumont PJ, Fraser IS, Llewellyn-Jones D. Body weight, exercise and menstrual status among ballet dancers in training. Br J Obstet Gynaecol. 1982;89(7):507–10.
18. Steinberg N, Hershkovitz I, Peleg S, Dar G, Masharawi Y, Zeev A, et al. Morphological characteristics of the young scoliotic dancer. Phys Ther Sport. 2013;14(4):213–20.
19. Steinberg N, Siev-Ner I, Zeev A, Dar G. The association between hallux valgus and proximal joint alignment in young female dancers. Int J Sports Med. 2015;36(1):67–74.
20. Steinberg N, Hershkovitz I, Zeev A, Rothschild B, Siev-Ner I. Joint hypermobility and joint range of motion in young dancers. J Clin Rheumatol. 2016;22(4):171–8.
21. Kadel N, Donaldson-Fletcher E, Gerberg LF, Micheli LJ. Anthropometric measurements of young ballet dancers: examining body composition, puberty, flexibility, and joint range of motion in comparison with nondancers controls. J Dance Med Sci. 2005;9(3&4):84–90.
22. Ravaldi C, Vannacci A, Zucchi T, Mannucci E, Cabras PL, Boldrini M, et al. Eating disorders and body image disturbances among ballet dancers, gymnasium users and body builders. Psychopathology. 2003;36(5):247–54.
23. Claessens AL, Beunen GP, Nuyts MM, Lefevre JA, Wellens RI. Body structure, somatotype, maturation and motor performance of girls in ballet schooling. J Sports Med Phys Fit. 1987;27 (3):310–7.
24. Bowerman E, Whatman C, Harris N, Bradshaw E, Karin J. Are maturation, growth and lower extremity alignment associated with overuse injury in elite adolescent ballet dancers? Phys Ther Sport. 2014;15(4):234–41.
25. Henry L. Leg length discrepancy in the professional dancer. J Back Musculoskelet Rehabil. 1995;5(3):209–17.
26. Beighton P, Grahame R, Bird HA. Hypermobility of joints. Berlin: Springer; 1983.
27. Briggs J, McCormack M, Hakim AJ, Grahame R. Injury and joint hypermobility syndrome in ballet dancers—a 5-year follow-up. Rheumatology. 2009;48(12):1613–4.
28. Hincapie CA, Morton EJ, Cassidy JD. Musculoskeletal injuries and pain in dancers: a systematic review. Arch Phys Med Rehabil. 2008;89(9):1819–29.
29. Klemp P, Chalton D. Articular mobility in ballet dancers. A follow-up study after four years. Am J Sports Med. 1989;17(1):72–5.
30. Scheper MC, de Vries JE, Juul-Kristensen B, Nollet F, Engelbert RH. The functional consequences of generalized joint hypermobility: a cross-sectional study. BMC Musculoskelet Disord. 2014;15:243.
31. Rietveld AB. Dancers' and musicians' injuries. Clin Rheumatol. 2013;32(4):425–34.
32. Sanches SB, Oliveira GM, Osorio FL, Crippa JA, Martin-Santos R. Hypermobility and joint hypermobility syndrome in Brazilian students and teachers of ballet dance. Rheumatol Int. 2015;35(4):741–7.
33. Grahame R. The hypermobility syndrome. Ann Rheum Dis. 1990;49(3):199–200.
34. Klemp P, Learmonth ID. Hypermobility and injuries in a professional ballet company. Br J Sports Med. 1984;18(3):143–8.
35. Foley EC, Bird HA. Hypermobility in dance: asset, not liability. Clin Rheumatol. 2013;32 (4):455–61.

36. McCormack M, Briggs J, Hakim A, Grahame R. Joint laxity and the benign joint hypermobility syndrome in student and professional ballet dancers. J Rheumatol. 2004;31(1):173–8.
37. Misigoj-Durakovic M, Matkovic BR, Ruzic L, Durakovic Z, Babic Z, Jankovic S, et al. Body composition and functional abilities in terms of the quality of professional ballerinas. Coll Antropol. 2001;25(2):585–90.
38. Tajet-Foxell B, Rose FD. Pain and pain tolerance in professional ballet dancers. Br J Sports Med. 1995;29(1):31–4.
39. Steinberg N, Tenenbaum S, Zeev A, Hershkovitz I, Siev-Ner I. Lower extremity and spine characteristics in dancers with and without patellofemoral pain. Res Sports Med. 2017 Jan;25(2):166–80.
40. Mouton C, Theisen D, Seil R. Objective measurements of static anterior and rotational knee laxity. Curr Rev Musculoskelet Med. 2016;9(2):139–47.
41. Siev-Ner I, Barak A, Heim M, Azaria M. The value of screening. J Dance Med Sci. 1997;1(3):87–92.
42. Liederbach MJ. Screening for functional capacity in dancers. J Dance Med Sci. 1997;1(3):93–106.
43. Steinberg N, Hershkovitz I, Peleg S, Dar G, Masharawi Y, Heim M, et al. Range of joint movement in female dancers and nondancers aged 8 to 16 years: anatomical and clinical implications. Am J Sports Med. 2006;34(5):814–23.
44. Anderson B, Burke ER. Scientific, medical, and practical aspects of stretching. Clin Sports Med. 1991;10(1):63–86.
45. Apostolopoulos N, Metsios GS, Flouris AD, Koutedakis Y, Wyon MA. The relevance of stretch intensity and position-a systematic review. Front Psychol. 2015 Aug 18;6:1128.
46. Koutedakis Y, Jamurtas A. The dancer as a performing athlete: physiological considerations. Sports Med. 2004;34(10):651–61.
47. Thompson WR, Gordon NF, Pescatello LS, editors. ACSM's guidelines for exercise testing and prescription, 8th ed. Baltimore, MD: Lippincott, Williams and Wilkins; 2010.
48. Lea RD, Gerhardt JJ. Range-of-motion measurements. J Bone Joint Surg Am. 1995;77(5):784–98.
49. Magee D. Orthopedic physical assessment. Philadelphia, PA: W.B. Saunders; 1997.
50. Roussel N, De Kooning M, Schutt A, Mottram S, Truijen S, Nijs J, et al. Motor control and low back pain in dancers. Int J Sports Med. 2013;34(2):138–43.
51. Gupta A, Fernihough B, Bailey G, Bombeck P, Clarke A, Hopper D. An evaluation of differences in hip external rotation strength and range of motion between female dancers and non-dancers. Br J Sports Med. 2004;38(6):778–83.
52. Bennell KL, Khan KM, Matthews BL, Singleton C. Changes in hip and ankle range of motion and hip muscle strength in 8–11 year old novice female ballet dancers and controls: a 12 month follow up study. Br J Sports Med. 2001;35(1):54–9.
53. Gamboa JM, Roberts LA, Maring J, Fergus A. Injury patterns in elite preprofessional ballet dancers and the utility of screening programs to identify risk characteristics. J Orthop Sports Phys Ther. 2008;38(3):126–36.
54. Steinberg N, Siev-Ner I, Peleg S, Dar G, Masharawi Y, Zeev A, et al. Joint range of motion and patellofemoral pain in dancers. Int J Sports Med. 2012;33(7):561–6.
55. Aalto TJ, Airaksinen O, Harkonen TM, Arokoski JP. Effect of passive stretch on reproducibility of hip range of motion measurements. Arch Phys Med Rehabil. 2005;86(3):549–57.
56. Khan K, Roberts P, Nattrass C, Bennell K, Mayes S, Way S, et al. Hip and ankle range of motion in elite classical ballet dancers and controls. Clin J Sport Med. 1997;7(3):174–9.
57. Myer GD, Ford KR, McLean SG, Hewett TE. The effects of plyometric versus dynamic stabilization and balance training on lower extremity biomechanics. Am J Sports Med. 2006;34(3):445–55.

58. Bennell K, Khan KM, Matthews B, De Gruyter M, Cook E, Holzer K, et al. Hip and ankle range of motion and hip muscle strength in young female ballet dancers and controls. Br J Sports Med. 1999;33(5):340–6.
59. Wiesler ER, Hunter DM, Martin DF, Curl WW, Hoen H. Ankle flexibility and injury patterns in dancers. Am J Sports Med. 1996;24(6):754–7.
60. Karim A, Millet V, Massie K, Olson S, Morganthaler A. Inter-rater reliability of a musculoskeletal screen as administered to female professional contemporary dancers. Work. 2011;40(3):281–8.
61. Kravitz SR. Pronation as a predisposing factor in overuse injuries. In: Solomon R, Minton SC, Solomon J, editors. Preventing dance injuries. 2nd ed. Champaign, IL: Human Kinetics; 2005. p. 185–9.
62. Kennedy JG, Collumbier JA. Bunions in dancers. Clin Sports Med. 2008;27(2):321–8.
63. Biz C, Favero L, Stecco C, Aldegheri R. Hypermobility of the first ray in ballet dancer. Muscles Ligaments Tendons J. 2012;2(4):282–8.
64. Motta-Valencia K. Dance-related injury. Phys Med Rehabil Clin N Am. 2006;17(3):697–723.
65. Davenport KL, Simmel L, Kadel N. Hallux valgus in dancers: a closer look at dance technique and its impact on dancers' feet. J Dance Med Sci. 2014;18(2):86–92.
66. Brown TD, Micheli LJ. Foot and ankle injuries in dance. Am J Orthop. 2004;33(6):303–9.
67. Modi H, Srinivasalu S, Smehta S, Yang JH, Song HR, Suh SW. Muscle imbalance in volleyball players initiates scoliosis in immature spines: a screening analysis. Asian Spine J. 2008;2(1):38–43.
68. Omey ML, Micheli LJ, Gerbino PG. 2nd. Idiopathic scoliosis and spondylolysis in the female athlete. Tips for treatment. Clin Orthop Relat Res. 2000;372:74–84.
69. Longworth B, Fary R, Hopper D. Prevalence and predictors of adolescent idiopathic scoliosis in adolescent ballet dancers. Arch Phys Med Rehabil. 2014;95(9):1725–30.
70. Kenanidis EI, Potoupnis ME, Papavasiliou KA, Sayegh FE, Kapetanos GA. Adolescent idiopathic scoliosis in athletes: is there a connection? Phys Sportsmed. 2010;38(2):165–70.
71. Dickson RA. Spinal deformity–adolescent idiopathic scoliosis. Nonoperative treatment. Spine (Phila Pa 1976). 1999 Dec 15;24(24):2601–6.
72. Bowerman EA, Whatman C, Harris N, Bradshaw E. A review of the risk factors for lower extremity overuse injuries in young elite female ballet dancers. J Dance Med Sci. 2015;19(2):51–6.
73. Liederbach M, Dilgen FE, Rose DJ. Incidence of anterior cruciate ligament injuries among elite ballet and modern dancers: a 5-year prospective study. Am J Sports Med. 2008;36(9):1779–88.
74. Orishimo KF, Kremenic IJ, Pappas E, Hagins M, Liederbach M. Comparison of landing biomechanics between male and female professional dancers. Am J Sports Med. 2009;37(11):2187–93.
75. Khan K, Brown J, Way S, Vass N, Crichton K, Alexander R, et al. Overuse injuries in classical ballet. Sports Med. 1995;19(5):341–57.
76. Negus V, Hopper D, Briffa NK. Associations between turnout and lower extremity injuries in classical ballet dancers. J Orthop Sports Phys Ther. 2005;35(5):307–18.
77. Arendt YD, Kerschbaumer F. Injury and overuse pattern in professional ballet dancers. Z Orthop Ihre Grenzgeb. 2003;141(3):349–56.
78. Coplan JA. Ballet dancer's turnout and its relationship to self-reported injury. J Orthop Sports Phys Ther. 2002;32(11):579–84.
79. Cimelli SN, Curran SA. Influence of turnout on foot posture and its relationship to overuse musculoskeletal injury in professional contemporary dancers: a preliminary investigation. J Am Podiatr Med Assoc. 2012;102(1):25–33.
80. Kushner S, Saboe L, Reid D, Penrose T, Grace M. Relationship of turnout to hip abduction in professional ballet dancers. Am J Sports Med. 1990;18(3):286–91.
81. Hodgkins CW, Kennedy JG, O'Loughlin PF. Tendon injuries in dance. Clin Sports Med. 2008;27(2):279–88.

82. Aujla IJ, Nordin-Bates SM, Redding E. Multidisciplinary predictors of adherence to contemporary dance training: findings from the UK Centres for Advanced Training. J Sports Sci. 2015;33(15):1564–73.
83. Maraz A, Kiraly O, Urban R, Griffiths MD, Demetrovics Z. Why do you dance? Development of the dance motivation inventory (DMI). PLoS ONE. 2015;10(3):e0122866.
84. Javed A, Tebben PJ, Fischer PR, Lteif AN. Female athlete triad and its components: toward improved screening and management. Mayo Clin Proc. 2013;88(9):996–1009.
85. Nagel DL, Black DR, Leverenz LJ, Coster DC. Evaluation of a screening test for female college athletes with eating disorders and disordered eating. J Athl Train. 2000;35(4):431–40.
86. McNulty KY, Adams CH, Anderson JM, Affenito SG. Development and validation of a screening tool to identify eating disorders in female athletes. J Am Dietet Assoc. 2001;101 (8):886–92 (quiz 93–4).
87. Black DR, Larkin LJ, Coster DC, Leverenz LJ, Abood DA. Physiologic screening test for eating disorders/disordered eating among female collegiate athletes. J Athl Train. 2003;38 (4):286–97.
88. Melin A, Tornberg AB, Skouby S, Faber J, Ritz C, Sjodin A, et al. The LEAF questionnaire: a screening tool for the identification of female athletes at risk for the female athlete triad. Br J Sports Med. 2014;48(7):540–5.
89. Ekegren CL, Quested R, Brodrick A. Injuries in pre-professional ballet dancers: Incidence, characteristics and consequences. J Sci Med Sport. 2014;17(3):271–5.
90. Luke A, Kinney S, D'Hemecourt PA, Baum J, Owen M, Micheli LJ. Determinants of injuries in young dancers. Med Probl Perform Art. 2002;17(3):105–12.

Chapter 3
A Screening Program for the Young Dancer: Perspectives on What and Why to Include in a Screen

Heather Southwick, PT, MSPT and Maribeth Crupi, PT

Pertinent Definitions

Screening: A preliminary procedure, such as a test or examination, performed on asymptomatic populations to detect the most characteristic signs of disorders that may require further investigation.
Evaluation: A comprehensive physical examination of the body and its functions, utilized as a means for diagnosing a previously detected problem. It generally includes objective tests and measurements that can be indicators of progress or change.

Background

Participating in dance classes and creative movement has tremendous physical and mental benefits for children and continues to increase in popularity in the USA; there are currently over 32,000 dance studios and an estimated 4 million children and adolescents studying some form of dance. Inevitably, this increase in participation brings with it a rising rate of injury [1], which mandates the need for specific health care related to the demands of all levels of dancers in training.

H. Southwick, PT, MSPT (✉)
Boston Ballet, 19 Clarendon Street, Boston, MA 02116, USA
e-mail: hsouthwick@bostonballet.org

M. Crupi, PT
Maribeth Crupi Physical Therapy LLC, 314 Main Street, Suite 101, Wilmington, MA 01997, USA
e-mail: mccrupi@comcast.net

R. Solomon et al. (eds.), *Prevention of Injuries in the Young Dancer*, Contemporary Pediatric and Adolescent Sports Medicine,
DOI 10.1007/978-3-319-55047-3_3

By way of injury prevention, preparticipation screenings have been utilized since the mid- to late 1980s in an effort to determine readiness for play and reduce injury in sports [2]. Given that participation in youth sports programs often requires at least a pre-participation physical examination by a physician, it is a matter of concern that dancers, who might be training at even higher levels of intensity, most often have no such requirement. In the dance medicine literature there is agreement that while screenings are not intended to substitute for a dancer's health care, they can be utilized to identify intrinsic risk factors for illness or injury. Screening allows for review of past and current issues that can impact future health and injury. It can also help healthcare practitioners establish baselines for a dancer in a variety of physical areas. As the majority of injuries in dance are musculoskeletal in nature, it makes sense that healthcare providers with a dance medicine background should be involved in the screening process.

Goals of Screening

There are many goals of screening in dance; however, the most important ones are to help improve safe participation in the more intense forms of training, like ballet, and determine whether an individual possesses the physical attributes necessary to progress in his or her chosen dance genre. A more specific goal is to gain an understanding of the baseline profile of a dancer's medical, psychological, nutritional, and physical status. The higher levels of dance, particularly in ballet, have unique requirements for flexibility and strength at end ranges of motion, and a screen in pre-adolescent and adolescent dancers can be instrumental in offering prudent training goals and recommendations during this period of accelerated growth. This supports another goal of educating the dancer on his/her individual strengths and weaknesses, promoting self-awareness with regard to what areas can be addressed with exercise to improve function and training. Ultimately, the most important objective of screening is to prevent potential injury, not predict injury, by identifying risk and underlying pathology that would not have otherwise been exposed. This has been debated in the literature, and the prevention of injury is difficult to measure even with a robust injury tracking method [3].

Benefits of Screening

There are many benefits to implementing a screening program. Allowing a dancer to meet and establish a relationship with a healthcare team of physicians, physical therapists, and athletic trainers who are knowledgeable in dance can have significant implications for creating trust and allowing for earlier problem recognition, reporting of injuries, and treatment. Removing the stigma of seeking health care, which is known to be a concern among collegiate and professional dancers [4], can help dancers feel more comfortable in accessing services for prevention, as opposed to waiting until they sustain an injury. A screening can also provide an opportunity for counseling and referral to specialties in fields like nutrition and sports psychology, and to educate young dancers on the importance of these areas to their overall health and performance. The education that accompanies the screening can serve to motivate young dancers to improve their overall fitness and performance on certain tests and measures. Most importantly, while the screening may be broad-based, it should always conclude with individual recommendations, a home exercise program to improve areas of weakness, and, if needed, referrals for further care.

Screening Versus Evaluation

A challenge with screenings, especially in a younger population, is how to keep an assessment that will help identify "red flags" from becoming a full-out musculoskeletal evaluation. The definition of screening includes the concept of a preliminary procedure to detect the most characteristic signs of disorders that may require further investigation. However, especially in the young, growing population, it is tempting for healthcare practitioners to revert to an evaluation format that is more formal, comprehensive, and analytical than a screen. It is also more time-consuming. Evaluation involves specific measurements of strength and range of motion or flexibility. While this can be very important information in a young dancer, a "screen" is often more of an assessment focused on gathering general information pertinent to the subject's age and motor development. In sports and in dance a comprehensive approach with "yes or no" categories offers the best opportunity to screen for health risk prior to participation.

Timing of a Screening Program

For a screening program to have the greatest impact the beginning of a school year, semester, or season is most beneficial to allow time for any identified issues to be addressed. Before a school year begins is arguably most effective, so there is time for deficits in strength and flexibility to be identified and targeted training initiated before the student dancer is too engaged in school activities. Incidentally, it is not appropriate to utilize screens as a test of acceptability into a company or school [5]. Following acceptance into a particular school, it may be beneficial to repeat the screening process throughout the year with young, growing dancers to track changes and improvements in strength and flexibility. If a screening program is implemented as an assessment for injury prevention, re-assessment during the year can also be helpful in motivating compliance with a home exercise program.

Location of Screening Assessments

Method and location for a screening varies depending on the needs and goals of the dance school and type of dance studied. Sometimes screens are performed in a physician's office or physical therapy clinic, which allows for consistency, privacy, and a setting outside of the dance studio. This may help dancers feel more comfortable about revealing themselves. More often screens are conducted at dance studios to promote convenience and compliance. Larger numbers are handled well in stations set up by a healthcare team that may be comprised of physicians, physical therapists, athletic trainers, sports psychologists, nutritionists, and a dance educator or healthcare provider with a background in dance and movement analysis. It is debatable whether the faculty or artistic staff directly involved with the dance students should be part of the screening team. Given the wide range of backgrounds of artistic staff, it is important that dance teachers in attendance have some knowledge of anatomy if asked to assist with the actual screening process. Their participation can be an advantage, exposing them to how healthcare professionals view dancers. Another advantage of having dance teachers involved who are well versed in anatomy is that they tend to be the most qualified expert on the screening team, where evaluating for potential issues with technique and movement patterns is concerned. The disadvantage is that some dancers may not feel comfortable with their teachers having access to their personal health information and musculoskeletal status.

Handling of Screening Information

For those conducting a screen it is important to ask why you want to employ particular screening tools, what you will do with the information collected, and how it will potentially improve the health of the dancers involved. The data collected must be treated as personal medical information to which total confidentiality and HIPAA laws apply. Before participating in a screen, dancers should be fully informed of its procedure, how the information collected will be used, and who will have access to it [5]. Parents should be part of the process when the dancers being screened are minors. Ultimately, the main purpose of a screen is to educate the dancers on their individual findings and offer interventions to address areas of concern. At the same time, an anonymous review of data from the group as a whole can be helpful for identifying trends, guiding programming, and promoting research [6].

Organization of the Screening Tool

With so many different forms of dance, levels of training, and a need to assess the areas of greatest risk for injury, there may be no single way to organize a screening tool for every situation. The proccss should be efficient and effective, addressing the most significant issues for the type of training in question. When the goals of the screening process are clear, then the tests and measures to be selected become more obvious. Regardless of the type of training, there are elements to healthy movement that are universal. Hence, screening tool assessments often include a comprehensive medical history and a combination of physical tests that look at a dancer's posture and structure, flexibility, strength, cardiovascular parameters, and issues with motor patterns and muscle recruitment. It should be noted that the use of validated tests allows for the kinds of comparisons that facilitate ongoing or future research.

Health History

One of the most comprehensive, and many would argue most significant, areas of the screen is the health history. This can be in a questionnaire format and should include dance background and exposure questions such as the following: How many years have you been dancing; how many hours a day/week do you dance; what types of dance do you study; are you en pointe; if so, at what age did you begin pointe work, and were there specific criteria used to determine readiness. The dancer should also be asked about participation in other sports, or if he/she engages in any kind of cross-training. General health questions and medical history can be brief or lengthy, but should at least inquire about asthma, allergies, diabetes, and history of concussion. Questions asking whether the dancer has had a medical illness or injury since last check up or if there is an ongoing or chronic illness can help identify the need for further information or referral. In pre-professional level students a few cardiac questions should be included, as over 95% of all sudden deaths in athletes under age 30 are due to structural cardiac problems [7]. Questioning of this kind is consistent with the Preparticipation Physical Evaluation published by the American College of Sports Medicine and used for athletes in high schools throughout the USA [8, 9].

In the dance population there is a higher-than-normal incidence of menstrual dysfunction, musculoskeletal injury, and lower bone density that is all interrelated (this is known as the "female athlete triad"). Including questions regarding the onset of menses and frequency of menstruation can help the healthcare practitioner uncover issues that can not only lead to injuries, but have other potentially serious and detrimental outcomes as well. A thorough history of past injuries is also important, as this is a risk factor for recurrent injury. Ankle sprains, which are often dismissed as insignificant by dancers, offer a perfect example of this requirement, as research provides ample evidence of future injury with history of prior ankle sprain [10, 11]. Another area that is important to include is prior stress injuries to bone, as there may be underlying issues with nutrition and energy deficiency that need to be further evaluated and addressed.

Physical Assessment

In terms of the physical assessment, what is included will depend on the overall goals of the screening process. Time constraints and resources may also be a factor. Unless there is the opportunity to spend 2–3 h screening each dancer all the tests and measurements discussed in this chapter may not be included in one screening assessment. Multiple screening test options, with indications and general rationale for use, are included to help the practitioner create a screen that meets the goals and constraints of a specific setting.

Height, Weight, and BMI

Obtaining anthropometric measurements such as height and weight provides a baseline for the young dancer and the information required to calculate body mass index (BMI). In growing children age needs to be included as a factor. Many young dancers face a major transition when they reach adolescence and their bodies begin to change. When height and weight measurements are taken, dancers should be asked about recent growth spurts. It is normal to gain weight right before a growth spurt or puberty, and dancers, parents, and teachers may need to be educated to this fact. It is important that clinicians and dancers understand that the purpose of obtaining these measurements is to help identify dancers who are at risk of injury because their BMI is too low and to help track if a young dancer is growing adequately. The approach to these measurements should be handled with sensitivity in this population, as adolescent girls who are focused on activities like ballet where thinness is the generally valued aesthetic are often preoccupied with weight and body image. A proper screening not only helps identify young dancers at risk due to a low BMI, but also assesses any issues with menstrual cycles, as this combination can lead to dangerous health issues and multiple injuries, such as stress fractures [12]. In cases where inadequate energy intake is a concern, or where the young dancer appears too thin, referral to a female athlete triad expert (with bone health emphasis) should be considered. Normative values in children and adolescents for skin-fold thickness assessment of body composition are now available [13].

Posture

Integral to all dance styles and aesthetic values is a dancer's technique and alignment. Faulty technique and compromised alignment may lead to injury [14]. Knowledge of a dancer's baseline posture and structure can be imperative to help understand these issues as they pertain to injury prevention. A quick observational review or the use of more comprehensive parameters to assess how a dancer is built can help highlight areas of weakness, unbalanced strength, or joint hyper/hypomobility. Since adolescent dancers may already be self-conscious about their changing appearance, it is important to put them at ease and assure them that it is very common to have postural asymmetries. The goal is to identify areas that may benefit from exercises or other interventions, or to facilitate referral for further evaluation.

The age of the dancer will help dictate the degree of and manner in which the findings are taken into consideration, and intense participation in activities such as dance may also have an effect on growth [15]. It is important to consider that chronological age versus physiologic age may vary [15]. In addition, screening the very young pre-pubescent dancer can result in typical developmental findings such as internal femoral rotation, valgus or "knock knees," anterior pelvic tilt, and hyperflexible joints [16]. Similar findings in the adolescent dancer might be more cause for concern or intervention.

It is necessary to view dancers from multiple perspectives to obtain a complete picture of their potential postural issues, generally from the rear, the side, and the front. As an example, screening from the rear offers a vantage point to view pelvic and shoulder girdle asymmetries, potential leg length discrepancies, and spinal alignment as a whole, including screening for scoliosis. When screening for scoliosis, the Adam's Forward Bend Test can be helpful to evaluate for rib hump and spinal asymmetry after a leg length discrepancy is ruled out or corrected. Tipped or winging scapulae will alert the skilled observer to potential weaknesses that could result in poor execution of port de bras in ballet, insufficient stability to execute handstands in contemporary or hip hop forms of dance, or safe performance of lifts during partnering work. Findings such as rear foot valgus and hyperpronated feet will have the trained observer thinking of how the impact of jump landings may strain the medial muscles of the ankle and foot and facilitate valgus moments at the knee. Conversely, a fixed high-arched cavus foot type should be recognized and noted, as this can be a risk factor for overuse injury in dancers, especially due to increased impact force with landing from jumps [17].

The benefit of screening for postural findings not only includes the correction of faults revealed, but can also be an opportunity to educate the developing dancer on preventing an overuse syndrome or future pathology caused by repetitive training in a dysfunctional manner. For the posture assessment to be fully appreciated, it needs to be compared and correlated with other areas of the screen. Any structural issue identified with a postural screen is likely to be more apparent when dance technique movement is added.

Hypermobility

In the literature it has been established that hypermobile dancers are at risk for increased injury [18], and assessment for hypermobility is a key component in the screening of an adolescent dancer. Joint hypermobility is a compound term for what could be a wide array of etiologies for excessive movement at a few or many joints. It may be bony in nature related to shallow joint sockets, the result of changes in collagen of joint capsules and ligaments, or neuropathic, resulting in muscle weakness or reduced joint proprioception [19]. Excessive joint mobility may be a product of a benign familial tendency toward increased laxity of the ligaments, or can represent a more serious condition such as Ehlers–Danlos or Marfan syndromes [19].

While the presence of joint hypermobility in a dancer is rather easy to assess in a screening, the ramifications of such findings are much more involved. It is estimated that 44% of dancers present with some type of joint hypermobility, depending on the screening tool that is used [18]. The most commonly used test is the 9-point Beighton Assessment of Hypermobility [20] (Fig. 3.1a, b). A dancer is considered hypermobile if the Beighton score is 4/9 or greater, and higher scores should be referred for physical therapy [18].

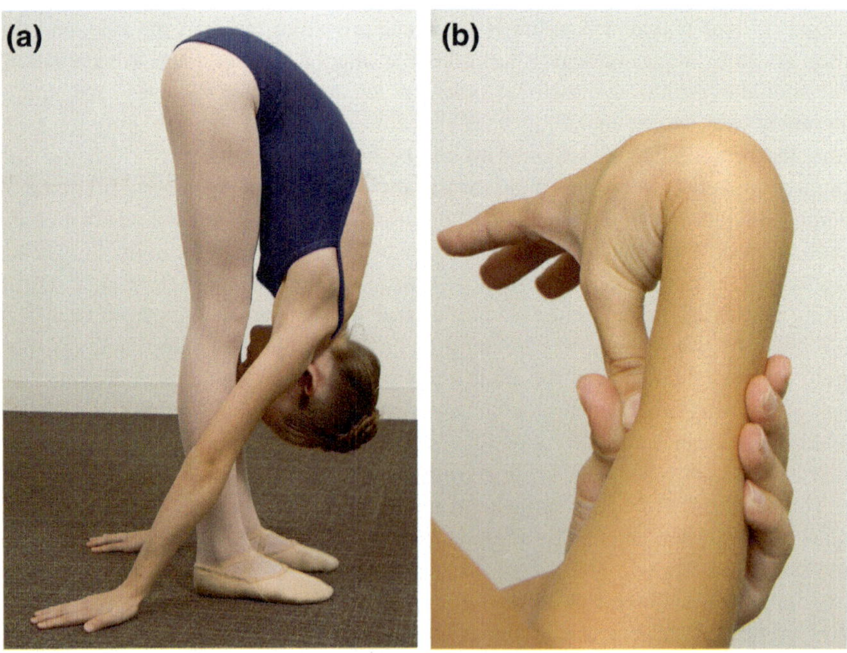

Fig. 3.1 Examples of Beighton test measures. **a** Positive Beighton forward bend. **b** Positive Beighton thumb to forearm. Photographs courtesy of James Koepfler

Hypermobile dancers must be educated on the need to increase strength and work on stability to reduce shearing forces at their joints. The hypermobile dancer will frequently complain of feeling "stiff." Their muscles may be tighter as they are working harder than the average individual just to stand and maintain postural stability at joints lacking adequate passive restraint of the ligaments. Screening for hypermobility offers the opportunity to assure that the dancer will be referred to a physical therapist who will teach her or him how safely to release stiffness in the muscles, rather than pushing into extreme ranges of motion where they are more likely to be overstretching already loose and compromised joint ligaments and capsules. Attention to promoting stability around the joints is paramount in helping the hypermobile dancer to avoid injury.

There are many characteristics of a hypermobile dancer that can affect multiple potential causes of injury. For example, due to altered joint proprioception hypermobile dancers may struggle at times to keep tempo with music. With a greater demand on their muscles to compensate for the lack of adequate ligament or capsular stability, they are working harder than their non-hypermobile peers, even during what might seem to be simple gestures and movements. This results in earlier onset of fatigue. With the known link between fatigue and injury for all dancers [21], it is not surprising that there is an even greater incidence of injury in the hypermobile dancer [16, 22].

Cardiovascular Fitness

Screening tests for cardiovascular fitness vary regarding parameters assessed and how the information can be applied. Research in this area has helped provide a better understanding of the physiological demands of dancing. In general, dance is categorized as a high intensity, intermittent form of exercise [23]. Cardiovascular testing in performance has shown that both the aerobic and anaerobic energy systems may be utilized, while dance class seems to stimulate only the anaerobic system, producing energy bursts for 10–12 s [24]. If class has lesser cardiovascular demands than performance, then a dancer's aerobic fitness may not be adequate for the demands of repetitive rehearsals or performance, leading to fatigue and injury. Screening tests looking at cardiovascular health, fitness, and recovery can be very helpful in establishing a baseline and helping to motivate young dancers to perform supplemental cardiovascular training.

The accelerated 3-min step test is utilized by many professional companies as a measure of cardiovascular fitness, as it is simple and quick to implement (Fig. 3.2). In addition to other parameters, physical fitness is characterized by the post-exercise heart rate, considered to be an indicator of cardiorespiratory fitness. Bronner and Rakov have compared an accelerated 3-min step test (112 beats min) to the well-studied YMCA step test (96 beats min) and a benchmark standard, the incremental treadmill test, using heart rate (HR) and oxygen consumption (VO2) as variables [25]. They have repeatedly found the accelerated 3-min step test to be an

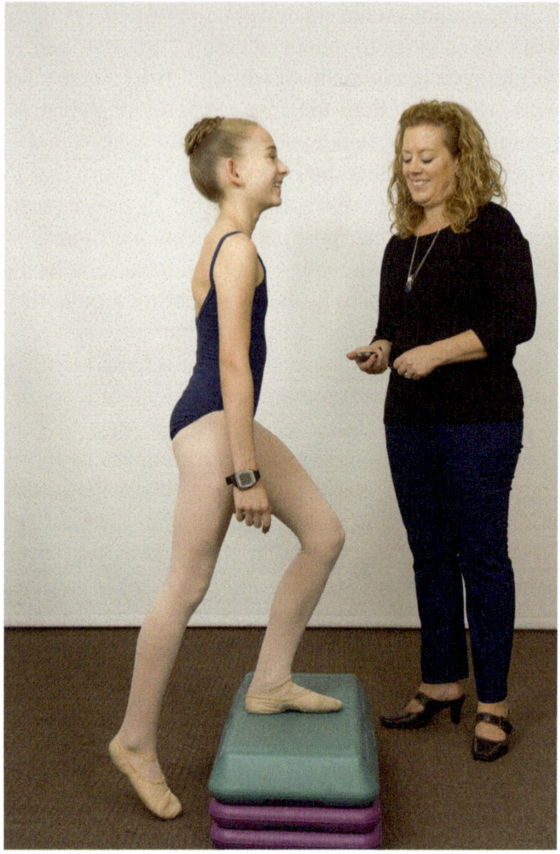

Fig. 3.2 3-min step test—forward step up. Photograph courtesy of James Koepfler

efficient, acceptable tool for testing cardiac recovery in dance populations when compared to other gold standards. In younger dancers the 3-min Kasch Pulse Recovery Test (KPR Test) could be indicated, as it delineates differences between children 6–9 and 10–12 years old [26]. The standard YMCA 3-min step test may be indicated for recreational dancers, while for pre-professional adolescents utilizing the 112 beat accelerated step test may be most appropriate.

There are many other screening tests that examine cardiovascular fitness that are useful for dance, such as the dance-specific aerobic fitness test (DAFT), that can also be implemented if the time and resources required to utilize them are available [27].

Range of Motion/Flexibility

Dancers generally work at the extremes of joint motion; many studies demonstrate greater range of motion than what is observed in the general population [28, 29].

When assessing range of motion in young dancers it can be helpful to screen for passive range of motion as it pertains to flexibility. In a still-growing population this can be very informative in helping a young dancer understand some of the limitations in motion that tight muscles can cause. As bone tends to grow faster than muscle, often a growing dancer will experience issues with flexibility along with strength of major muscle groups. Changes also occur in proprioception and biomechanics, impacting performance and increasing risk for injury. In general, injury reported during growth spurts may be due to a period of "relearning" when previously learned technique no longer relates to the new body structure. Many screens tend to observe technique only in evaluating some of these issues, but screening for passive range of motion can help establish whether the dancer possesses enough flexibility to achieve proper technique. Some screens will actually measure range with a goniometer to track changes, but full measurements constitute an evaluation, not a screening. A screening that includes flexibility should only have yes or no answers when establishing whether there is enough flexibility present. Generally, when range of motion tests are performed to establish flexibility they are done passively and stopped at the "first end feel," defined as the first onset of resistance or compensatory adjacent joint movement.

Hip motion and its effect on the spine and lower extremities is imperative to proper technique, especially in ballet. Screening for tightness in the iliopsoas with a Thomas test will generally show that most dancers are tight in the deep hip flexors, which can make it difficult to correct an anterior pelvic tilt, increase lumbar lordosis, place lower abdominals in an efficient position, and affect height of the arabesque. The Ely test for the quadriceps and Ober tests for the iliotibial band are also often positive and tight, especially in growing male dancers. Passive straight leg raise (SLR) helps establish the length of the hamstrings. In technique, if a young dancer is expected to flex the hip forward with knee extension higher than 90°, to accomplish this he or she needs at least 90° passive range of motion in order to maintain proper pelvic alignment. At the professional level a passive SLR of greater than 120° is expected. Clinically, tightness in the hamstring muscles can contribute to anterior hip pain and pathology, as the hip flexors overwork to achieve a leg height that is not possible with restrictions in hamstring flexibility.

Screening passive range of motion for external and internal rotation can be very helpful in ballet students, in particular when the hip is in extension, to establish baseline motion. Screening for motion in this area can indicate whether a dancer is using all the motion that is available. Evaluating internal rotation can also be very helpful to either establish that the motion is excessive in dancers who may have femoral anteversion, or very limited, as many professional level dancers present with 10° or less of internal rotation. This also provides the opportunity to educate the adolescent dancer on the importance of incorporating internal rotation stretches and strengthening exercises to balance rotation around the hip joint. Lack of internal rotation can lead to various injuries in the lower back, SI joint, and hips. Also, screening for significant asymmetries in hip rotation is important, as many dancers will present with differences between hips. With external rotation, to reduce the risk of injury dancers should work to equalize the lesser side. If the dancer consistently forces the lesser turned out hip to match the one with more turnout, problems may result around the hip joint of the lesser one and possibly also further up or down the kinetic chain in the lower back, knee, or ankle and foot.

Screening for tightness in the lower leg at the ankle and foot is also extremely important to assess for areas that demonstrate imbalance or lack of sufficient motion for proper technique. The most common injuries in dance are often at the ankle, due to limitations in dorsiflexion or plantar flexion. Studies have shown that dorsiflexion range decreases with increasing dance experience and ability, while plantar flexion is observed to increase with enhanced dance proficiency [30]. Adequate ankle dorsiflexion is important to achieve proper demi-plié (hip and knee flexion with ankle dorsiflexion) as it provides shock absorption in both preparation for and recovery from jumps and turns [31].

Screening to determine whether a dancer has enough plantar flexion to achieve proper alignment can be one significant factor in assessing the safety of pointe work. The motion required to achieve that technique is greater than the normative data reported in the general population [32, 33]. To attain the correct position en pointe requires more than 90° of combined motion in the talocrural, subtalar, and midtarsal joints. Proper alignment is demonstrated when the line of the metatarsals (top surface of the forefoot) is parallel to the line of the tibia (front of the shin) when the foot is pointed. During a screen, asymmetry en pointe and/or in demi-pointe in parallel can indicate differences in strength as well as range of motion that may need to be addressed with further evaluation.

Screening for ROM at the 1st metatarsal phalangeal (MTP) joint can be very important to see whether there are deficits in motion that will cause issues when weight bearing in demi-pointe (Fig. 3.3a–c). The demi-pointe position is the movement between the extremes of plié (end-range dorsiflexion) and pointe (end-range plantar flexion), where the foot is less stable. It is used in static balance poses for dancers, is the position that male dancers generally use for turning, and requires 90° of dorsiflexion in the 1st MTP joint. The demi-pointe position also forms the transitional phase when taking off and landing from jumps. In demi-pointe all the toes should be relaxed. If clawed toes or gripping of the toes is observed, it is often a sign of weakness in the deep intrinsic foot muscles. Decreased range of motion into dorsiflexion of this joint, along with foot type, can lead to alignment issues, as the dancer can not be fully over the 1st and 2nd rays due to lack of motion, and generally compensates with inversion (sickling) or winging (eversion) of the foot, increasing the risk of injury.

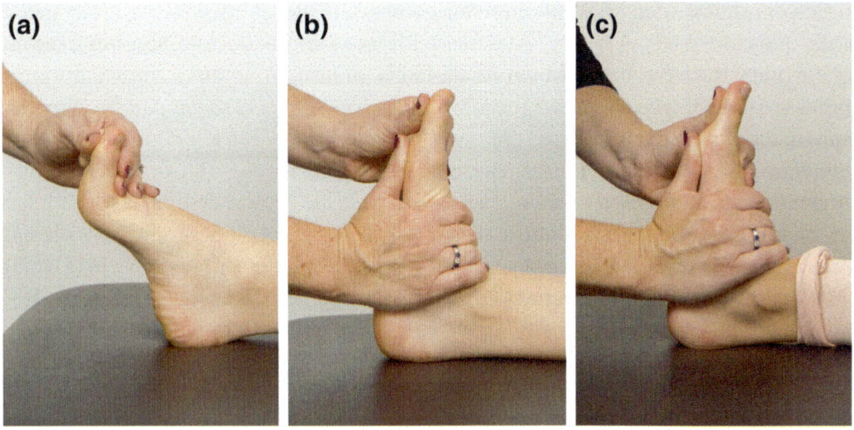

Fig. 3.3 Assessing 1st metatarsal phalangeal (MTP) joint motion. **a** 1st MTP joint extension accurately measured with ankle in plantar flexion. **b** Restricted 1st MTP extension with ankle dorsiflexed and first ray fixed, suggesting limited excursion of the flexor hallicus longus (FHL) muscle. **c** Approximately 20 degrees of MTP extension indicating normal excursion of the FHL as in Fig. 3.3b

Strength

In all sports, poor core stability has been identified as a risk factor for both upper and lower extremity injury, along with inadequate neuromuscular control. Assessing core strength and pelvic stability both with muscle testing and functional testing is probably the most important aspect of any screening process, and should be the first priority. Adolescent dancers commonly use their global stabilizers to maintain stability of the trunk, underutilizing the local core spinal stabilizers. This encourages imbalanced use of iliopsoas and thigh musculature, which may lead to multiple issues in the lower back and hip. Proximal control of the hip and trunk is an important indicator of lower extremity stability, as a dancer needs to be able to control his or her center of gravity over a small base of support. Screening should focus on strength and recruitment of the transversus abdominis and lower abdominal area, as most young dancers are surprisingly weak there. Weakness can be exacerbated by standing in a lordotic posture (sway back) with tight deep hip flexors and an anterior pelvic tilt compromising the mechanical efficiency of the lower abdominals and efficient recruitment of the transversus abdominis, along with the pelvic floor and multifidi in the spine, which can affect alignment of the entire spine. The gold standard for testing lower abdominal strength is the Kendall and Kendall double-leg-lowering test, but its reliability of grading has been called into question [34]. It is imperative that this test not only be done correctly, but also that young dancers and dance teachers know it is a test and never to be used as an exercise.

Screening for strength at the hip can be instrumental in identifying areas that if weak can contribute to injury. Athletes with weak hip abductors and hip external rotator muscles have been shown to be likely to sustain an ankle injury during a sports season [35]. Weakness in the hip abductors and adductors can be screened with functional testing such as the step down test or Trendelenburg test. When screening certain muscle groups, strength in the end range, with the muscle at its shortest length, can be significant, as that is where the muscle will be most utilized. For example, the external rotators of the hip need to be very strong at their end range, which is not typical for the strength–tension relationship of muscle. Testing hip external rotation strength provides an opportunity to compare active turnout to passive range. In addition, many lower extremity injuries have been shown to be related to lack of external rotator strength, in particular patellofemoral pain syndromes [36, 37].

Balance

The ability to control balance during activity is critical for preventing lower extremity injury. Screening for postural control and the ability to balance can be very helpful in discovering areas of weakness, lack of range of motion, and decreased proprioception. Testing can also help the practitioner detect residual deficits that remain following a previous injury. With training, dancers learn to adjust postural responses (achieve and maintain balance) to different conditions. The systems involved in balance include the visual system, the vestibular system located in the inner ear, and the somatosensory system, which includes touch, nociception (which senses pain or harm), and proprioception. Screening to evaluate balance can involve decreasing the input of one of these systems, such as vision, in the single leg stance with eyes closed. The age of the dancers being evaluated may help determine the type of testing utilized, as children 12 years and under rely predominantly on vision for balance, while the other systems mentioned above are added with increasing maturity [38]. In pre-professional adolescents and the professional dancer, a single leg balance test with eyes closed for 60 s is the gold standard. Screening with a movement-based test, such as the Star Excursion Test, may be more beneficial in younger dancers, or when dynamic balance is being tested. It should also be recognized that growth spurts often affect motor development, as changes occurring in body mass, limb length, proportions, flexibility, and strength will cause variability in balance and coordination.

Functional Testing

The use of functional tests can be an efficient way to combine the elements of flexibility, strength, balance, and technique. Functional testing can help establish a baseline, but also be utilized as a measure to allow for return to dance, or progression to more vigorous dancing such as jumping, following an injury. Generally, functional testing is performed in parallel position, as the goal is to find deviations from functional movement that are common in anatomical neutral. The ability to perform at least 20–25 repetitions of single leg elevé (heel rise) in parallel with two fingers on the barre and proper alignment and technique is one test that can be useful to establish sufficient strength, endurance, and proprioception for jumping and pointe work. Testing such as the single leg step down test, performed in parallel off a 9" step to the depth of the dancer's deepest plié, can be an efficient way to screen for neuromuscular control (Fig. 3.4a). Observing five repetitions of this test with attention to pelvic alignment, excessive hip adduction or internal rotation, knee valgus, and foot pronation can disclose many risks for injury that need to be addressed with physical therapy intervention and conditioning to avoid future issues [39] (see Fig. 3.4a–c).

The Airplane test is another functional measure that is often included to screen for neuromuscular control [40] (Fig. 3.5a, b). The triplanar nature and combined dynamic movement allow for quick assessment of cervical stability, lumbopelvic control, ability to maintain lower limb alignment, and compensations at the ankle and foot.

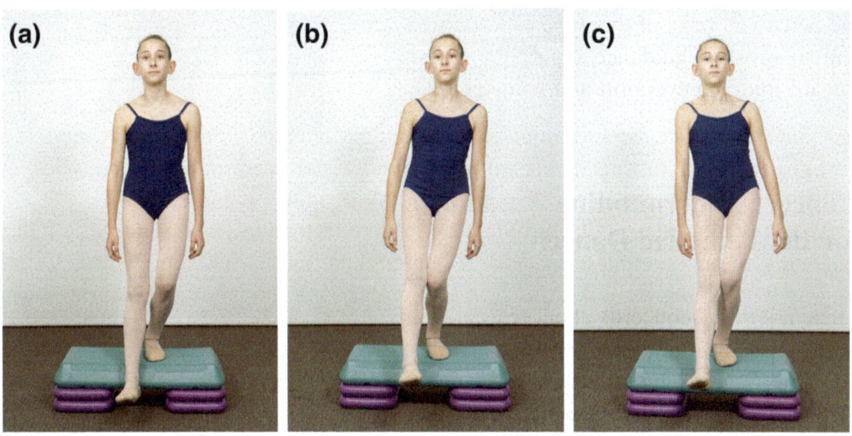

Fig. 3.4 Proper alignment and movement dysfunctions with step down test. **a** Proper alignment. **b** *Left* knee valgus collapse. **c** Positive *left* Trendelenburg (hip drop). Photographs courtesy of James Koepfler

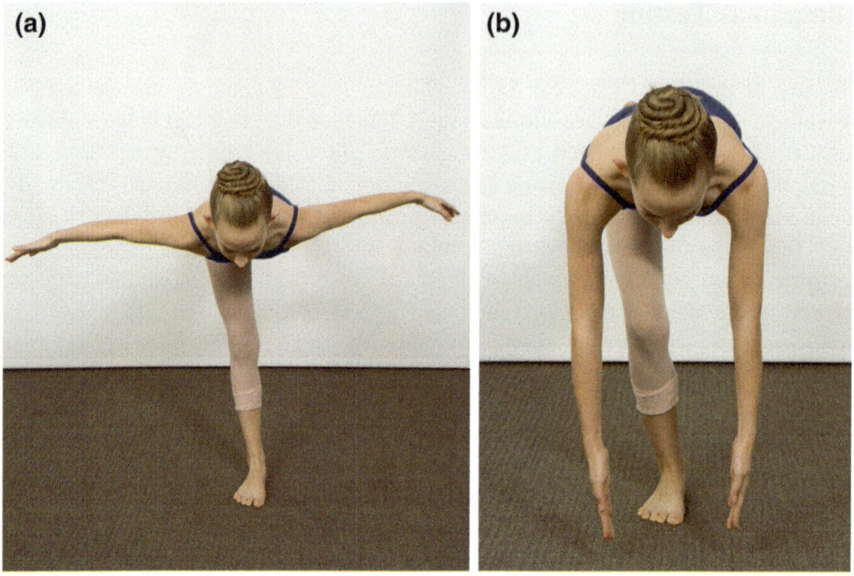

Fig. 3.5 Airplane test. **a** Proper alignment of starting position with leg extended. **b** Proper alignment into plié with arms coming down and together. Photographs courtesy of James Koepfler

Technique

Assessing technique as part of a screening is also a form of functional testing. While it is generally the most subjective aspect of the screen, it can yield important information regarding areas that need to be addressed to prevent injury. Technique is often assessed from two distinct points of view: To the dancer, dance teacher, or choreographer, attaining the optimal aesthetic is the primary focus; for the healthcare provider, how the optimal aesthetic is attained is the top priority. If a gesture, leap, or turn is executed with suboptimal recruitment of muscles or unhealthy skeletal movement or posturing, risk of injury is increased.

With the requirements of turnout so prevalent in many forms of dance, a quick screening of this technique should be undertaken, as this is a movement where forcing beyond the natural limits of the hip joint, with compensations at the lower back, knee, and foot, is both damaging and common. Current research has confirmed that active turnout can be improved with training in the collegiate level dancer [41], so a screening measure for this has merit for offering a successful intervention if forced turnout is the result of weakness.

Virtually all forms of dance require some need to hold balance on one limb, whether in flat or on the ball of the foot. With knowledge that the majority of dance injuries in the adolescent dancer occur at the foot and ankle [1, 3], and likely derive from lack of adequate core and hip girdle strength, a simple elevé in coupé or passé (or in flat in the very young dancer) can easily expose qualities of proper weight shift and ability to maintain pelvic alignment. A physical therapist can readily determine the muscles that may be weak or overactivated just by observing the deviation from neutral alignment. To dancers who may appear to be holding their balance well, observation of excessive toe gripping can be noted as a sign they are not truly on balance, just as can tense shoulders and overactive neck musculature. With very young dancers, it can be effective to use single leg balance in turned out position as a technique assessment by observing how they move into the position and maintain it before adding any tests that incorporate a gesture or elevé.

Recommendations

Providing timely feedback for dancers on the results of the screen significantly affects the success of the program. Dancers as a group tend to be perfectionistic, so results of a screen should be delivered positively, sensitively, and without judgment. There are special considerations when making recommendations to young dancers. Helping them understand that all elite athletes need to have a good understanding of their own strengths and weaknesses can be empowering and useful. Imparting the idea that no one is perfect, and revealing that all elite professional dancers have some issues they also need to address to perform optimally and avoid injury, can help young dancers understand and apply the information they receive. In adolescence this can be difficult to comprehend, as young dancers and athletes are always comparing themselves to others as they work out their own identities. The focus of the recommendations should be on exploring options and enhancing abilities, rather than obstacles to performance or greater risk of injury. It is also important to instruct them and their parents/dance teachers that some findings are likely temporary in nature related to where they are in their growth and development. Also, encouragement should emphasize that the goal of any exercises recommended is to address these areas so they will improve their dance technique. Some findings from the screen will have influence on their overall health beyond their dance training.

It should be recognized that the recommendations from a screen are designed to raise "red flags," so referral to appropriate practitioners can be made as indicated. From the health history section there may be issues identified that should be further addressed by the primary care physician or a sports medicine specialist (preferably with experience in dance). Depending on the areas addressed by the screen, referral to a sports psychologist or nutritionist may be warranted. Most often from the physical assessment, there may be areas identified that require a comprehensive physical therapy evaluation and treatment. There are also issues that when noted should be referred to the dance teacher. As part of the planning process it is important to identify a group of practitioners in the community who can be helpful in dealing with areas of risk identified with the screening.

Screening Potential for Research and Standardization

It must be emphasized again that a plethora of screens has been developed by now, and what is included in a screening assessment should be guided by the overall goals of the process, the age group being screened, and the intensity of dance training involved. One of the exciting aspects of screening is that an abundance of information can be collected and integrated, creating an excellent opportunity for research. The primary goal of screening is generally not research, but that does not mean that the information collected cannot be analyzed. When that is the intention, the tests and measurements selected need to be objective and to have demonstrated reliability and validity in the current literature. Another challenge is standardizing one screening tool for multiple school populations and goals. In professional dance this is currently being explored by the Dance/USA Task Force on Dancer Health, but it is more realistic with this relatively homogenious professional dance population. Age group, the dance focus of the school, intensity of dance training, available resources, time restrictions, and overall goals are likely to vary tremendously between schools and colleges. Regardless, utilizing a standardized screen is the ideal goal for the future so that the dance medicine community can more fully identify and understand the various attributes that are needed for optimal function and safety of dance training. Of course, to truly establish the value of identifying characteristics in dancers that are thought to be risk factors for injury a comprehensive and standardized injury tracking system also needs to be established and studied. Until such a system is available and widely utilized, focusing on tests that have been studied in the literature can help with comparisons within dance and other populations.

Screening tools need to be adaptable to change in the evolving research. As more evidence-based work is produced in dance medicine and sports medicine, there are often changes proposed for previously validated tests or new tests and measures that are shown to explore a musculoskeletal issue more accurately. Research is constantly being produced that promotes adaptations in sports screening tests to make them more specific to dancers. Currently, the literature does not identify any data to support one definitive screen or to establish the best practices for risk factor identification [2]. In some cases screening has been abandoned, as it has not been shown to be either predictive or preventative in reducing injury [3]. Nonetheless, screenings can unquestionably be valuable in the training, education, and care of dancers. The potential benefits have been discussed here, and if one injury is prevented or a single life-threatening situation such as an eating disorder is diagnosed, then helping even one young dancer is beneficial.

Conclusion

A comprehensive, extensive screen, or even a simple screen can be effective as an initial step in understanding a dancer's strengths and weaknesses and providing education and recommendations to help reduce injury and maximize a young dancer's capabilities. It has been well established that screening programs are most effective when coupled with ongoing educational programs and interventions [6]. It is evident that screening will continue to be a significant area for study and research, especially if the intrinsic factors identified can be linked to the prevention of future injuries.

References

1. Roberts K, Nelson N, McKenzie N. Dance-related injuries in children and adolescents treated in US emergency departments in 1991–2007. J Phys Act Health. 2013;10(2):143–50.
2. Sanders B, Blackburn T, Boucher B. Clinical commentary: pre-participation screening the sports physical therapy perspective. Int J Sports Phys Ther. 2013;8(2):180–93.
3. Gamboa J, Roberts L, Fergus M. Injury patterns in elite pre-professional ballet dancers and the utility of screening programs to identify risk characteristics. J Orthop Sports Phys Ther. 2008 Mar;(38)3:126–36.
4. Lai R, Krasnow D, Thomas M. Communication between medical practitioners and dancers. J Dance Med Sci. 2008;12(2):47–53.
5. Potter K, Galbraith G, Baas J. Screening for improved dance function. The IADMS Bulletin for Teachers. 2011;3(1):14–7.
6. Clark T, Gupta A, Chester H. Developing a dancer wellness program employing developmental evaluation. Front Psychol. 2014;5:731.
7. Van Camp S. Sudden death in athletes. In: Grana WA, Lombardo JA, editors. Advances in sports medicine and fitness. Chicago: Year Book Medical Publishers; 1988. p. 121–42.
8. Riebe D, Franklin B, Thompson P, Garber C, Whitfield G, Magal M, Pescatello L. Updating ACSM's recommendations for exercise preparticipation health screening. Med Sci Sports Exerc. 2015;47(11):2473–9.
9. Pre-Participation Screening. https://www.aap.org/en-us/professionalresources/practice-support/Documents/Preparticipation-Physical-Exam-Form.pdf.
10. Brinkman R, Evans T. History of ankle sprain as a risk factor of future lateral ankle sprain in athletes. J Sport Rehabil. 2011;20(3):384–8.
11. Mandarakas M, Pourkazemi F, Sman A, Burns J, Hiller C. Systematic review of chronic ankle instability in children. J Foot Ankle Res. 2014;7(1):21–31.
12. Stokic E, Srdic B, Barak O. Body mass index, body fat mass and the occurrence of amenorrhea in ballet dancers. Gynecol Endocrinol. 2005;20(4):195–9.
13. Addo O, Himes J. Reference curves for triceps and subscapular skinfold thicknesses in US children and adolescents. Am J Clin Nutr. 2010;91(3):635–42.
14. Howse J, McCormack M. Dance technique and injury prevention. 3rd ed. London: A & C Black Publishers; 2000. p. 190–3.
15. Rogol A, Clark P, Roemmich J. Growth and pubertal development in children and adolescents: effects of diet and physical activity. Am J Clin Nutr. 2000;72(2 Suppl):521S–8S.
16. Penha P, João S, Casarotto R, Amino C, Penteado D. Postural assessment of girls between 7 and 10 years of age. Clinics (Sao Paulo). 2005 Jan–Feb;60(1):9–16.
17. Manoli A, Graham B. The subtle cavus foot, "the underpronator". Foot Ankle Int. 2005;26 (3):256–63.
18. Day H, Koutedakis Y, Wyon M. Hypermobility and dance: a review. Int J Sports Med. 2011;32(7):485–9.
19. Knight IA. A guide to living with hypermobility syndrome; bending without breaking. London: Kingsley Publishers; 2011. p. 22–3.
20. Smits-Engelsman B, Klerks M, Kirby A. Beighton score: a valid measure for generalized hypermobility in children. J Pediatr. 2011;158(1):119–23.

21. Liederbach M, Schanfein L, Kremenic I. What is known about the effect of fatigue on injury occurrence among dancers? J Dance Med Sci. 2013;17(3):101–8.
22. Wyon MA, Koutedakis Y. Muscular fatigue: considerations for dance. J Dance Med Sci. 2013;17(2):63–9.
23. Wyon M, Redding E. Physiological monitoring of cardiorespiratory adaptations during rehearsal and performance of contemporary dance. J Strength Cond Res. 2005;19(3):611–4.
24. Wyon M, Redding E, Head A, Sharp C, Craig S. Oxygen uptake during modern dance class, rehearsal, and performance. J Strength Cond Res. 2004;18(4):646–9.
25. Bronner SJ, Rakov S. An accelerated step test to assess dancer pre-season aerobic fitness. J Dance Med Sci. 2014;18(1):12–21.
26. Janokowski M, Niedzielska A, Brzezinski M, Drabik J. Cardiorespiratory fitness in children: a simple screening test for population studies. Pediatr Cardiol. 2015;36(1):27–32.
27. Wyon M, Redding E, Head A, Craig S. Development, reliability, and validity of a multistage dance specific aerobic fitness test (DAFT). J Dance Med Sci. 2003;7(3):80–4.
28. Gannon LM, Bird HA. The quantification of joint laxity in dancers and gymnasts. J Sports Sci. 1999;17(9):743–50.
29. Steinberg N, Hershovitz I, Peleg S, Dar G, Masharawi Y, Helm M, Siev-Ner I. Range of joint movement in female dancers and non-dancers aged 8–16 years: anatomical and clinical implications. Am J Sports Med. 2006;34(5):814–23.
30. Russell JA, Kruse DW, Nevill AM, Koutedakis Y, Wyon MA. Measurement of the extreme ankle range of motion required by female ballet dancers. Foot Ankle Spec. 2010;3(6):324–30.
31. Dickson D, Hollman-Gage K, Ojofeitimi S, Bornner S. Comparison of functional ankle motion measures in modern dancers. J Dance Med Sci. 2012;16(3):116–25.
32. Russell J. Is goniometry suitable for ankle range of motion measurements in female ballet dancers? Initial comparison with radiographical measurement. Foot Ankle Spec. 2011;4 (3):151–6.
33. Hamilton WG, Hamilton LH, Marshall P, Molnar M. A profile of the musculoskeletal characteristics of elite professional ballet dancers. Am J Sports Med. 1992 May–Jun;20 (3):267–73.
34. Zannotti CM, Bohannon RW, Tiberio D, Dewberry MJ, Murray R. Kinematics of the double-leg-lowering test for abdominal muscle strength. J Orthop Sports Phys Ther. 2002 Sep;(32)9:432–6.
35. Leetun DT, Ireland ML, Willson JD, Ballantyne BT, McClay I. Core stability measures as risk factors for lower extremity injury in athletes. Med Sci Sports Exerc. 2004;36(6):926–34.
36. Dolak K, Silkman C, Medina McKeon J, Hosey R, Lattermann C. Hip strengthening prior to functional exercises reduces pain sooner than quadriceps strengthening in females with patellofemoral pain syndrome: a randomized clinical trial. J Orthop Sports Phys Ther. 2011;41(8):560–70.
37. Khayambashi K, Mohammadkhani Z, Ghaznavi K, Lyle MA, Powers CM. The effects of isolated hip abductor and external rotator muscle strengthening on pain, health status, and hip strength in females with patellofemoral pain. J Orthop Sports Phys Ther. 2012;42(1):22–9.
38. Krasnow DH, Wilmerding MV. Motor learning and control for dance. Champaign, IL: Human Kinetics; 2015. p. 24–41.
39. Park K, Cynn H, Choung S. Musculoskeletal predictors of movement quality for the forward step-down test in asymptomatic women. J Orthop Sports Phys Ther. 2013;43(7):504–10.
40. Richardson M, Leiderbach MJ, Sandow E. Functional criteria for assessing pointe readiness. J Dance Med Sci. 2010;14(3):6–7.
41. Sherman A, Mayall E, Tasker S. Can a prescribed turnout conditioning program reduce the differential between passive and active turnout in pre-professional dancers? J Dance Med Sci. 2014;18(4):159–68.

Chapter 4
Physical Therapy Rehabilitation for the Young Dancer

Heather Southwick, PT, MSPT and Maribeth Crupi, PT

Pertinent Definitions

Intrinsic risk factors: Specific characteristics of an individual that have the potential to precipitate injury, but are controllable or preventable. Examples include previous injury, bone structure, muscle weakness, poor conditioning, inflexibility, and ligamentous laxity.
Extrinsic risk factors: Forces from outside the body that can cause injury. Examples include floor surface, shoes, training schedule, costume, and sets.
Periodization: The systematic planning of athletic or physical training with the goal of attaining optimal performance. Conditioning programs break up training into sections of off-season, pre-season, in-season, and post-season, with each phase focused on different goals.

Introduction

In general, it has been observed that all youth sports are increasing in training intensity [1]. Dancers have historically and traditionally adhered to an intense and disciplined training schedule from a very young age. Many dancers will report that they started some form of training as young as age three. The advantages of early

H. Southwick, PT, MSPT (✉)
Boston Ballet, 19 Clarendon Street, Boston, MA 02116, USA
e-mail: hsouthwick@bostonballet.org

M. Crupi, PT
Physical Therapy LLC, 314 Main Street, Suite 101, Wilmington, MA 01887, USA
e-mail: mccrupi@comcast.net

R. Solomon et al. (eds.), *Prevention of Injuries in the Young Dancer*,
Contemporary Pediatric and Adolescent Sports Medicine,
DOI 10.1007/978-3-319-55047-3_4

training include the progressive development of strength and flexibility necessary to excel in all forms of dance. The disadvantage is that intense training at a young age can create more opportunity for injury [2]. In the period from 1991 to 2007 annual emergency room visits for dance-related injuries in 3–19 year olds increased 37.2%, and given the other options available for care dance injury rates were likely significantly higher during that period of time [3].

Risk Factors for Injury

Understanding and awareness of both intrinsic and extrinsic risk factors that can lead to injuries in young dancers are paramount to preventing injuries. Young dancers frequently strive for the aesthetic and performance level achieved by adult professional dancers. Furthermore, young students are consistently pushed by their teachers to the end of their range of motion and expected to have the strength required to function there even when developmentally they lack the ability to attain and hold those positions because they are still growing children. Compensations in alignment and technique often occur when young bodies are not ready to meet the challenges of moving and holding many end range positions. As there is currently no accreditation process for dance teachers in the USA, their knowledge of the growth and developmental factors that can affect their students may vary greatly. A better understanding of motor development would allow teachers to structure classes that assure the desired skill acquisition is attainable. For example, barre work before the age of 7 or 8 is not to be encouraged [4]. Improving the methods of educating dance teachers would allow them to appreciate and likely alter the demands they place on young dancers, thus promoting safer training and injury reduction.

Adolescent Growth Factors

The adolescent growth spurt and its effect on bone and muscle can also be a risk factor for injury [2]. This accelerated growth often coincides with the age at which dancers begin to train more intensely; it generally occurs between ages 11 and 14 for girls and 13 and 21 for boys, and lasts for 18–24 months. An adolescent may grow several inches in a few months, followed by a period of very slow growth, and then another spurt months later.

Changes with puberty (sexual maturation) may occur gradually, or several signs may become visible all at once. There is a substantial amount of variation in the rate and timing of the changes that occur, and they tend to have a large emotional impact on adolescents.

Rapidly elongating bones may exceed muscular growth, creating muscle tightness. Muscle strength can be compromised, and there is generally a period of weakening with increased susceptibility to stress-related bone injuries. Decreased coordination and balance also accompany a growth spurt, making turns and balancing on one leg more difficult and increasing the risk of strain or sprain. Physicians customarily record height measurements upon examination. Rehabilitation professionals are encouraged to employ this practice as well. Identifying significant growth may put the dancer's mind at ease if it is likely contributory to the condition for which they are being treated.

There is pressure to increase flexibility at a time when it is most compromised; thus, care must be taken with stretching during the adolescent growth spurt. With seven apophyses about the hip and pelvis corresponding to areas of attachment of muscles used frequently in dance, caution must be taken to avoid injury to these growth sites. In some instances such injuries can take a considerable time to heal [5]. Reducing impact work and keeping gestures out of extreme ranges of motion during adolescence presents an opportunity to focus on activities that develop higher levels of balance and joint proprioception. This promotes adaptation to more advanced positions of the body that cause it to be placed out of vertical alignment during dance training [4].

Training and Technique

Significant risk factors for injury throughout a dancer's lifetime are poor alignment and faulty technique. Issues with alignment are generally congruent with faulty posture, and examples observed in ballet include: forward head and shoulders; increased lumbar lordosis; forced turnout or excessive external rotation in first or fifth position, causing the knee to be medial to the ankle and foot (Fig. 4.1 a, b); and pronation of the feet. Proper alignment allows for more efficient movement and is less likely to cause increased strain and tension on ligaments, tendons, and muscles around a joint. All injuries in dancers need to be evaluated for faulty alignment and technique as potential contributors. Faults must be corrected to avoid reoccurrence as the dancer works to return to full dance activity. The age of the dancer should be considered when making postural corrections. It is quite normal and developmentally appropriate for dancers under 6–7 years of age to have postural findings of anterior pelvis, hyper extended valgus knees, and limited turnout [6]. Frustrating a very young dancer with corrections his or her body is not ready to accept can be detrimental. Dance should be fun and creative at those early ages.

Anatomical Limitations

Anatomical limitations are another risk factor for injury in all dancers, but young dancers can be educated on how to work with their body as their artistic instrument and learn what they can improve. Truly understanding their own body and their own strengths and limitations can be paramount to avoiding injury. No one has a perfect body, and every dancer's body is different. Dancers and their teachers need to understand an individual student's unique anatomical advantages and limitations and how to work within those physical capabilities. For example, dancers who are very flexible tend to have to work harder to build strength and those who are very strong generally need constantly to address flexibility issues. Given the nature of dance and the need to execute gestures in extreme ranges of motion, it is important for the rehabilitation professional to have knowledge of the dancer's bony architecture if imaging has been done or is advised. For example, it is important to know if any hip dysplasia is present, as it has been demonstrated in the literature that those with dysplastic hips have labrum that supports more of the total load across the hip joint (4–11%) than those with normal hips (1–2%) [7], thus increasing the risk of labral injury [7]. These measures reflect components of the normal gait cycle and ascending and descending stairs, so it is likely the force transmissions are substantially greater with dance [7].

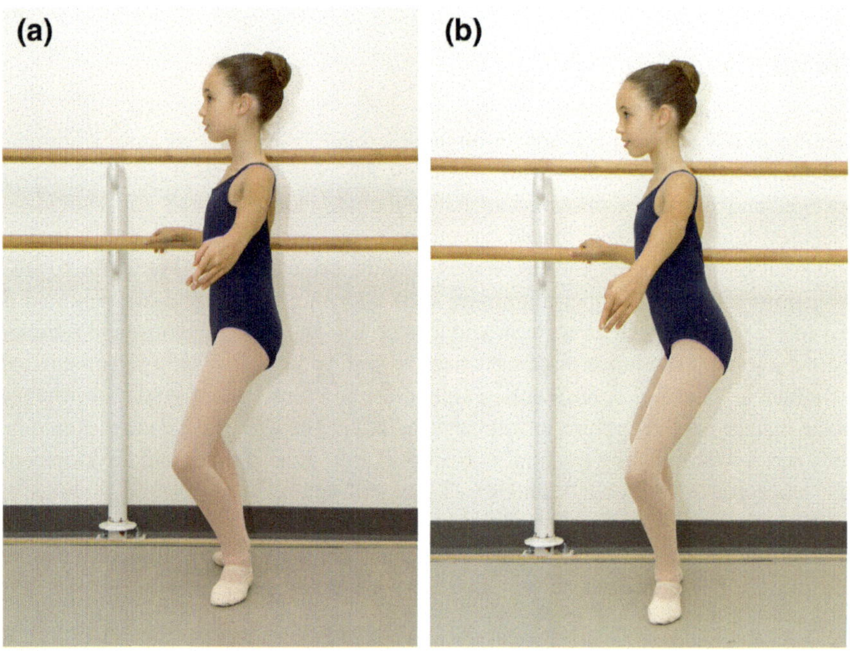

Fig. 4.1 Demi-plié in first position demonstrating challenges to proper alignment. **a** Knee slightly forward of foot in lieu of optimal position with knee centered over second toe. **b** Further compensation with excessive hip flexion. Photographs courtesy of James Koepfler

Hypermobility

Understanding hypermobility and the presence of benign or more serious heritable connective tissue disorders (HCTD) is important, as ligamentous laxity can lead to injury. An easy and basic test for assessing joint hypermobility is the Beighton Scale, which while widely used has only recently been tested for validity [8]. More and more dancers are being selected into different forms of dance due to their hypermobility. The laxity of their ligaments can make it harder to control the end range of movement in a joint, so there is often a presentation of instability around the joint with the paradox of tight muscles because they are working harder than non-hypermobile individuals to keep the joint stable. Addressing core and pelvic stability and teaching how properly to stretch without compromising ligaments is extremely important for the hypermobile dancer.

Muscle Imbalances

Reviewing and correcting muscle imbalances can be critical to preventing injuries in young dancers. In order to avoid injury the muscles surrounding a joint should be relatively equal in strength and flexibility. This helps prevent one side of the joint, for example, the plantar flexors at the ankle, from being more stressed and over used than the dorsiflexors. This is a typical imbalance seen in ballet because of the emphasis on demi-pointe and pointe work. An imbalance like this can make a dancer more susceptible to shin pain and tibial stress, as when jumping she or he does not have the posterior chain flexibility to land with a deep plié and then enough eccentric strength in the dorsiflexors to control the landing motion.

Encouraging proper technique and facilitating optimal muscle strength and use are extremely important. The deep outward rotators of the hip should be trained for turnout. Healthy length and strength of the iliopsoas is necessary for its role as both a trunk stabilizer and hip flexor. The often weak gluteus maximus needs to be recruited and contracted before the hamstrings for safer movement of the femoral head in gestures such as arabesque.

Fatigue

Fatigue is another well known and documented precursor of injuries seen in practice and supported in the literature [9]. In students pursuing intense dance training there is often little to no periodization provided for minimal rest time. Generally with dance students injuries are more likely to occur at the beginning of a season when they return to a demanding schedule after having time off from dance, which in itself is becoming a shorter period of time. Injuries are also becoming more common mid-year, as many young dancers are performing in "Nutcracker" or other seasonal productions while also auditioning for summer dance intensives. Following this, many multidiscipline dancers move on to competitions and then right on to their year-end training with added rehearsals and final performances. While periodization has traditionally been reserved for training at the elite level, as just illustrated the young dancers of today are now keeping schedules that are similar to those of their professional adult counterparts. Guidelines are needed to promote schedules that offer the required time for musculoskeletal repair and recovery between intense periods of dance.

Lack of Warm Up

Lack of a proper warm up before class or rehearsal is another potential risk factor for injury. As every dancer has different needs, warming up should be individualized, but must include movement and exercises that will help increase body temperature and heart rate, and lubricate the joints [10]. Static stretching in a split is commonly misconceived by younger dancers as warming up. While research is ongoing as to what methods of stretching are best, it is generally agreed that before dancing a combination of controlled warm-up exercises followed by dynamic stretching is beneficial for addressing both the need for increased muscle flexibility and joint range of motion. Long periods of static stretching are best reserved for after dancing, and more advanced forms of stretching, such as contract-and-release techniques, are for the more mature dancer. Dancers should be encouraged to keep themselves warm during rehearsals and breaks in performances when they are not dancing for extended periods of time.

Psychological Factors

During adolescence psychological factors can be more of a risk for injury than at any other age in a dancer. Pressure and expectations from parents, peers, and teachers can all lead to increased stress. Stress and anxiety can affect concentration, making injury more likely. Fear of injury, not achieving goals or being picked for a role, letting down your competition team due to inability to perform, or teacher criticism are all examples of potential stressors in the dancer's life. As a practitioner, attending to who is answering intake questions, whether it is the young dancer or his/her parent or guardian, and how the questions are answered can be revealing. It is important for the healthcare provider to educate and offer objective criteria for safe return to dance. Having some resources to help address psychological factors, and when needed referring to a dance/sports psychologist, can facilitate the healthiest return to dancing.

Nutrition

Finally, nutrition is an enormous component of injury prevention and rehabilitation. As young dancers mature, concerns about their changing bodies and maintaining the thin aesthetic characteristic of most dancers can lead to poor nutritional practices and eating habits. In the USA there is also a tendency for young dancers just not having enough time to eat well due to their demanding schedules, and processed food becoming the easy mainstay. Teaching dancers about proper nutrition and that at such a high level of peak performance our bodies need fuel can be paramount to preventing and treating injury. In particular, understanding adequate vitamin D and calcium intake in the adolescent years is a significant component for good bone health, not only while training but also in a dancer's adult life [11]. In areas where there are four seasons of climate change, often the dancer experiences little to no natural sunlight during a day filled with academic and dance study. Educating young female dancers on how poor nutrition can affect their menstrual cycles and lead to hormone imbalances that can then cause lower bone density and reproductive issues is vital to preventing and treating injuries when they are young, and has significance for when they are older. While this may be taken for granted by healthcare providers and well-informed dancers/dance educators, in practice many dancers and their parents receive such information as new and surprising.

Components of Rehabilitation

Many of the risk factors for injury are common to all young athletes and are not unique to dancers. In rehabilitating an injury in a young dancer, the initial treatment and education may therefore be very similar to that of any young athlete. A comprehensive rehabilitation program should include incorporation of the young dancer's goals; emphasis on education and communication with the dancer, parent, and dance teacher to help ensure a safe and successful return to dancing [12]; use of objective and functional protocols to determine readiness to progress in rehab; cross training; relative rest; task-specific rehab while addressing motor learning and motor control to change long-standing habitual ways of moving: and review of dance technique that might contribute to injury. The overall goal should always be to return the dancer to optimal performance, and more confidence than prior to the injury. Dancers are generally anxious to return to classes, rehearsal, and performance too quickly following an injury [13]. Premature return not only increases the risk of reinjury, but also places the dancer at risk for a new injury as compensatory movement patterns emerge.

Rehabilitation should begin immediately following an injury and should not end until the dancer has returned safely to full activity. Initially, any rehabilitation program should focus on how to maximize the dancer's abilities while protecting the existing injury. It is important to educate healthcare providers, dance teachers, and parents on the importance of an immediate referral to therapy, especially for dancers who will need to significantly limit or refrain from dance activity. Having a few early visits to establish a comprehensive home program that can also be done at the dance studio will allow the dancer to maintain or improve optimal condition and can help prevent depression and other issues due to the injury. It also allows the later phases of rehab to be focused on the area of specific injury without concern that the rest of the body is conditioned well enough to initiate the return to dance. Dancers with injuries that require limited weight bearing or more gradual progression of therapeutic exercise may benefit from water or floor barre exercise therapy. The buoyancy of water allows the dancer to replicate dance movements typically done at the barre with much greater ease and less impact as compared with on-land training. The hydrostatic benefits of water include reduction in pain and edema, which can facilitate an increase in joint range of motion [14]. Depending on the exercise, water can provide assistance or resistance to muscles. It is effective in challenging the cardiorespiratory system to maintain aerobic capacity, and there is research to support that it does not increase risk of infection postsurgically [15]. Without access to a pool, or in addition to water therapy, floor barre exercises allow the dancer to avoid weight bearing positions by lying on all sides of their body (injury permitting) to replicate many of the dance movements they perform in standing, such as passé or développé. Pilates matwork serves as a wonderful compliment to floor barre work, especially since entry-level Pilates matwork teaches the young dancer how properly to engage their local core stabilizers: the pelvic floor, transversus abdominus, and multifidi [16]. Use of equipment-based Pilates such as a reformer or cadillac also serves to reduce weight bearing impact (Fig. 4.2a, b, c). Similar to Pilates is the Gyrotonic method of exercise, which also offers a beneficial method to improve pelvic and core stability. The primary difference between the two is that in Gyrotonic the equipment offers more diagonal and rotational movement as opposed to Pilates equipment, which is more linear in nature.

Dancers thrive on movement, so starting core and pelvic stability exercises, for example, while a dancer is in a boot for a foot injury can help the dancer to feel that he/she is an active participant in the healing process. It is crucial that dancers be fully evaluated for weakness and muscle imbalances that may be separated from the area of injury, but contribute to overall control and stability. For example, weakness and muscle imbalance around the hips and core muscles are often contributory to injury at the knee, foot, and ankle [14, 17].

Addressing the uninjured side of the body along with the effected side is critical in any patient to insure improved quality and strength of movement, and can give excellent feedback to the injured side. Prior studies in the literature have indicated that dancers tend to lack strength in certain muscle groups such as lower abdominals, posterior hips and trunk, and pelvic stabilizers [13, 18]. As dance is an intense, very repetitive, and high-impact activity, strength and endurance are critical

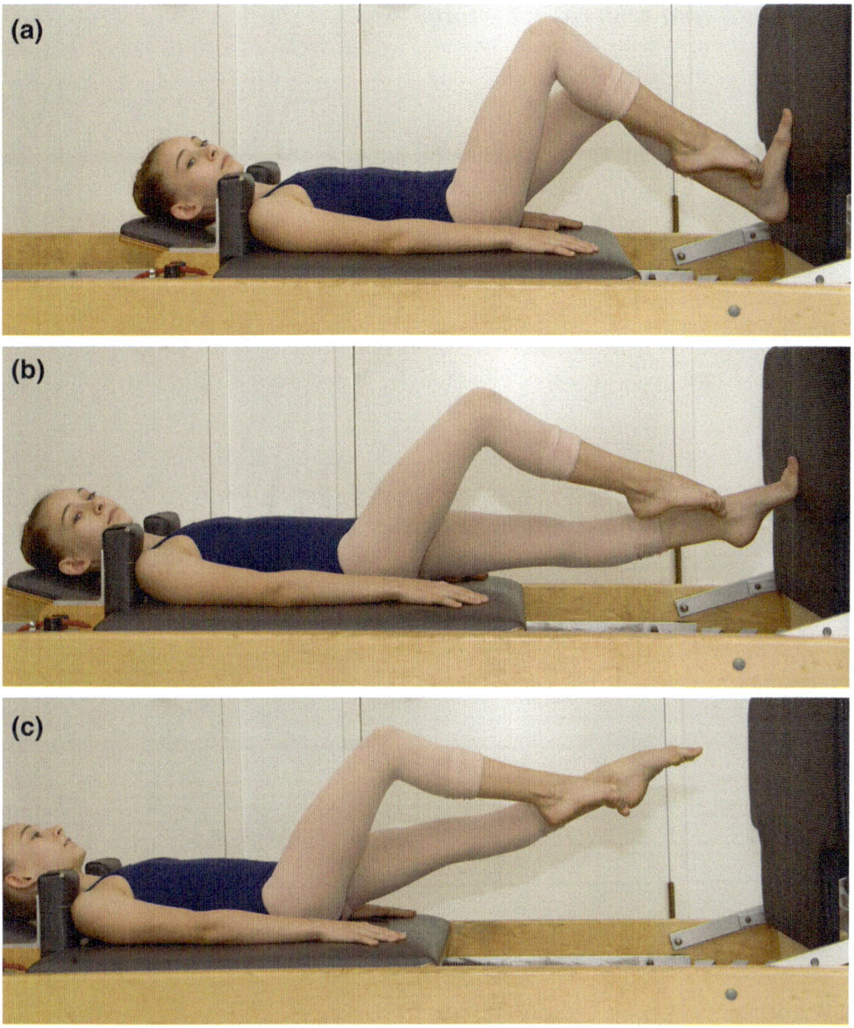

Fig. 4.2 Use of a Pilates reformer to facilitate dancer-specific rehabilitation. **a** Single leg plié. **b** Single leg elevé. **c** Single leg jump in parallel. Photographs courtesy of James Koepfler

for joint and postural stability, motor control, absorption of shock when landing, and stamina. Immediately focusing on some of these areas that have a tendency to demonstrate weakness when not consistently addressed can improve overall conditioning and make return to dancing a healthier and smoother process [13]. Young dancers should always be given a home exercise program to address areas contributing to the injury and to supplement dance activity. With poor postural habits becoming increasingly prevalent in this age of constant computer and cell phone use, a home program can provide an opportunity to work on strengthening and encouraging improved posture in the cervico-thoracic and shoulder regions.

Functional and Objective Testing

The use of functional/objective testing to determine and progress the effectiveness of rehabilitation is very important to allow for safe and timely return to dancing. Objective testing needs to incorporate the different demands the dancer will face upon return to full activity. Utilizing functional tests that address agility, balance, proprioception, concentration, trunk strength and endurance, transfer of weight and direction, and lower extremity strength and power, is essential [13] (Fig. 4.3a, b). Use of functional testing helps the practitioner evaluate the effectiveness of treatment throughout the rehabilitation process. This also allows a practitioner to direct treatment based on deficits observed with testing and to make sound recommendations for return to dance, especially at higher levels such as return to pointe work [19].

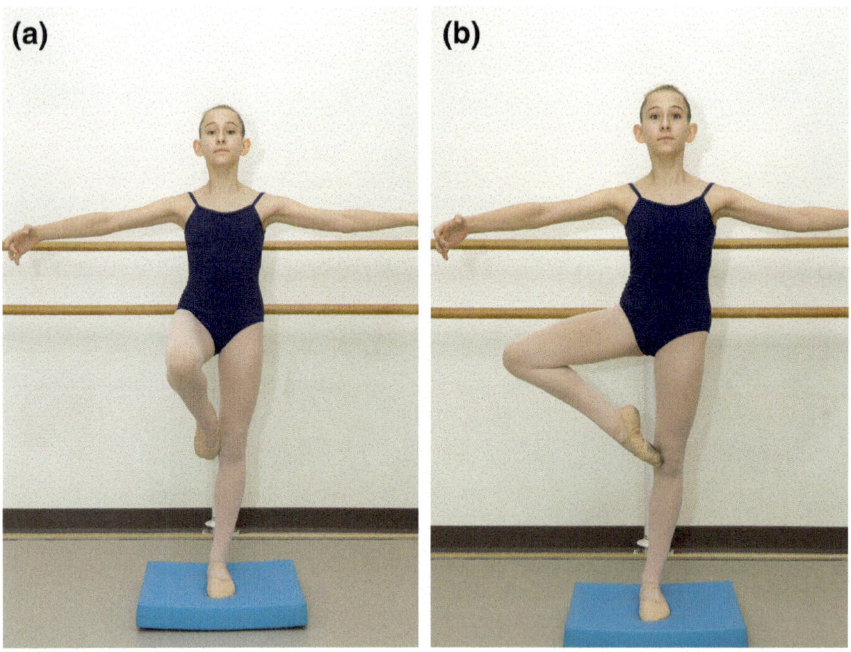

Fig. 4.3 Use of foam balance pad to challenge alignment and balance. **a** Parallel passé. **b** Open passé. Photographs courtesy of James Koepfler

Cross Training

Educating dancers, physicians, and dance teachers on the concept that they cannot use dance training alone to improve fitness and be "in shape" is a challenge, but it is a critical component of injury prevention and treatment. Often dancers are told to rest completely for a period, and then just return to full dance. This is time wasted that could have served as an opportunity for rehabilitation. In this situation, the pain or disability usually returns quickly once activity is resumed, and the dancer is often further deconditioned and their psych more bruised as a result of time away from dance. With this type of scenario in mind, cross training should always be a part of a dancer's conditioning regimen, for injury prevention purposes as much as for injury recovery. Aerobic exercise should be introduced as early as possible in the rehabilitation process to increase energy expenditure and allow for maintenance of healthy body weight. Enhancing cardiovascular conditioning can be paramount to preventing injury by reducing fatigue [13, 20], and is a necessary adjunct to skill acquisition in the training dancer [21]. Use of a stationary bike, swimming, and low-impact cardiovascular exercise like an elliptical trainer can be incorporated as appropriate for 30–40 min a day, with frequency per week determined by stage of healing and patient presentation.

Relative Rest and Restrictions in Dance

With certain injuries young dancers may be able to continue to participate in dance with modifications until healing and full strength and control are achieved through physical therapy [22]. Educating young dancers and their teachers on the concept of "relative rest" can help keep a dancer training safely while allowing an injury time to heal. Dance activity can be modified to avoid pain or for injury protection by curtailing specific exercises such as grand plié or jumps. Decreasing the amount of external rotation (turnout) at the hips can offload stress from a number of joints and lowering the height of the gesture leg (elevated leg performing the movement) in extension can reduce stress on the iliopsoas muscle (Fig. 4.4), promote control of the standing leg, and improve hip and lumbopelvic alignment. Using relative rest and modifying movements can be challenging for many dancers, as it can interfere with their drive to constantly push themselves physically. However, such restrictions allow the young dancer to participate safely as much as possible in class or rehearsal before returning to full activity.

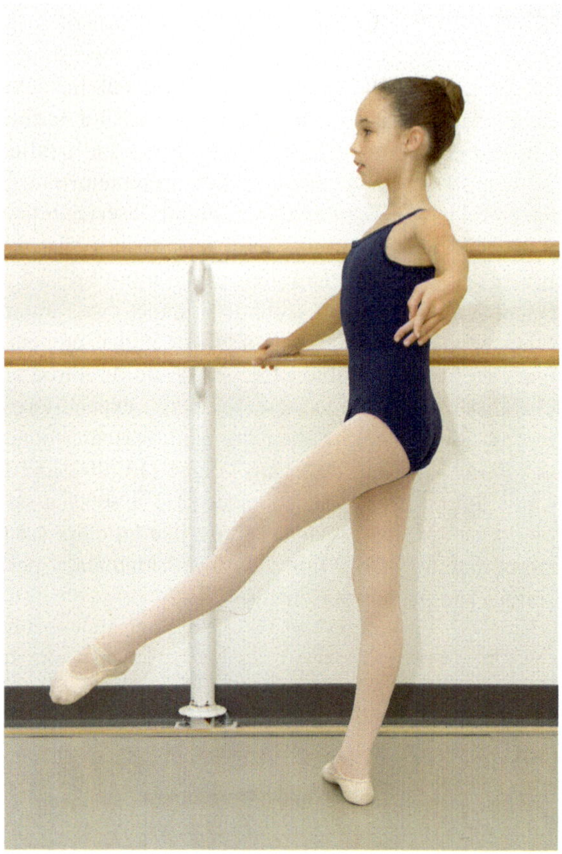

Fig. 4.4 Relative rest of iliopsoas by reducing height of dégagé. Photograph courtesy of James Koepfler

In order to assure continuity of what is recommended by the rehabilitation professional and what actually takes place in the dance studio, it is suggested that a system of communication be established by use of a form the caregiver can fill out and have the dancer give to his or her teacher (Fig. 4.5).

Return to Dance-Specific Activity

To return a young dancer safely to dance after an injury, employing task-specific rehabilitation exercises and activities can help to restore the desired function.

Dear Dance Educator,

______________________________________ **is receiving physical**

therapy for: ______________________________________

Participation in classes and /or rehearsals should to be modified as follows:

- ☐ **Observe class and work on exercises prescribed by PT**
- ☐ **Modify participation in class as follows:**
  - ☐ **Barre only** ______________________________
  - ☐ **No Grande Plie'**
  - ☐ **No Turning**
  - ☐ **No Leaping/Jumping**
  - ☐ **No work en pointe**
  - ☐ **No lifting**
  - ☐ **No cambré, back extension or arabesque past tendu**
  - ☐ **Limit turnout**______________________________
  - ☐ **Limit height of gestures/working leg** ____________________
  - ☐ **Other**______________________________

Special Notes:______________________________________

____

Thank You,

____
Therapist Signature **Date**

Fig. 4.5 Dance teacher communication sheet. *Credit* Maribeth Crupi, PT, Maribeth Crupi Physical Therapy, LLC. Heather Southwick, MSPT, Director of Physical Therapy, Boston Ballet

Dance-specific exercises can be incorporated into the rehabilitation program as the dancer demonstrates adequate healing, range of motion, flexibility, strength, and balance. Progressive strength training and volume should be managed by varying number of repetitions and load. Restoring balance and proprioception is critical after any injury in dancers, and can be accomplished by progressing through stable and unstable surfaces and varying vision, speed, acceleration and deceleration (all important variables of dynamic balance) to simulate the demands of dancing. Working at end ranges of motion and promoting a balance between mobility and stability are other areas that exercises and tasks should address. This can be challenging, but dancers need to be strongest at the end ranges of motion, and working in those ranges can help. In dance, choreography varies widely; the possibilities are endless. Therapeutic exercise should reflect those varied demands by focusing on agility, reaction time, speed of weight shifting, and point of contact between foot and floor, whether it be full foot, demi-pointe, or full pointe relevé.

Motor Learning and Motor Control

Promoting appropriate motor learning and control is critical in the young dancer population. Often dancers need to relearn movement strategies to move in a healthier way. Helping the young dancer make changes in movement patterns and control can be a little easier than with the adult professional, who may have years of potentially dangerous movement patterns and habits ingrained. The process of rehabilitation and the exercises employed as part of a plan of care should address how to give a young dancer the tools needed to meet the strength and flexibility demands of his or her training. For example, focus on motor control has been proven to be beneficial for improving such components as narrowing the difference between active and passive turnout range of motion in pre-professional dancers [23].

Dance Technique

Evaluation of dance technique involves addressing alignment, quality of movement, proper muscle recruitment, and the prevention of compensation habits. For practitioners with no background in dance who have dancers in their care, focusing on proper alignment and biomechanics common to all movement and postural patterns can be helpful. Employing a team approach to technique with the dancer and dance teacher is vital. Some approaches to technique will vary and may deviate from the most healthy patterns of movement. Regardless, it is essential to establish clear communication and to be sure that the student is given consistent information from both the practitioner and dance teacher to avoid confusion and frustration.

Research and Resources

Fully preventing dance injuries may never be possible, but as the field of dance medicine and science grows and more research emerges, great progress continues to be made. Practitioners with a background in dealing with dancers have much anecdotal knowledge to contribute to this progression. There are organizations that focus on more formalized education and sharing of information between healthcare practitioners and dance teachers, and hopefully in the future this practice will become more common as the body of knowledge grows and is increasingly valued. Young dancers can often find information in books and online to help them navigate medical issues and understand their bodies more fully. However, dancers are often reticent to seek health care when appropriate for a number of reasons, and to rely too heavily on teachers and peers for guidance. As more and more educational resources become available hopefully dancers will grow to understand that seeking medical help early is the best way to handle injury.

Conclusion

For rehabilitation to be successful all dance-related injuries must be evaluated for technique concerns or the injury will almost certainly reoccur due to the faulty habits. Creating an effective rehabilitation program for a young dancer requires a physical therapist who has knowledge of the patient's type of dance and level of intensity, and understands the intrinsic and extrinsic factors that can cause and contribute to injuries in dancers. The therapist should also have the ability to determine an accurate differential diagnosis, and be attentive to basic principles that promote a successful and long lasting rehabilitation, reducing the risk of injury recurrence. This will assure optimal recovery and outcome, with the overarching goal of return to dance better than before the injury and protecting the body from residual lifelong pain or disability.

References

1. DiFiori JP, Benjamin HJ, Brenner J, Gregory A, Jayanthi N, Landry GL, Luke A. Overuse Injuries and burnout in youth sports: a position statement from the American Medical Society for Sports Medicine. Clin J Sports Med. 2014;24(1):3–20.
2. Micheli L, Solomon R. Training the young dancer. In: Ryan AJ, Stephens RE, editors. Dance medicine: a comprehensive guide. Chicago: Plurbius Press; 1987. pp. 51–72.
3. Roberts K, Nelson N, McKenzie N. Dance-related injuries in children and adolescents treated in US emergency departments in 1991–2007. J Phys Act Health. 2013;10(2):143–50.
4. Krasnow D, Wilmerding D. Motor learning and control for dance. Champaign, IL: Human Kinetics; 2015. p. 60.

5. Kivel CG, d'Hemecourt CA, Micheli LJ. Treatment of iliac crest apophysitis in the young athlete with bone stimulation: report of 2 cases. Clin J Sport Med. 2011;21(2):144–7.
6. Penha P, João S, Casarotto R, Amino C, Penteado D. Postural assessment of girls between 7 and 10 years of age. Clinics (Sao Paulo). 2005;60(1):9–16.
7. Turner R, O'Sullivan E, Edelstein J. Hip dysplasia and the performing arts: is there a correlation? Curr Rev Musculoskelet Med. 2012;5(1):39–45.
8. Smits-Engelsman B, Klerks M, Kirby A. Beighton score: a valid measure for generalized hypermobility in children. J Pediatr. 2011;158(1):119–23 e1-4.
9. Liederbach MJ, Schanfein L, Kremenic I. What is known about the effect of fatigue on injury occurrence among dancers? J Dance Med Sci. 2013;17(3):101–8.
10. Critchfield B. Stretching for dancers IADMS www.DanceScience.org. 2011; www.iadms.org.
11. Ducher G, Kukulian S, Hill B, Garnham A, Nowson C, Kimlin M, Cook J. Vitamin D status and musculoskeletal health in adolescent male ballet dancers a pilot study. J Dance Med Sci. 2011;15(3):99–107.
12. Ruanne L, Krasnow D, Thomas M. Communication between medical practitioners and dancers. J Dance Med Sci. 2008;12(2):47–53.
13. Liederbach MJ. General considerations for guiding dance injury rehabilitation. J Dance Med Sci. 2000;4(2):54–64.
14. Kravitz L, Jayo J. The physiological effects of aquatic exercise. Aqua Exercise Review. https://www.unm.edu/~lkravitz/Article%20folder/aqua.html.
15. Villalta E, Peiris C. Early aquatic physical therapy improves function and does not increase risk of wound-related adverse events for adults after orthopedic surgery: a systematic review and meta-analysis. Arch Phys Med Rehabil. 2013;94(1):138–48.
16. Kloubec J. Pilates: how does it work and who needs it? Muscles Ligaments Tendons J. 2011;1(2):61–6.
17. Powers CM. The influence of abnormal hip mechanics on knee injury: a biomechanical perspective. J Orthop Sports Phys Ther. 2010;40(2):42–51.
18. Hamilton WG, Hamilton LH, Marshall P, Molnar M. A profile of the musculoskeletal characteristics of elite professional ballet dancers. Am J Sports Med. 1992;20(3):267–73.
19. Richardson M, Leiderbach MJ, Sandow E. Functional criteria for assessing pointe readiness. J Dance Med Sci. 2010;14(3):6–7.
20. Twitchett E, Brodrick A, Nevill AM, Koutedakis Y, Angioi M, Wyon M. Does physical fitness affect injury occurrence and time loss due to injury in elite vocational ballet students? J Dance Med Sci. 2010;14(1):26–31.
21. Wyon MA, Redding E. Physiological monitoring of cardiorespiratory adaptations during rehearsal and performance of contemporary dance. J Strength Cond Res. 2005;19(3):611–4.
22. Bryan N, Smith BM. Back school programs. The ballet dancer. Occup Med. 1992;7(1):67–75.
23. Sherman A, Mayall E, Tasker S. Can a prescribed turnout conditioning program reduce the differential between passive and active turnout in pre-professional dancers? J Dance Med Sci. 2014;18(4):159–68.

Chapter 5
Resistance Training for Pediatric Female Dancers

Andrea Stracciolini, MD, FAAP, FACSM, Gregory D. Myer, PhD, FACSM, CSCS*D and Avery D. Faigenbaum, EdD

Pertinent Definitions

Pediatric: For the purposes of this paper the term pediatric is used to depict prepubertal (skeletally immature) and pubertal (approaching skeletal maturity) dancers.

A. Stracciolini, MD, FAAP, FACSM (✉) · G.D. Myer, PhD, FACSM, CSCS*D
The Micheli Center for Sports Injury Prevention, Waltham, MA, USA
e-mail: andrea.stracciolini@childrens.harvard.edu

A. Stracciolini, MD, FAAP, FACSM
Division of Sports Medicine, Department of Orthopaedics,
Boston Children's Hospital, 300 Longwood Avenue,
Boston, MA 02115, USA

A. Stracciolini, MD, FAAP, FACSM
Division of Emergency Medicine, Department of Medicine,
Boston Children's Hospital, Boston, MA, USA

A.D. Faigenbaum, EdD
Department of Health and Exercise Science, The College of New Jersey,
2000 Pennington Rd, Ewing, NJ 08628, USA
e-mail: faigenba@tcnj.edu

G.D. Myer, PhD, FACSM, CSCS*D
Division of Sports Medicine, The SPORT Center, Cincinnati Children's
Hospital Medical Center, Cincinnati, OH, USA
e-mail: greg.myer@cchmc.org

G.D. Myer, PhD, FACSM, CSCS*D
Departments of Pediatrics and Orthopaedic Surgery, University of Cincinnati,
Cincinnati, OH, USA

G.D. Myer, PhD, FACSM, CSCS*D
Department of Orthopaedics, University of Pennsylvania, Philadelphia, PA, USA

R. Solomon et al. (eds.), *Prevention of Injuries in the Young Dancer*,
Contemporary Pediatric and Adolescent Sports Medicine,
DOI 10.1007/978-3-319-55047-3_5

Concentric muscle contraction: The external force on the muscle is less than the force the muscle is generating—a muscle and joint angle *shortening* contraction.
Eccentric muscle contraction: Active contraction of a muscle occurring simultaneously with lengthening of the muscle and increasing joint angle.
Muscular fitness: An inclusive term that refers to muscle strength, muscular power, and local muscular endurance.
Plyometrics: A type of exercise characterized by hops, jumps, and throws; it involves a rapid stretch of a muscle-tendon unit immediately followed by shortening of the muscle unit (called the "stretch shortening cycle") [1].
Resistance training: A method of conditioning, also called "strength training," that involves the progressive use of a wide range of resistive loads, different movement velocities, and a variety of training modalities, including body weight, free weights (barbells and dumbbells), weight machines, resistance bands, suspension systems, and medicine balls, to improve muscle strength, muscular power, and local muscular endurance.
Weightlifting: A competitive sport that involves the performance of the snatch and clean and jerk lifts. Weightlifting training refers to a variety of explosive multi-joint exercises that are performed as controlled movements, requiring a high degree of technical skill and qualified instruction.
Q angle: The angle formed by a line drawn from the anterior superior iliac spine to the central patella and a second line drawn from the central patella to the tibial tubercle; an increased Q angle is a risk factor for patellar subluxation; the normal Q angle is 14° for males and 17° for females.

Introduction

It is estimated that approximately 3.5 million children receive dance instruction from dance specialists in the USA alone [2]. Because of the incredible physical demands of the discipline, dancers sustain a high rate of injury [3–7]. There is now a call to action for those caring for and training pediatric dancers to support a paradigm shift toward injury prevention and away from reliance solely on post-injury treatment [3, 8, 9].

Adult dancers experience various musculoskeletal injuries throughout their careers; however, the pediatric dancer may be even more vulnerable to injury due to the physiological growth process [10, 11]. Several epidemiological studies report that the injury incidence of pediatric to pre-professional dancers ranges between 0.77 and 1.55 per 1000 dance hours [12–15]. This incidence is significantly higher than the 0.60–0.62 per 1000 dance hours noted for both adult professional ballet and modern dancers [16, 17]. Furthermore, the rate of injury requiring an emergency room evaluation is exceptional for pediatric dancers. A retrospective study reported that between 1991 and 2007 a total of 113,084 children and adolescents were treated in US emergency departments due to dance-related injuries [5]. (With regard to all of the studies referenced here it should be noted that the interpretation of injury incidence data is difficult due to lack of uniformity in injury definition among studies.)

Resistance training usually is not an inherent component of current training for female pediatric dancers. This is likely because muscular strength has not historically been considered an essential ingredient for success in dance. In part, this may also reflect the unfounded view that supplemental training and consequent gains in muscle strength and mass would diminish the female dancer's aesthetic appearance and gracefulness [18]. To the contrary, an early study by Fitt [19] found that dancers who participated in a well-designed resistance training program were able to increase muscle strength without building muscle bulk. This same study demonstrated improved effects of resistance training on dance performance. The pediatric dancer in training requires sufficient lower extremity strength for power generation during leaps and jumps, and muscle endurance for prolonged periods of use. Ankle sprains are a leading cause of traumatic injury to pediatric dancers [14]. Stabilization of the lower extremity during landing is therefore important to prevent such injuries. Data on female ballet dancers have indicated that supplemental resistance training for hamstrings and quadriceps can lead to improvements in leg strength without interfering with key artistic and physical performance requirements [18, 20, 21]. Similar findings exist in contemporary dance, showing that dancers improve in muscle power and endurance and aesthetic competence with supplemental circuit training [22].

Much like research in other athletic activities, the process of injury prevention in dance includes investigations that seek to identify individual risk factors for injury, followed by interventions targeted at the prevention of injuries unique to dance [23]. In pediatric dancers one risk factor for injury unquestionably involves inappropriate progression of the rate, intensity, and duration of dance training, with inadequate periods of rest and recovery [24]. Muscle-tendon imbalances of strength, endurance, or flexibility that develop during growth and maturation, as well as those resulting from focused training in one dance mode alone, are other risk factors for pediatric dancers [11, 25, 26]. It has been said that by addressing such risk factors acute and overuse injuries in youth participating in dance training could be reduced by up to, and possibly even more than, 50% [27, 28]. Hence, it can be argued that greater emphasis needs to be placed on strength-specific exercises for pediatric dancers to decrease injury and resulting time loss. Rickman et al. [29] report that there is limited comprehensive literature examining the multiple components of core strength as they relate to injury in dancers. Incorporating a resistance training program that develops core stability and strength should be considered fundamental to the training of the pediatric dancer with the goal of injury prevention [23].

It is important to note that many fallacies exist with regard to resistance training in children. Perhaps the most well known of these is the notion that strength-building exercises are injurious to the immature skeleton. Actually, concerns associated with resistance training in children have not been supported in the literature. In fact, resistance exercise for children can be safe and effective and can provide a multitude of benefits, including improved performance, injury prevention, and increased bone health. As a multidisciplinary team comprised of pediatric exercise specialists, athletic trainers, fitness specialists, and dance/sport medicine physicians, the current authors' goals are to provide readers with a review of the benefits of resistance training for pediatric female dancers, to discuss and reconcile the perceived risks of this type of training on growing skeletally immature dancers, and to provide guidance regarding a resistance training regimen that is geared toward injury prevention and enhanced dance performance.

Concerns Surrounding Resistance Training for the Pediatric Dancer

There are many concerns about resistance training in children and adolescents. The purpose of the following section is to discuss these issues as they pertain to the pediatric female dancer. One of the primary concerns involves safety. There is no evidence that resistance training will negatively impact growth and maturation in children and adolescents [30]. In fact, resistance training can be a safe part of training and injury prevention for pediatric dancers when conducted with qualified guidance and supervision. Growth cartilage injuries historically have been one of the largest concerns among pediatricians and athletic trainers relative to resistance training in youth; however, injury to the growth cartilage has not been reported in any prospective youth resistance training research study [31]. Growth cartilage injuries described in case reports from the 1970s to 1980s typically resulted from improper lifting techniques, poorly chosen training loads, or lack of qualified adult supervision [32]. A recent review of the literature indicated that there is a relatively low risk of injury in children and adolescents who follow age-appropriate resistance training guidelines, including: qualified and targeted instruction, constructive feedback on exercise technique, and a sensible progression of training loads and volume [32]. In ten studies that systematically monitored injuries in this population, only three injuries were reported, with estimated injury rates of 0.176, 0.053, and 0.055 per 100 participant hours in the respective programs [30].

Data from patients presenting to US emergency departments revealed that many injuries related to resistance training were largely due to accidents and poor technique rather than to the actual resistance training activities; notably, two-thirds of the injuries sustained by 8- to 13-year-old patients were to the hand and foot and were most often related to "dropping" and "pinching" (based on injury descriptions) [33]. Quatman et al. [34] found that adolescent and young adult males may suffer more exertional-type resistance injuries to the trunk, while females in the same age category may be more susceptible to lower extremity injuries resulting from accidents during resistance training. The recently published "Position statement on youth resistance training: the 2014 International Consensus" is an excellent resource for dance practitioners, as it describes resistance training guidelines for children and adolescents and emphasizes considerations for young females [35].

Another significant concern of young dancers themselves is the development of bulky muscles and alteration of the "sleek and stealth" appearance generally preferred in their art form. Results of studies on muscle hypertrophy in children with regard to resistance training have been mixed and inconclusive to date [36]. Muscular strength development is a multidimensional fitness component that is influenced by a combination of muscular, neural, and biomechanical factors. For example, a potential factor for increasing strength during childhood may be related to maturation of the central nervous system, improvements in motor unit recruitment, firing frequency, synchronization, and neural myelination [35]. In preadolescents, proper resistance training can enhance strength without concomitant muscle hypertrophy. Such gains in strength can be attributed to the aforementioned neurologic mechanisms [37]. These mechanisms are factors in increases of strength in populations with low androgen concentrations, including females and pre-adolescent boys [38].

Assessments of muscular strength in children and adolescents indicate that strength increases in a relatively linear fashion throughout childhood for both boys and girls. As children reach the onset of puberty they experience rapid skeletal growth, along with observable nonlinear gains in muscular strength. During this period sex differences in muscular strength begin to emerge, with boys demonstrating accelerated gains due to increased hormonal concentrations, including testosterone, growth hormone, and insulin-like growth factors. Girls appear to continue to develop in a more linear fashion [35].

Physical education teachers and dance instructors may start early (during primary school) to educate novice dancers and their parents about the benefits of resistance training and reasonable adaptations that are likely to occur with regular training. Thought needs to be given to how resistance training is explained and offered to dancers. While some teenage girls may shy away from weightlifting with American football players in a high school program, dancers may be interested in fitness activities that emphasize neuromuscular control and coordination that can be introduced in familiar environments, like the dance studio (Fig. 5.1).

Many people feel that resistance training will not increase muscle strength in girls. Recent scientific studies have demonstrated that this is not true. Malina [30] reviewed 22 reports dealing with experimental resistance training protocols in both males and females before and during early puberty. He found that most programs used weight machines and free weights (i.e., dumbbells and barbells), 2- to 3-day protocols, and 8- to 12-week durations. Significant improvements in muscular strength during childhood and early adolescence were achieved in both sexes.

There is not one optimal combination of sets, repetitions, and exercises that will result in favorable adaptations in muscular strength, fitness performance, and body composition in all youth [39, 40]. By periodically altering the training variables over time the training stimulus will remain effective, and adaptations to the training program will be maximized [1, 41–43]. Nor is there a "minimal age" requirement for participation in a youth resistance training program provided participants are able to

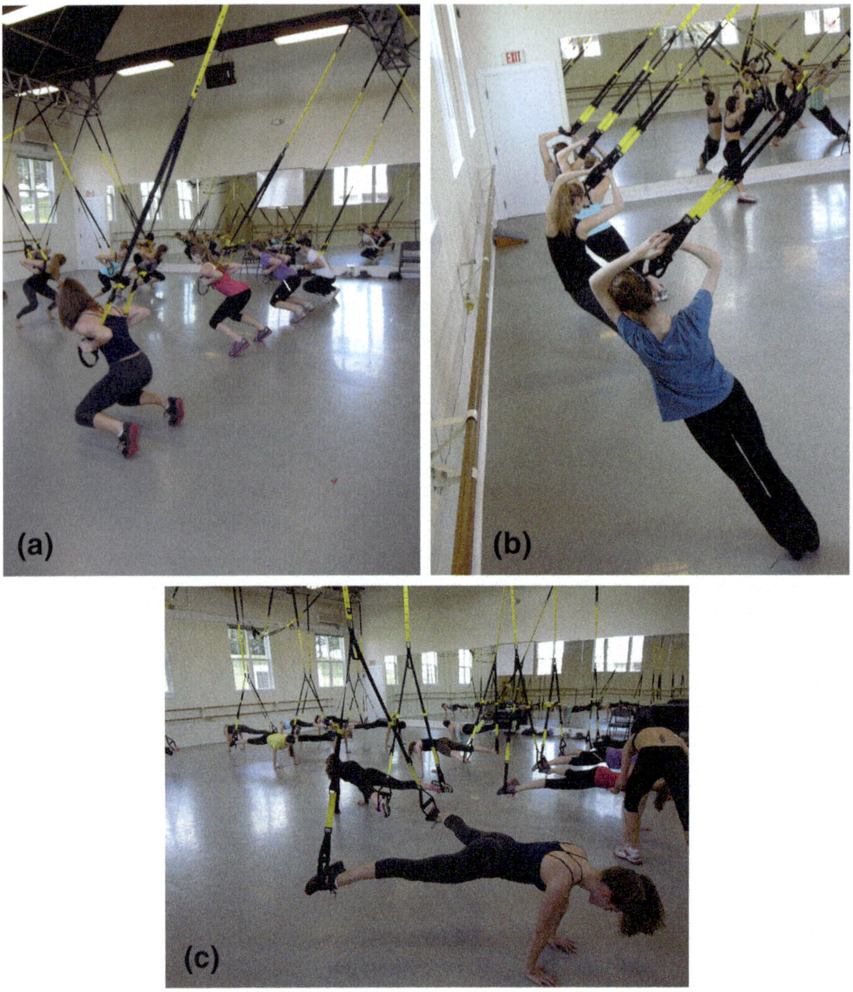

Fig. 5.1 **a**, **b**, **c** Adolescent dancers participating in resistance training in the dance studio as part of dance training

follow directions and pay attention to safety rules, and by 7 or 8 years of age most girls are ready for some type of resistance exercise [32]. Resistance training with free weights, medicine balls, elastic bands, and one's own body weight is beneficial for pediatric dancers for multiple reasons. As part of an integrative neuromuscular training program resistance training may help to enhance motor skill performance and motor coordination, improve balance, and increase muscle strength and power [31, 41, 44, 45]. These same factors are critical components of dance training.

There is a paucity of published data on the strength characteristics of ballet dancers. Micheli et al. found female professional dancers (mean age 27 years) to have strong lower extremities (quadriceps, hamstrings, dorsiflexors, and plantarflexors) and relatively weak upper extremities (elbow flexors and extensors) [46]. Muscle groups about the hip and pelvis were not isolated in this study, and there was no control group for comparison. In other studies, female dancers demonstrated only 77% of weight-predicted norms when compared to other groups of athletes [47]. Relative to peak in-season performance, Kirkendall and Calabrese [48] reported the mean quadriceps strength in female ballet dancers was the lowest among the athletic groups reviewed, at around 70% of the weight-predicted normal for athletes. Gupta et al. [49] found that dancers demonstrated an adaptive training response with a shift in the strength curve toward the inner range of hip external rotation as opposed to a true difference in strength, as compared to non-dancer controls. More specific to pediatric dancers, Bennell et al. compared hip muscle strength in 8- to 11-year-old novice female ballet dancers versus non-dancing age matched controls. After controlling for body weight controls had stronger overall hip muscles than dancers, with the exception of their hip abductor strength, which was similar between groups [50]. Further study in this same age group revealed that 12 months of dance activity produced greater muscular strength improvement in female dancers compared to that of controls over the same period of time [51]. Supplementary resistance training programs for professional dancers have been shown to be beneficial in improving both muscular endurance and anaerobic power [20]. Finally, Koutedakis and Sharp [21] reported that after strength training professional dancers demonstrated enhanced knee extension and flexion torques without altering dance aesthetics.

Resistance Training During Growth and Maturation in Dancers

A basic understanding of child and adolescent development as it relates to injury profile is critical when caring for or training pediatric dancers. Overall body mass and height may increase at a dramatic rate in the preadolescent and adolescent years. The rapid increase in bone length often results in a decrease in muscle-tendon unit flexibility, leading to greater injury risk from either a single traumatic event, such as a sudden forced muscle elongation, or repetitive stress and micro-trauma [11]. The biomechanical changes that occur during growth may predispose the dancer to a host of injuries. Prime examples include coxa saltans externa or snapping hip, and posterior column stress injury or spondylolysis. These quintessential dance injuries may, in part, be attributed to strength, flexibility, and neuromuscular deficits that are typically associated with growth and often magnified during the growth process. Specifically, the combination of relatively weak abdominal and posterior chain musculature, tight overused and weak hip flexors and quadriceps, and the anterior tilt of the widened pelvis may place female pediatric dancers at risk for injury [52]. Tursz et al. [53] demonstrated that following rapid growth and development female athletes sustain a higher rate of "sprains" than males, and this trend continues into maturity.

There is a tendency toward an increasingly early age of menarche for girls across the USA, with the average age of 12.6 years [54], and girls tend to reach their peak height and body mass at approximately 15 years of age [55]. Notably, the onset of puberty in the child dancer may be delayed, extending both the dancer's growth period and duration of increased vulnerability to injury [56, 57]. In general, female dancers appear to have greater ligamentous laxity than their male counterparts following the onset of puberty [58, 59]. It is hypothesized that this increased laxity (alterations in passive joint restraints) combined with the physiological changes (i.e., neuromuscular control) that occur during puberty may affect the type, severity, and incidence of injuries in the maturing female adolescent population [60, 61]. It has also been suggested that cyclic changes in the hormonal milieu of females may play a role in injury patterns [62–66]. Parents, teachers, and the dancers themselves need to be aware of the physiological changes, psychological issues, nutritional considerations, and the need for training modifications during this vulnerable time in the dancer's career.

Strength deficits unique to the discipline of dance need to be aggressively addressed with individualized training protocols that target actively growing females [46, 49]. Anatomical changes during growth and development include the aforementioned widening of the pelvis, increase in the Q angle, and changes in center of gravity [67]. Researchers have hypothesized that following the onset of puberty and the initiation of peak height velocity, increases in tibia and femur length, overall body mass, and height of the center of mass lead to decreased core stability. A key tenet of this decrease in core stability is that this change occurs in the absence of increases in strength and muscle recruitment at the hip and trunk [68, 69]. As female athletes reach maturity, decreased core stability and deficient core strength may underlie their tendency to demonstrate increased dynamic lower extremity valgus load during sport specific tasks, placing them at increased risk for injury [70–72].

Intervention efforts with targeted training that includes increasing strength and improving neuromuscular control while incorporating skill development can be implemented in a timely and effective manner [43]. Quatman-Yates and colleagues investigated the longitudinal trajectories of lower extremity strength across maturational stages for females. They found that hip abduction and hamstring-quadriceps strength ratio decreased from prepubertal to pubertal stages, lending further support to the need for strength training during preadolescence with the goal of injury prevention [73]. Evidence currently supports the implementation of injury prevention programs that focus on strength and neuromuscular control of the lower extremity [74–82]. The window of opportunity is open to maximizing training during preadolescence, when children are more responsive to interventions that promote strength, flexibility, and peri-pelvic stabilization. This is especially important before neuromuscular deficits become engrained, and before the pediatric dancer succumbs to injury [83]. Finally, and importantly, new research has shown that intervention with an individualized conditioning program based on injury history and functional movement screening is effective in preventing dance injuries [84].

Resistance Training and Bone Mineral Density (BMD)

A recent meta-analysis by Amorin et al. [85] evaluating 35 studies of BMD in dancers concluded that based on the current available research it is unclear whether low BMD is prevalent among female dancers. Childhood through late adolescence is the most critical time period for bone mass accrual [86]. The literature on BMD and sports participation continues to evolve. Physical activities characterized by considerable loading have been shown to have the greatest osteogenic effects on the growing skeleton [87]. Resistance training for females during this time period may be an important component of exercise when considering future bone health and risk for stress related bone injury [88]. Bass et al. [89] have reported that prepubertal female gymnasts, whose training mainly involves high-impact and resistance training, had significantly higher lumbar spine bone mass, volume, and volumetric BMD than a control group. Morris et al. explored lean mass, strength, and bone mineral response to a 10-month, high-impact, strength-building exercise program in premenarchal girls. The exercise group gained significantly more lean mass, strength, and BMD versus controls, and had less body fat content. Although a large proportion of bone mineral accrual in the premenarchal skeleton was related to growth, an osteogenic effect was also found to be associated with the exercise protocol in this young female cohort [90].

It is important to note, especially for the dancer population, that resistance training begun at a young age is associated with a decreased risk of osteoporotic fractures later in life [91]. Evaluation of bone mass relative to muscle strength and reproductive hormone concentration in elite endurance athletes supports the theory that muscle forces are significant osteogenic factors. Research findings also indicate that in female athletes muscle forces acting on bone potentially counteract a negative effect of reproductive hormonal disorders on BMD [92]. To et al. sought to compare BMD between regularly exercising dancers and age matched non-exercising females between the ages of 17 and 19 years to assess the impact of weight-bearing exercises and menstrual status on bone density. Results from this study were notable in that young women undergoing regular intensive weight-bearing exercise, as in the dancers under study, had higher BMD than the non-exercising females of the same age, but only if they remained eumenorrheic during their training. This advantage was lost when they developed oligo/amenorrhea [93]. Furthermore, Benson and colleagues reported that very lean dancers are more prone to injury than their less lean counterparts [94]. The evidence now appears strong in support of resistance training and weight-bearing physical activities that promote strength development to ensure the greatest osteogenic potential in young females [95]. This may be particularly critical for female athletes at high risk for bony injury, including dancers.

Resistance Training Programs for the Pediatric Female Dancer

Resistance training for pediatric dancers may be particularly challenging given what may appear to be opposing goals in the dancers' eyes. The need to build strength may seem to contrast with the aesthetic requirements of the discipline, specifically the desire to appear thin and sleek. In this context, designing resistance training protocols that are conducted in environments familiar to the dancer (e.g., the dance studio) while dispelling the myths often associated with lifting weights is encouraged. Training protocols should be designed to correct strength imbalances unique to the discipline. For the ballet dancer this may mean conducting resistance training in the parallel, as opposed to the turned out, position. This technique encourages improving the strength of the relatively weaker adductor and internal rotator muscles of the lower extremity. Resistance training in this population should include dynamic concentric and eccentric muscle actions, and be performed through full ranges of motion in keeping with the unique demands of dance.

Liederbach and colleagues evaluated the incidence of anterior cruciate ligament (ACL) injuries in dancers and found that dancers suffer considerably fewer ACL injuries than athletes participating in team ball sports. Notably, the incidence of ACL injury was not statistically different between sexes. The authors hypothesize that the training dancers utilize to perfect lower extremity alignment, jump, and balance skills may serve to protect them against ACL injury [96]. As a result, the training protocol for the dancer may not need to target balance and landing as intensely as athletes who play soccer and basketball. More recent research on ACL injury biomechanics in dancers has shown that although they take longer to reach fatigue of the lower extremities when compared to team athletes, once fatigue is reached for both dancers and team athletes their landing mechanics place them at greater risk for ACL injuries than before the onset of fatigue [97]. This research supports the need for resistance training for dancers to improve muscle endurance, as well as strength, to reduce injury risk. More specifically, pelvic stabilization (targeting strength and neuromuscular control of the deep hip stabilizers) and strengthening of the abdominal and gluteal muscles should be a cornerstone of training for this active group of females.

Conclusion

Resistance training in pediatric dancers is safe and effective for improving muscle strength, power, and endurance without effecting dance aesthetics. Research continues to evolve supporting the multitude of benefits to be derived from resistance training for female dancers, along with a well-balanced diet and adequate rest and recovery time. The call to action for all those caring for pediatric dancers is shifting focus from injury treatment to injury prevention. A discipline-wide approach to injury prevention is needed, and might well begin with educating the dance community about the benefits, safety, and effectiveness of resistance training programs that are designed, supervised, and taught by qualified professionals who understand the physical and psychosocial uniqueness of active children and adolescents.

References

1. Chu D, Myer G. Plyometrics. Champaign, IL: Human Kinetics; 2013.
2. Organization NDE. Statistics: general US education and dance education. 2014; http://www.ndeo.org/content.aspx?page_id=22&club_id=893257&module_id=55774. Accessed 17 Feb 2014.
3. Ramkumar PN, Farber J, Arnouk J, Varner KE, McCulloch PC. Injuries in a professional ballet dance company: a 10-year retrospective study. J Dance Med Sci. 2016;20(1):30–7.
4. Jacobs CL, Cassidy JD, Cote P, Boyle E, Ramel E, Ammendolia C, et al. Musculoskeletal injury in professional dancers: prevalence and associated factors: an international cross-sectional study. Clin J Sport Med. 2017;27(2):153–60.
5. Roberts KJ, Nelson NG, McKenzie L. Dance-related injuries in children and adolescents treated in US emergency departments in 1991-2007. J Phys Act Health. 2013;10(2):143–50.
6. Garrick JG, Requa RK. Ballet injuries. An analysis of epidemiology and financial outcome. Am J Sports Med. 1993;21(4):586–90.
7. Hincapie CA, Morton EJ, Cassidy JD. Musculoskeletal injuries and pain in dancers: a systematic review. Arch Phys Med Rehabil. 2008;89(9):1819–29.
8. Koutedakis Y, Pacy PJ, Ray RJ. Carson, Dick F. Health and fitness in professional dancers. Med Prob Perform Art. 1997;12(1):23–7.
9. Koutedakis Y, Stavropoulos-Kalinoglou A, Metsios G. The significance of muscular strength in dance. J Dance Med Sci. 2005;9(1):29–34.
10. Flachsmann R, Broom ND, Hardy AE, Moltschaniwskyj G. Why is the adolescent joint particularly susceptible to osteochondral shear fracture? Clin Orthop Rel Res. 2000;381:212–21.
11. Micheli LJ. Overuse injuries in children's sports: the growth factor. Orthop Clin North Am. 1983;14(2):337–60.
12. Ekegren CL, Quested R, Brodrick A. Injuries in pre-professional ballet dancers: incidence, characteristics and consequences. J Sci Med Sport. 2014;17(3):271–5.
13. Gamboa JM, Roberts LA, Maring J, Fergus A. Injury patterns in elite preprofessional ballet dancers and the utility of screening programs to identify risk characteristics. J Orthop Sports Phys Ther. 2008;38(3):126–36.
14. Leanderson C, Leanderson J, Wykman A, Strender LE, Johansson SE, Sundquist K. Musculoskeletal injuries in young ballet dancers. Knee Surg Sports Traumatol Arthrosc. 2011;19(9):1531–5.
15. Steinberg N, Aujla I, Zeev A, Redding E. Injuries among talented young dancers: findings from the UK centres for advanced training. Int J Sports Med. 2014;35(3):238–44.
16. Nilsson C, Leanderson J, Wykman A, Strender LE. The injury panorama in a Swedish professional ballet company. Knee Surg Sports Traumatol Arthrosc. 2001;9(4):242–6.
17. Shah S, Weiss DS, Burchette RJ. Injuries in professional modern dancers: incidence, risk factors, and management. J Dance Med Sci. 2012;16(1):17–25.
18. Koutedakis Y, Jamurtas A. The dancer as a performing athlete: physiological considerations. Sports Med. 2004;34(10):651–61.
19. Fitt S. Conditioning for dancers: investigating some assumptions. Dance Res J. 1981–2;14(1–2):32–8.

20. Stalder M, Noble, Wilkinson JG. The effects of supplemental weight training for ballet dancers. J Appl Sport Sci Res. 1990;4(3):95–102.
21. Koutedakis Y, Sharp NC. Thigh-muscles strength training, dance exercise, dynamometry, and anthropometry in professional ballerinas. J Strength Cond Res. 2004;18(4):714–8.
22. Angioi M, Metsios G, Twitchett EA, Koutedakis Y, Wyon M. Effects of supplemental training on fitness and aesthetic competence parameters in contemporary dance: a randomised controlled trial. Med Probl Perform Art. 2012;27(1):3–8.
23. Russell JA. Preventing dance injuries: current perspectives. Open Access J Sports Med. 2013;4:199–210.
24. Luke A, Lazaro RM, Bergeron MF, Keyser L, Benjamin H, Brenner J, et al. Sports-related injuries in youth athletes: is overscheduling a risk factor? Clin J Sport Med. 2011;21(4):307–14.
25. Kenny SJ, Whittaker JL, Emery CA. Risk factors for musculoskeletal injury in preprofessional dancers: a systematic review. Br J Sports Med. 2016;50(16):997–1003.
26. Micheli LJ. Lower extremity overuse injuries. Acta Med Scand. 1986;S711:171–7.
27. Micheli LJ. Preventing injuries in team sports: what the team physician needs to know. In: Chan K, Micheli L, Smith A, Rolf C, Bachl N, Frontera W, Alenabi T, editors. FIMS team physician manual. Hong Kong: CD Concepts; 2006. p. 555–72.
28. Valovich McLeod TC, Decoster LC, Loud KJ, Micheli LJ, Parker JT, Sandrey MA, White C. National athletic trainers' association position statement: prevention of pediatric overuse injuries. J Athl Train. 2011;46(2):206–20.
29. Rickman AM, Ambegaonkar JP, Cortes N. Core stability: implications for dance injuries. Med Probl Perform Art. 2012;27(3):159–64.
30. Malina RM. Weight training in youth-growth, maturation, and safety: an evidence-based review. Clin J Sport Med. 2006;16(6):478–87.
31. Faigenbaum AD, Myer GD. Resistance training among young athletes: safety, efficacy and injury prevention effects. Br J Sports Med. 2010;44(1):56–63.
32. Faigenbaum AD, Kraemer WJ, Blimkie CJ, Jeffreys I, Micheli LJ, Nitka M, et al. Youth resistance training: updated position statement paper from the national strength and conditioning association. J Strength Cond Res. 2009;23(5 Suppl):S60–79.
33. Myer GD, Quatman CE, Khoury J, Wall EJ, Hewett TE. Youth versus adult "weightlifting" injuries presenting to United States emergency rooms: accidental versus nonaccidental injury mechanisms. J Strength Cond Res. 2009;23(7):2054–60.
34. Quatman CE, Myer GD, Khoury J, Wall EJ, Hewett TE. Sex differences in "weightlifting" injuries presenting to United States emergency rooms. J Strength Cond Res. 2009;23 (7):2061–7.
35. Lloyd RS, Faigenbaum AD, Stone MH, Oliver JL, Jeffreys I, Moody JA, et al. Position statement on youth resistance training: the 2014 international consensus. Br J Sports Med. 2014;48(7):498–505.
36. Behm DG, Faigenbaum AD, Falk B, Klentrou P. Canadian society for exercise physiology position paper: resistance training in children and adolescents. Appl Physiol Nutr Metab. 2008;33(3):547–61.
37. Granacher U, Goesele A, Roggo K, Wischer T, Fischer S, Zuerny C, Gollhofer A, Kriemler S. Effects and mechanisms of strength training in children. Int J Sports Med. 2011;32(5):357–64.
38. Ozmun JC, Mikesky AE, Surburg PR. Neuromuscular adaptations following prepubescent strength training. Med Sci Sports Exerc. 1994;26(4):510–4.
39. Faigenbaum AD, Lloyd RS, Myer GD. Youth resistance training: past practices, new perspectives, and future directions. Pediatr Exerc Sci. 2013;25(4):591–604.
40. Faigenbaum AD, Lloyd RS, MacDonald J, Myer GD. Citius, Altius, Fortius: beneficial effects of resistance training for young athletes: marrative review. Br J Sports Med. 2016;50(1):3–7.
41. Faigenbaum A. Youth strength training: programs for health, fitness and sport. Champaign, IL: Human Kinetics; 2009.
42. Faigenbaum AD. Resistance training for overweight and obese youth: beyond sets and reps. Obes Weight Manag. 2009;5(6):282–5.

43. Myer GD, Faigenbaum AD, Chu DA, Falkel J, Ford KR, Best TM, et al. Integrative training for children and adolescents: techniques and practices for reducing sports-related injuries and enhancing athletic performance. Phys Sportsmed. 2011;39(1):74–84.
44. Faigenbaum AD, Farrell A, Fabiano M, Radler T, Naclerio F, Ratamess NA, et al. Effects of integrative neuromuscular training on fitness performance in children. Pediatr Exerc Sci. 2011;23(4):573–84.
45. Faigenbaum ADMG, Farrell A, Radler T, Fabiano M, Kang J, et al. Integrative neuromuscular training and sex-specific fitness performance in 7-year-old children: an exploratory investigation. J Athl Train. 2014;49(2):145–53.
46. Micheli LJ, Gillespie WJ, Walaszek A. Physiologic profiles of female professional ballerinas. Clin Sports Med. 1984;3(1):199–209.
47. Reid DC. Prevention of hip and knee injuries in ballet dancers. Sports Med. 1988;6(5):295–307.
48. Kirkendall DT, Calabrese LH. Physiological aspects of dance. Clin Sports Med. 1983;2(3):525–37.
49. Gupta A, Fernihough B, Bailey G, Bombeck P, Clarke A, Hopper D. An evaluation of differences in hip external rotation strength and range of motion between female dancers and non-dancers. Br J Sports Med. 2004;38(6):778–83.
50. Bennell K, Khan KM, Matthews B, et al. Hip and ankle range of motion and hip muscle strength in young female ballet dancers and controls. Br J Sports Med. 1999;33(5):340–6.
51. Bennell KL, Khan KM, Matthews BL, Singleton C. Changes in hip and ankle range of motion and hip muscle strength in 8–11 year old novice female ballet dancers and controls: a 12 month follow up study. Br J Sports Med. 2001;35(1):54–9.
52. Janda V. Muscles and motor control in low back pain: assessment and management. In: Twomey LT, editor. Physical therapy of the low back. New York: Churchill Livingstone; 1987. p. 253–78.
53. Tursz A, Crost M. Sports-related injuries in children. A study of their characteristics, frequency, and severity, with comparison to other types of accidental injuries. Am J Sports Med. 1986;14(4):294–9.
54. Euling SY, Herman-Giddens ME, Lee PA, Selevan SG, Juul A, Sørensen TI, et al. Examination of US puberty-timing data from 1940 to 1994 for secular trends: panel findings. Pediatrics. 2008;121(Suppl 3):S172–91.
55. Malina B, Bar-Or. Growth, maturation and physical activity. 2nd ed. Champaign, IL: Human Kinetics; 2004.
56. Pigeon P, Oliver I, Charlet JP, Rochiccioli P. Intensive dance practice. Repercussions on growth and puberty. Am J Sports Med. 1997;25(2):243–7.
57. Brooks-Gunn J, Warren MP. The effects of delayed menarche in different contexts: dance and nondance students. J Youth Adolesc. 1985;14(4):285–300.
58. Rozzi SL, Lephart SM, Gear WS, Fu FH. Knee joint laxity and neuromuscular characteristics of male and female soccer and basketball players. Am J Sports Med. 1999;27(3):312–9.
59. Rosene JM, Fogarty TD. Anterior tibial translation in collegiate athletes with normal anterior cruciate ligament integrity. J Athl Train. 1999;34(2):93–8.
60. Quatman CE, Ford KR, Myer GD, Paterno MV, Hewett TE. The effects of gender and pubertal status on generalized joint laxity in young athletes. J Sci Med Sport. 2008;11(3):257–63.
61. Myer GD, Ford KR, Paterno MV, Nick TG, Hewett TE. The effects of generalized joint laxity on risk of anterior cruciate ligament injury in young female athletes. Am J Sports Med. 2008;36(6):1073–80.
62. Stijak L, Kadija M, Djulejic V, Aksić M, Petronijević N, Marković B, et al. The influence of sex hormones on anterior cruciate ligament rupture: female study. Knee Surg Sports Traumatol Arthrosc. 2015;23(9):2742–9.
63. Hohmann E, Bryant AL, Livingstone E, Reaburn P, Tetsworth K, Imhoff A. Tibial acceleration profiles during the menstrual cycle in female athletes. Arch Orthop Trauma Surg. 2015;135(10):1419–27.

64. Heitz NA, Eisenman PA, Beck CL, Walker JA. Hormonal changes throughout the menstrual cycle and increased anterior cruciate ligament laxity in females. J Athl Train. 1999;34(2):144–9.
65. Wojtys EM, Huston LJ, Lindenfeld TN, Hewett TE, Greenfield ML. Association between the menstrual cycle and anterior cruciate ligament injuries in female athletes. Am J Sports Med. 1998;26(5):614–9.
66. Slauterbeck JR, Fuzie SF, Smith MP, Clark RJ, Xu KT, Starch DW, Hardy DM. The menstrual cycle, sex hormones, and anterior cruciate ligament injury. J Athl Train. 2002;37 (3):275–8.
67. Hewett TE, Myer GD. The mechanistic connection between the trunk, hip, knee, and anterior cruciate ligament injury. Exerc Sport Sci Rev. 2011;39(4):161–6.
68. Myer GD, Chu DA, Brent JL, Hewett TE. Trunk and hip control neuromuscular training for the prevention of knee joint injury. Clin Sports Med. 2008;27(3):425–8, ix.
69. Ford KMG, Hewett TE. Increased trunk motion in female athletes compared to males during single leg landing. Med Sci Sports Exerc. 2007;39(5):S70.
70. Hewett T, Snyder-Mackler L, Spindler KP. The drop-jump screening test: difference in lower limb control by gender and effect of neuromuscular training in female athletes. Am J Sports Med. 2007;35(1):145; author reply 146–7.
71. Hewett TE, Myer GD, Ford KR, Slauterbeck JR. Preparticipation physical examination using a box drop vertical jump test in young athletes: the effects of puberty and sex. Clin J Sport Med. 2006;16(4):298–304.
72. Ford KR, Shapiro R, Myer GD, Van Den Bogert AJ, Hewett TE. Longitudinal sex differences during landing in knee abduction in young athletes. Med Sci Sports Exerc. 2010;42 (10):1923–31.
73. Quatman-Yates CC, Myer GD, Ford KR, Hewett TE. A longitudinal evaluation of maturational effects on lower extremity strength in female adolescent athletes. Pediatr Phys Ther. 2013 Fall;25(3):271–6.
74. Zebis MK, Andersen LL, Brandt M, Myklebust G, Bencke J, Lauridsen HB, et al. Effects of evidence-based prevention training on neuromuscular and biomechanical risk factors for ACL injury in adolescent female athletes: a randomised controlled trial. Br J Sports Med. 2016;50 (9):552–7.
75. Hewett TE, Lindenfeld TN, Riccobene JV, Noyes FR. The effect of neuromuscular training on the incidence of knee injury in female athletes. A prospective study. Am J Sports Med. 1999;27(6):699–706.
76. Myklebust G, Engebretsen L, Braekken IH, Skjolberg A, Olsen OE, Bahr R. Prevention of anterior cruciate ligament injuries in female team handball players: a prospective intervention study over three seasons. Clin J Sport Med. 2003;13(2):71–8.
77. Gilchrist J, Mandelbaum BR, Melancon H, Ryan GW, Silvers HJ, Griffin LY, et al. A randomized controlled trial to prevent noncontact anterior cruciate ligament injury in female collegiate soccer players. Am J Sports Med. 2008;36(8):1476–83.
78. Myer GD, Ford KR, Brent JL, Hewett TE. Differential neuromuscular training effects on ACL injury risk factors in"high-risk" versus "low-risk" athletes. BMC Musculoskelet Disord. 2007;8(8):39.
79. Myer GD, Ford KR, Palumbo JP, Hewett TE. Neuromuscular training improves performance and lower-extremity biomechanics in female athletes. J Strength Cond Res. 2005;19(1):51–60.
80. Myer GD, Ford KR, Brent JL, Hewett TE. The effects of plyometric versus dynamic balance training on power, balance and landing force in female athletes. J Strength Cond Res. 2006;20 (2):345–53.
81. Myer GD, Ford KR, McLean SG, Hewett TE. The effects of plyometric versus dynamic stabilization and balance training on lower extremity biomechanics. Am J Sports Med. 2006;34(3):445–55.

82. Myer GD, Stroube BW, DiCesare CA, Brent JL, Ford KR, Heidt RS Jr, Hewett TE. Augmented feedback supports skill transfer and reduces high-risk injury landing mechanics: a double-blind, randomized controlled laboratory study. Am J Sports Med. 2013;41(3):669–77.
83. Myer GD, Sugimoto D, Thomas S, Hewett TE. The influence of age on the effectiveness of neuromuscular training to reduce anterior cruciate ligament injury in female athletes: a meta-analysis. Am J Sports Med. 2013;41(1):203–15.
84. Allen N, Nevill AM, Brooks JH, Koutedakis Y, Wyon MA. The effect of a comprehensive injury audit program on injury incidence in ballet: a 3-year prospective study. Clin J Sport Med. 2013;23(5):373–8.
85. Amorim T, Wyon M, Maia J, Machado JC, Marques F, Metsios GS, et al. Prevalence of low bone mineral density in female dancers. Sports Med. 2015;45(2):257–68.
86. Bailey DA, McKay HA, Mirwald RL, Crocker PR, Faulkner RA. A six-year longitudinal study of the relationship of physical activity to bone mineral accrual in growing children: the university of Saskatchewan bone mineral accrual study. J Bone Miner Res. 1999;14 (10):1672–9.
87. Gunter KB, Almstedt HC, Janz KF. Physical activity in childhood may be the key to optimizing lifespan skeletal health. Exerc Sport Sci Rev. 2012;40(1):13–21.
88. Nattiv A, Kennedy G, Barrack MT, Abdelkerim A, Goolsby MA, Arends JC, et al. Correlation of MRI grading of bone stress injuries with clinical risk factors and return to play: a 5-year prospective study in collegiate track and field athletes. Am J Sports Med. 2013;41 (8):1930–41.
89. Bass S, Pearce G, Bradney M, Hendrich E, Delmas PD, Harding A, Seeman E. Exercise before puberty may confer residual benefits in bone density in adulthood: studies in active prepubertal and retired female gymnasts. J Bone Miner Res. 1998;13(3):500–7.
90. Morris FL, Naughton GA, Gibbs JL, Carlson JS, Wark JD. Prospective ten-month exercise intervention in premenarcheal girls: positive effects on bone and lean mass. J Bone Miner Res. 1997;12(9):1453–62.
91. Heinonen A, Sievanen H, Kannus P, Oja P, Pasanen M, Vuori I. High-impact exercise and bones of growing girls: a 9-month controlled trial. Osteoporos Int. 2000;11(12):1010–7.
92. Wulff H. BMD in elite female triathletes is related to isokinetic peak torque without any association to sex hormone concentrations. J Sports Med Phys Fitness. 2012;52(5):489–500.
93. To WW, Wong MW, Lam IY. Bone mineral density differences between adolescent dancers and non-exercising adolescent females. J Pediatr Adolesc Gynecol. 2005;18(5):337–42.
94. Benson JE, Geiger CJ, Eiserman PA, Wardlaw GM. Relationship between nutrient intake, body mass index, menstrual function, and ballet injury. J Am Diet Assoc. 1989;89(1):58–63.
95. Smith JJ, Eather N, Morgan PJ, Plotnikoff RC, Faigenbaum AD, Lubans DR. The health benefits of muscular fitness for children and adolescents: a systematic review and meta-analysis. Sports Med. 2014;44(9):1209–23.
96. Liederbach M, Dilgen FE, Rose DJ. Incidence of anterior cruciate ligament injuries among elite ballet and modern dancers: a 5-year prospective study. Am J Sports Med. 2008;36 (9):1779–88.
97. Liederbach M, Kremenic IJ, Orishimo KF, Pappas E, Hagins M. Comparison of landing biomechanics between male and female dancers and athletes, part 2: influence of fatigue and implications for anterior cruciate ligament injury. Am J Sports Med. 2014;42(5):1089–95.

Chapter 6
Spine Conditions in the Young Dancer

Joana L. Fraser, MBChB, BSc

Pertinent Definitions

Apophysitis: Irritation and inflammation of the apophysis, a secondary ossification center which acts as an insertion site for a tendon.
Hyperlordosis: Excessive inward curvature, or arch, of the low back.
Kyphosis: Outward curvature of the spine, causing hunching of the back.
Pars interarticularis: Part of the vertebra found between the inferior and superior articular processes of the facet joint.
Spondylolysis: Bony defect or fracture in the pars interarticularis of the vertebral arch in the spinal column.
Spondylolisthesis: Forward displacement of a vertebral bone in relation to the natural curve of the spine, most commonly due to a fracture and most often at the fifth lumbar vertebrae.
Scoliosis: Abnormal lateral curvature of the spine.

Introduction

Back pain is a common complaint in the young dancer; the overall prevalence of back pain in children and adolescents is reported to be anywhere from 12 to 50% [1]. Studies of pre-professional and professional dancers have found that between

J.L. Fraser, MBChB, BSc (✉)
Division of Sports Medicine, Department of Orthopedics, Boston Children's Hospital, 319 Longwood Avenue, Boston, MA 02115, USA
e-mail: Joana.fraser@childrens.harvard.edu

R. Solomon et al. (eds.), *Prevention of Injuries in the Young Dancer*, Contemporary Pediatric and Adolescent Sports Medicine,
DOI 10.1007/978-3-319-55047-3_6

9.4 and 23% of injuries occur in the back [2–4]. Age of the dancer is also important to keep in mind, as age ≥ 12 years has been shown to be associated with an increased risk of spine injuries compared to even younger dancers [5].

It is perhaps not surprising that many dancers suffer from back pain. Classical training aims for both excessive external rotation at the hip joint—"turnout"—and high extension of the leg(s) above 90°. These movements require significant contribution from the spine, especially in all movements of the leg to the rear, such as with arabesque. Deficiencies in strength or incorrect technique can all too quickly lead to tension and stress on the spine and resultant pain and injury. Musculoskeletal factors such as postural lordosis, tight extensor musculature, and weak abdominal musculature are often contributors to back problems.

In this chapter several of the most common causes of back pain in the young dancer will be discussed. In addition, the specific management of scoliosis will be reviewed.

Dance Technique in Relation to Back Pain

Dance technique is an important factor to consider when assessing the young dancer with back pain. Lack of mobility in the iliofemoral ligament (or Y ligament) at the anterior hip joint can restrict both hyperextension and external rotation, for which the dancer may try to compensate by lifting the hip to the side [6], thereby increasing stress on the low back. Similarly, if the dancer attempts to keep the back in too upright a position, this will limit anterior tilt of the pelvis as the leg is raised to the rear, again placing increased load on the low back. It has been estimated that almost half of cases of low back pain in dancers are related to lifting the hip in arabesque, while another 25% are due to forcefully trying the raise the leg above 90° while keeping the back too straight [6].

Initial Evaluation of Low Back Pain in the Dancer

The initial evaluation of any musculoskeletal complaint should focus on history. Duration of symptoms, any inciting factors, and injury and pain descriptors are important to elucidate. These include intensity, character, severity, location, exacerbating and relieving factors, and any radiation of the pain. In the female athlete menstrual history and nutritional status should also be assessed, as abnormalities involving these factors increase the risk for stress fracture.

Evaluation should also focus on alignment. With respect to the spine, hyperlordosis may result from dancers trying to force turn out by "rolling in" or pronating the foot, or by flexing the knee when attempting to turn out the foot. Weak abdominal muscles can also contribute to hyperlordosis [7]. While a certain amount of hyperlordosis is necessary for the positions required of the young dancer, excessive training, poor technique, muscle imbalance, or underlying musculoskeletal defects can increase the risk of back injury.

During the evaluation, "red flag" symptoms that may indicate underlying serious systemic or musculoskeletal etiology should be sought. These include unintentional weight loss, fevers, or night sweats, which can indicate infection or malignancy. Severe, recalcitrant pain should also heighten the awareness of these possibilities. Neurological deficits including radicular pain, bowel or bladder dysfunction, or new onset scoliosis or kyphosis should prompt urgent evaluation.

Spondylolysis and Spondylolisthesis

Spondylolysis is a bony defect in the pars interarticularis of the vertebral arch, while spondylolisthesis is the forward translation of one vertebra on another and can occur in cases of bilateral defects. The pars are bony bridges connecting the upper with the lower facet joints of the vertebrae (Figs. 6.1 and 6.2). The incidence of this defect in the general population is around 6% [8, 9], whereas there is a fourfold increase in these conditions in dancers [7]. They occur more frequently in females, and this may be due to the fact that females tend to begin their training earlier than males, prior to the union of the pars interarticularis [10]. In the pediatric dance population a 4.5% frequency of spondylolysis was seen in a group of injured dancers [2], and all of these injuries were seen in patients ≥ 12 years old [2].

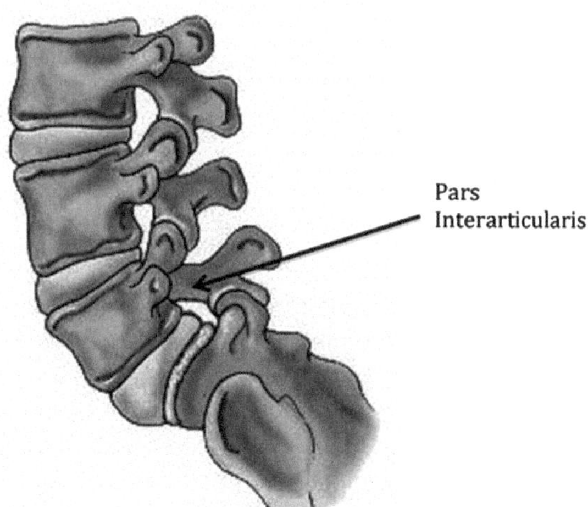

Fig. 6.1 Anatomy of vertebral body showing location of pars interarticularis. Reprinted from D'Hemecourt [11]

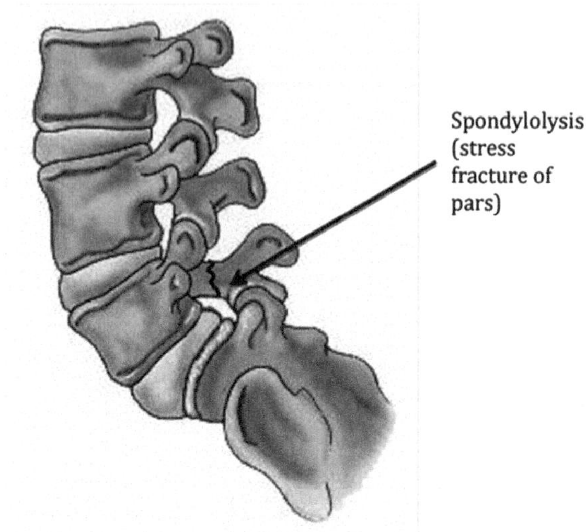

Fig. 6.2 Fracture of pars interarticularis in spondylolysis. Reprinted from D'Hemecourt [11]

The defect can either be asymptomatic or associated with significant low back pain. The hyperlordosis practiced by dancers with either weak abdominal muscles, tight thoracolumbar fascia, or incorrect technique increases the stress on the L5-S1 joint [12]. There are likely several other contributing risk factors, although ultimately symptomatic spondylosis is a condition of overuse of the spine. While there are certain hereditary risk factors, an increased prevalence is seen in individuals who participate in sports, especially those that place increased stress on the lower spine as a result of repeated extension and rotation, such as gymnastics, figure skating, and dance [13]. The majority of defects occur at the L5 level (85–95%), with the next most commonly affected level being L4 (5–15%) [14].

Physical Examination and Diagnosis

The most common complaint in patients suffering from symptomatic spondylolysis is low back pain. This is typically unilateral, although it can be bilateral and may radiate to the buttock, around to the lateral aspect of the hip, or into the proximal lower limb. The onset of pain may be acute or gradual and is typically worsened after prolonged exertion. Activities that involve lumbar hyperextension, particularly while standing on one foot as in arabesque, are often known to exacerbate pain.

Tenderness to palpation is not always present. If significant spondylolisthesis is present, a step-off may be palpated. The most significant finding on examination is pain reproduced by the one-legged extension maneuver. During this test the patient stands on one leg and is directed by the examiner to lean backward in an attempt to recreate the pain (Fig. 6.3).

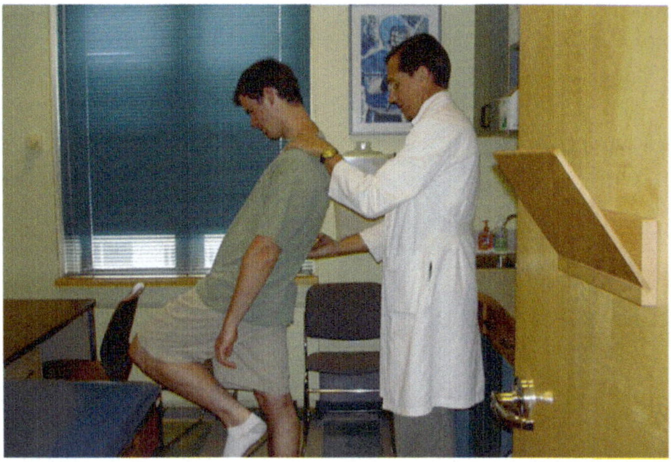

Fig. 6.3 Single-leg extension known as the "stork test" can reproduce the pain in spondylolysis. Reprinted from D'Hemecourt [11]

Radiographic and advanced imaging modalities assist in the diagnosis. Plain radiographs are helpful in ruling out underlying specific diagnoses and can also help to describe degenerative spine changes. Spondylolisthesis is often visible on plain X-ray [1]. However, only about 20% of pars defects can be seen on oblique view [14]. Advanced imaging modalities such as MRI and CT are more sensitive in picking up the pars defect and can also detect other musculoskeletal causes of back pain. MRI is preferable over CT in the younger population, given its lack of radiation exposure. On MRI, the injury is visualized as bony edema, and in more advanced cases a distinct fracture line can often be seen (Fig. 6.4). In cases of spondylolisthesis, MRI will also determine the condition of the intervertebral disk at the affected level and evaluates for canal or foraminal stenosis that can result in neural compression [12] (Fig. 6.5).

Treatment

Treatment always begins with conservative measures, including modification of activity, rest, and physical therapy. Exercises should concentrate on relieving spasm and tightness in the hip flexors, quadriceps, and hamstrings, as well as avoiding any extension stresses on the spine. Core strengthening of the abdominal, trunk, and multifidus muscles is also essential. The use of nonsteroidal anti-inflammatory drugs (NSAIDs) should be discouraged due to their propensity to slow down bony healing [8].

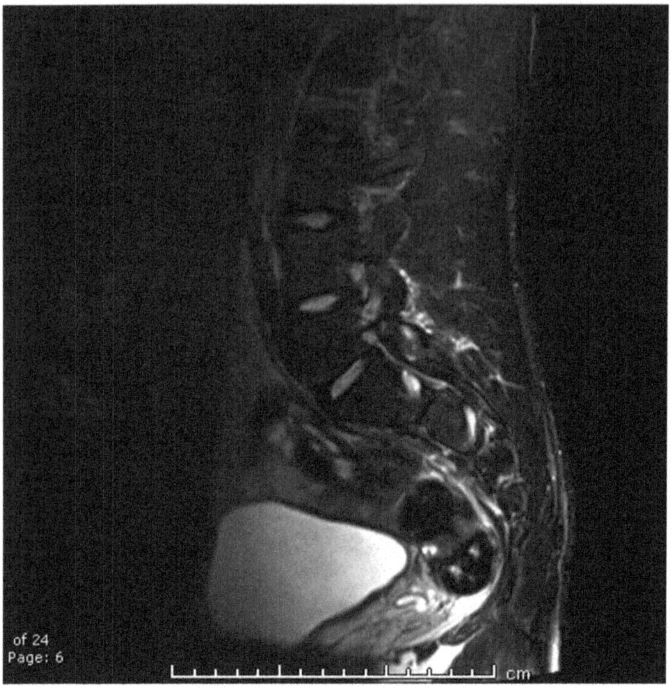

Fig. 6.4 Edema of the pars interarticularis on T2-weighted MRI indicating stress reaction of the bone

Bracing treatment is required in the initial period, until the patient becomes pain-free. The effect of bracing unloads the posterior elements of the spine and reduces the amount of shear stress across the pars [12]. Patients with spondylolisthesis should be followed clinically and with radiographs every 6–12 months to monitor for progression of the slip.

Management of spondylolysis is often done clinically, with the resolution of pain and ability to return to prior activities indicative of successful healing. Repeated imaging, either with MRI or CT, may be indicated in patients who do not have the expected course of symptomatic improvement. Healing may not always produce a solid bony union, but the patient will often become pain-free as a result of fibrous healing. Minimum treatment time in the brace of six weeks is often needed, after which the patient can be progressed slowly back to dance activity if pain-free. This is often started initially in the brace and advanced as guided by symptoms.

Persistent pain after a six-month period of nonoperative management should be considered for surgical intervention [12]. Approximately 9–15% of cases of spondylolysis will undergo surgery [8]. Other indications for surgical treatment include the development of neurological deficits and segmental spine instability.

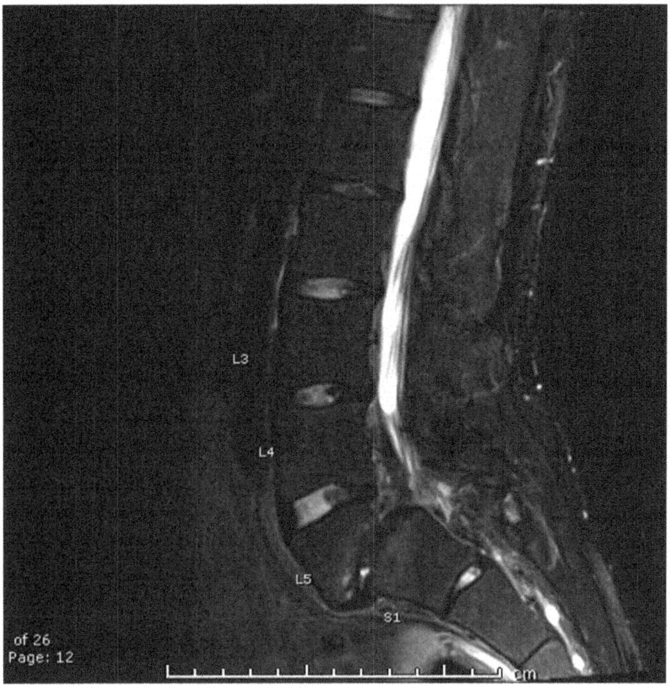

Fig. 6.5 Anterior slippage of L5 on S1 vertebrae in spondylolisthesis

Scheuermann's Kyphosis (Juvenile Kyphosis)

Scheuermann's kyphosis is a rigid kyphotic deformity of the thoracic or thoracolumbar spine occurring in adolescents [15]. It is an abnormality of the vertebral epiphyseal growth plates. Typically, it involves anterior wedging of three consecutive vertebral bodies of at least 5° each. The etiology of this condition is multifactorial and includes genetic factors, repetitive microtrauma, necrosis ring apophysis, and tight hamstrings. The incidence is reported as 1–8%, affecting males and females equally [15]. A severe roundback deformity may also be seen in the adolescents. This is less of a fixed deformity than a secondary reaction to muscular imbalances and poor posture [16]. The characteristic findings on imaging noted below will not be seen in this condition.

Physical Examination and Diagnosis

The most common complaint is poor posture or cosmetic deformity. Hamstring tightness and flattening of the thoracolumbar spine are often seen. In 80% of patients, the disease is asymptomatic [15]. When pain is present it is often exacerbated by forward flexion and located in the thoracic area over the kyphotic deformity. The onset of pain is usually gradual exacerbated by activity, and improves with rest. In true Scheuermann's kyphosis the curvature is not correctable by hyperextension or lying supine.

Imaging

On plain radiographic imaging, a thoracic kyphosis of greater than 35° is diagnostic, with the apex commonly seen between T7 and T9 [1]. Other features that may be noted are as follows: irregular upper and lower endplates with Schmorl's nodes, disk-height loss, and associated apophyseal ring fractures (Figs. 6.6 and 6.7).

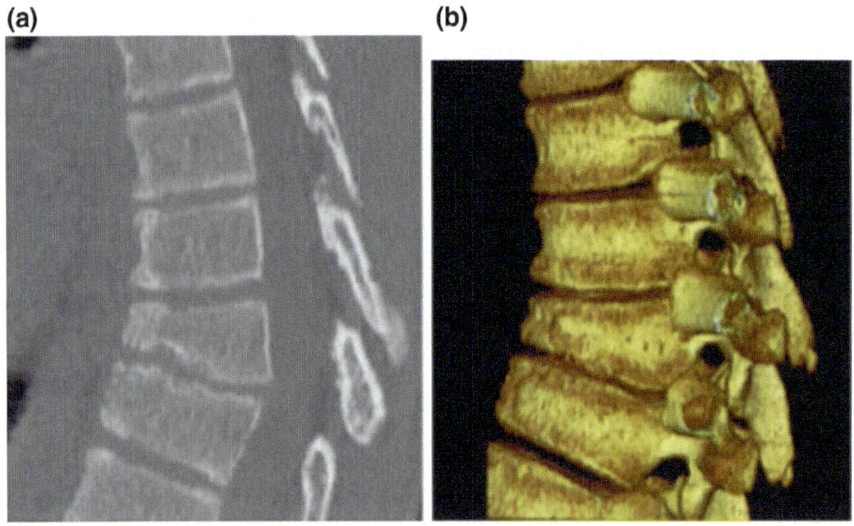

Fig. 6.6 Scheuermann's kyphosis in a 15-year-old boy. **a** Sagittal 2D CT reconstruction image demonstrates midthoracic kyphosis with anterior wedging of at least three consecutive vertebrae with presence of Schmorl nodes. **b** Sagittal 3D CT reconstruction image demonstrates midthoracic kyphosis with anterior wedging of at least 3 consecutive vertebrae and the presence of Schmorl nodes. Republished with permission of Rodriguez and Poussaint [1]

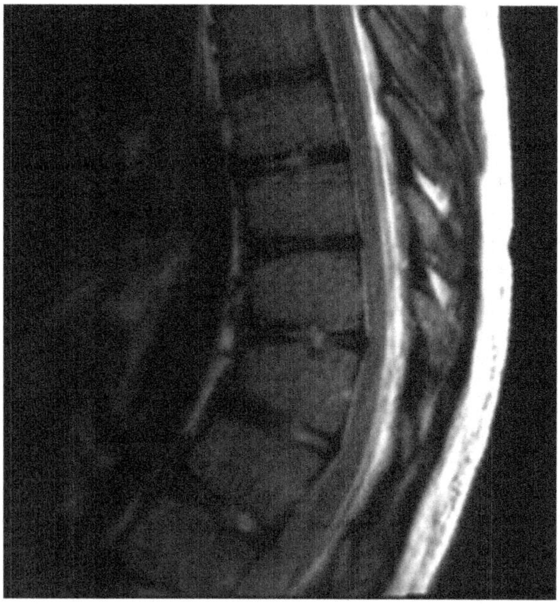

Fig. 6.7 Scheuermann's kyphosis in a 14-year-old boy. Sagittal T2-weighted image demonstrates thoracic kyphosis with mild anterior wedging of the T10–T12 vertebral bodies, slight disk space irregularity, and Schmorl nodes. Minimal annular bulges slightly indent the ventral aspect of the thecal sac. Republished with permission of Rodriguez and Poussaint [1]

Treatment

Treatment should entail postural exercises as well as trunk extensor strengthening and pectoralis stretching. Hamstring tightness should be addressed, as one biomechanical theory presumes that tight hamstrings prevent anterior pelvic tilt on forward bending, transmitting the bending stresses to the thoracic spine [16].

When the kyphotic curve reaches 60°, thoraco-lumbo-sacral orthosis (TLSO) bracing is instituted [17]. The kyphotic curve does not then tend to progress further, and bracing with a gradual return to activities can help to alleviate the pain during exercise.

Sacroiliac (SI) Dysfunction

The function of the SI joint(s) is to transfer forces from the legs and pelvis to the trunk. This requires rotational motion of the posterior hemipelvis [14]. As the pelvis develops from childhood through puberty, this joint transitions from flat and hypermobile to being rougher, more undulated, and less mobile.

Due to the requirement for turnout in the dancer, there is an increased amount of stress translated across the pelvis. SI dysfunction is often multifactorial, resulting from a combination of asymmetry in strength and flexibility between sides. For example, a tight psoas muscle will result in relative downward and anterior deviation of the pelvis on the affected side. This stresses the SI joint and can also load and tighten the contralateral iliotibial (IT) band.

Physical Examination and Diagnosis

SI joint pain is typically located over the area of the joint itself and may radiate into the buttocks, groin, or posterior thigh. Pain is usually exacerbated by jumping, hyperextension, and abduction positions, especially if accompanied by forced turnout.

Physical examination may reveal tenderness to palpation at the site of the SI joints. Weakness or tightness in the psoas and/or tightness in the ITB with a positive Ober's test (often on the contralateral side) may also be present. Specific SI joint loading maneuvers may reproduce the pain. These include thigh thrust, sacral distraction, sacral compression, and iliac torque testing. The flexion-abduction-external rotation, or FABER test, can also be used to assess hip joint or SI pathology. This is performed with the dancer lying supine with the leg being tested placed in a "figure 4" position. The examiner then applies force to the bent knee and a positive test occurs when the dancer's pain is reproduced or range of motion is restricted.

Imaging

Imaging with plain films of the pelvis is helpful to evaluate the bony morphology of the hip and pelvis complex, but the SI joints almost always appear normal. MRI can also be used, which may show inflammation at the SI joints and help to evaluate for other potential causes of pain, such as stress injuries of the pelvis or lumbar disk pathology.

Treatment

Treatment involves a biomechanical evaluation to identify causative and aggravating factors. Attention should be focused on ensuring symmetrical mobility of the hip flexors and ITB. Activation of the transverse abdominal stabilizing muscles (transverse abdominus, lower portions of the internal oblique) has been shown to have a stabilizing effect on the SI joint [18].

For acute pain, a period of rest, NSAIDs, and physical therapy to address these factors is helpful. Manual therapy can also help to mobilize the joint. In recalcitrant cases, cortisone injection into the SI joints can also be considered.

Spinous Process Apophysitis

Skeletally immature dancers differ from mature dancers because of their open growth plates (physes). The physes are at risk of injury either during an acute traumatic event or as a result of repeated stress, in which case the pain may present more insidiously. An apophysitis occurs when a tuberosity is stressed in traction [19]. Due to the different rates of maturation of the male and female skeletons, male athletes tend to present with physical injuries one to two years later than female athletes. In addition, dancers may show delayed skeletal maturity and therefore may present at a later age than athletes in other sports.

Physical Examination and Diagnosis

Spinous process apophysitis may mimic the symptoms of spondylolysis. Presentation often involves diffuse low back pain reproduced with hyperextension maneuvers, but it is not localized to one side or the other. Tenderness to palpation on the spinous process may be present. Resisted extension from a flexed position may cause pain, as this results in traction stress on the dorsal spinous process [19]. Radiographs are usually unremarkable. Bone or SPECT scans may be required to differentiate spinous process apophysitis from spondylolysis [19].

Treatment

Treatment involves avoiding hyperextension, and bracing can often be helpful. A time period of four to six weeks of rest and immobilization is usually sufficient to allow full return to activities.

Discogenic Back Pain

The intervertebral disks primarily act as shock absorbers in the spine. They are composed of a central soft, gelatinous ring called the nucleus pulposus and an outer ring of annulus fibrosus (Fig. 6.8). This outer ring is heavily infused with pain fibers.

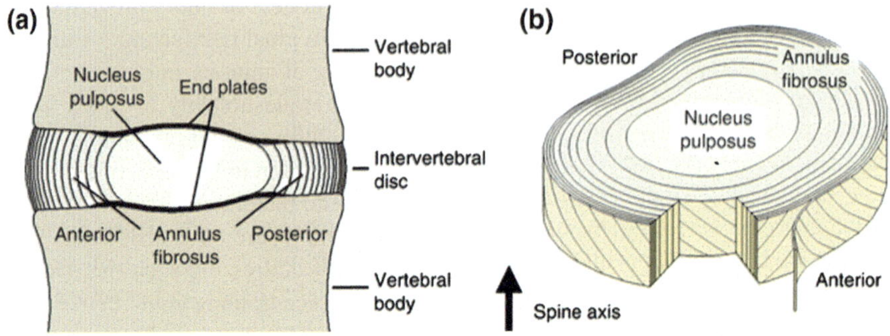

Fig. 6.8 Diagrammatic representation of the intervertebral disk. Reprinted from Cortes [20]

Discogenic back pain results when the disk degenerates and there is tearing and fissuring of the annulus fibrosis. This type of pain is seen more frequently in male than female dancers, due to the demands of lifting. With more advanced degeneration whereby herniated elements of the disk impinge on exiting nerve roots, the patient will describe shooting pains in the lower limb(s) along the distribution of the affected nerve. Discogenic pain is usually in the lumbar area, may be central, unilateral, or bilateral, and (barring nerve impingement) is dull in character. It is exacerbated by flexion, sitting, rotation, axial loading, and/or Valsalva maneuvers. Onset may be acute or insidious.

Physical Examination and Diagnosis

On examination, a hesitant, stiff gait may be noted. Pain is increased with forward flexion movements of the spine, which load the intervertebral disk and anterior column; therefore, pain with these movements can indicate disk pathology. A straight leg raise test is performed with the patient lying supine, whereby the examiner raises the patient's leg with the knee extended (Fig. 6.9). Pain either in the back or radiating down the leg suggests disk herniation or nerve root impingement [15]. Sensory and motor functions should also be assessed. When sacral nerve root involvement is suspected, it may be necessary to test anal sphincter tone.

Imaging

Plain radiographs are helpful for looking at alignment of the spine. In cases of severe or recalcitrant pain, or nerve root impingement signs or symptoms, MRI can be performed. This modality has the benefits of avoiding radiation exposure as well as better imaging of soft tissue structures and intervertebral disks, and assessing for bony edema in the acute reaction phase of a stress fracture, which at times is also on the differential.

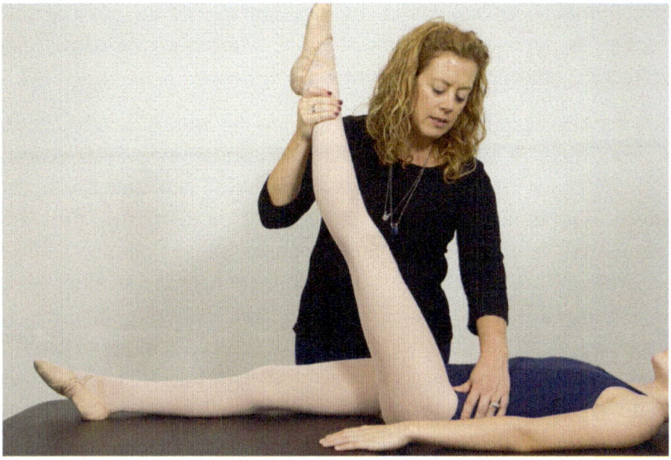

Fig. 6.9 Straight leg raise. Photograph courtesy of James Koepfler

Treatment

Most cases will resolve within 4–6 weeks of conservative treatment, which includes rest, NSAIDs, modification of physical activities, and physical therapy. In cases that do not resolve, more invasive measures such as epidural steroid injections or surgical discectomy can be considered.

Prevention efforts should focus on core strengthening, specifically of the transversus abdominus and multifidus. Changes in the recruitment of these local stabilizer muscles have been shown to occur in cases of low back pain, limiting their ability to stabilize the spine effectively [21]. Strengthening efforts should also target hip abductor and external rotators.

Scoliosis

Scoliosis is the most common spine disorder among children and adolescents, with an overall prevalence of 0.47–5.2% [22]. The defect involves both a side-to-side curvature and a rotational component, making it a three-dimensional deformity. There are two major groups of scoliosis: idiopathic and nonidiopathic. The diagnosis of idiopathic scoliosis is only made if nonidiopathic causes have been ruled out.

Nonidiopathic causes include the following:

I. Congenital scoliosis: caused by malformation of vertebrae. Examples of this are hemivertebra, unilateral bar, or block vertebra.
II. Neuromuscular scoliosis, caused by insufficiency of the active muscular stabilizers of the spine, is seen in disorders such as cerebral palsy, spina bifida, spinal muscular atrophy, or spinal cord injuries.

III. Mesenchymal scoliosis, caused by insufficiency of the passive stabilizers of the spine, is seen in disorders such as Marfan's syndrome, osteogenesis imperfection, and certain inflammatory diseases.

Idiopathic scoliosis is classified depending on the age of development. Infantile refers to development at the age of 0–3 years, juvenile at 4–10 years, and adolescent at 11–18 years. The adolescent variety (AIS) accounts for approximately 90% of cases of idiopathic scoliosis in children [22], and because of its high degree of prevalence it will be the focus of the remainder of this chapter.

The measurement used to determine the severity of the curvature in scoliosis is called the Cobb angle. This is measured on anterior–posterior standing radiographs and is the angle between the superior endplate of the vertebra at the proximal end of the curvature and the inferior endplate of the vertebra at the distal end of the curvature. The overall prevalence of AIS is anywhere from 0.35 to 13%, depending on the threshold of the Cobb angle used [23]. Typically, scoliosis is defined as a lateral spinal curvature with a Cobb angle of 10° or more. For curves of <10° there is equal incidence between sexes. The female-to-male ratio increases with the severity of the curve. The ratio rises to 1.4:1.0 for curves between 11° and 20°, and up to 7.2:1.0 for curves requiring treatment [24]. Females have up to a 10-fold greater risk of curve progression, and therefore close monitoring is especially important. As curve magnitude increases with skeletal growth, the more skeletally immature a patient is, the greater the likelihood of curve progression. Patients with curves >20° at presentation and who are skeletally immature are at the greatest risk for curve progression [25].

Risk Factors for AIS

AIS has been found in up to 30% of nonprofessional and professional dancers [26–28]. Proposed reasons for increased incidence in dancers compared to the general population include a higher incidence of hypermobility in this population, delayed menarche, and low body mass index.

The relationship between delayed menarche and scoliosis is unclear. In one study of 75 female dancers an increased incidence of scoliosis was found in those with delayed menarche, defined as age 14 years or older (83% vs. 54%) [24], while other studies of young nonprofessional dancers did not find a relationship between the mean age of onset of menarche and the presence of scoliosis [26]. Similarly, dancers with scoliosis have been shown to have a higher prevalence of secondary amenorrhea than dancers without (44% vs. 31%) [27]. It is worth noting that hours of practice per week, age at beginning of dance training, and duration of dance practice have not been associated with the presence of scoliosis [26].

Physical Examination

Physical examination for scoliosis begins with inspection. Shoulder asymmetry with the patient standing may be noted. The key examination maneuver is the Adam's forward bend. During this test the patient stands and bends forward at the waist. The examiner then assesses for asymmetry of the back from behind and the side. If scoliosis is present there will be lateral curvature of the spine, producing a rib hump. The degree of curvature can be roughly quantified using a scoliometer. An angle of <5° is usually insignificant; however, a measurement of 5°–9° should be re-evaluated in 6 months. Any measurement over 10° requires radiographic evaluation.

Imaging

Radiographic evaluation for scoliosis should consist of a standing posterior–anterior (PA) and lateral radiograph of the whole spine, including the hip joints in a single 3-ft film. A low-dose system for scoliosis imaging has recently been developed (EOS Imaging, Paris, France) which eliminates the need for two separate images by capturing frontal and sagittal views simultaneously and reducing the overall radiation dose [15] (Fig. 6.10).

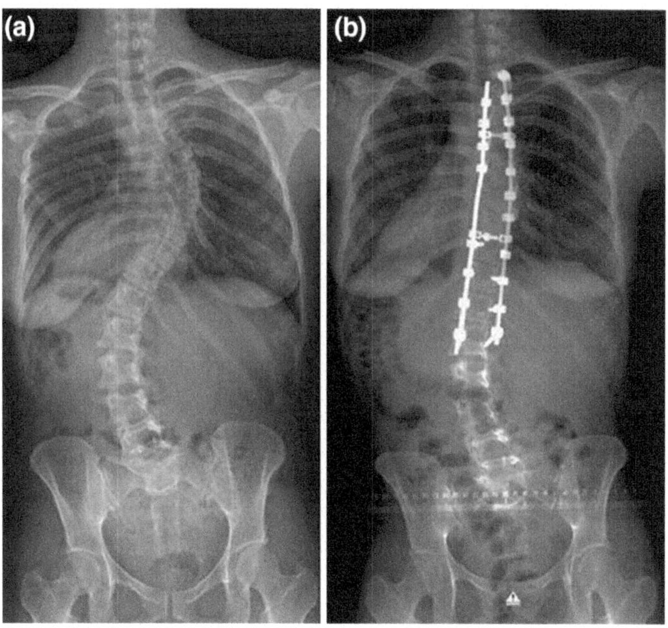

Fig. 6.10 Female with adolescent idiopathic scoliosis **a** pre- and **b** post-surgical correction with thoracolumbar anterior spinal fusion. Reprinted from Studer et al. [29]

Screening for Scoliosis

Screening for scoliosis has been a controversial issue. However, at this point the Scoliosis Research Society, the Pediatric Orthopedic Society of North America, the American Academy of Orthopedic Surgeons, and the American Academy of Pediatrics agree that girls should be screened twice, at 10 and 12 years of age, and boys should be screened once for the condition at 13 or 14 years of age [25].

Treatment

Observation is recommended for curves 25° or less, regardless of the stage of skeletal maturity. Close follow-up every 3–6 months of patients in this group is required for monitoring of curve progression. The frequency of follow-up should reflect the stage of both skeletal maturity and degree of curvature, with patients who are less mature and/or with greater curvatures requiring closer monitoring.

Bracing treatment is instituted for curves between 25° and 45° who are Risser 2 or less on the skeletal maturity scale (Fig. 6.11). The purpose of bracing is not to

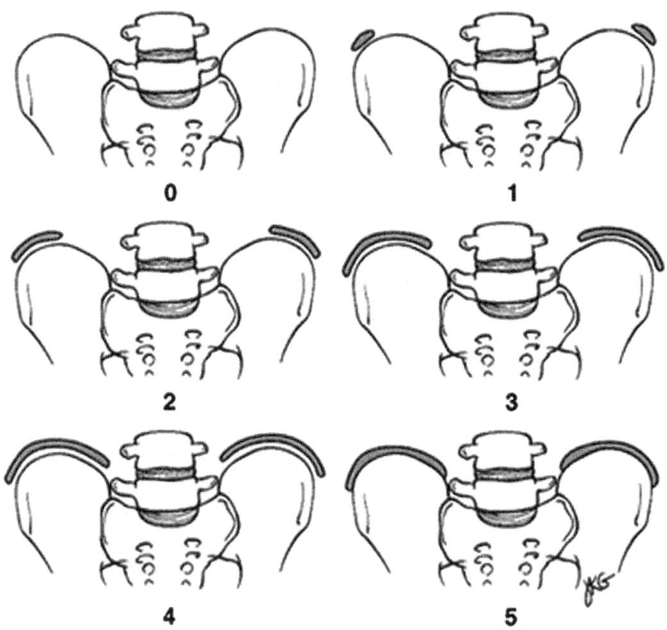

Fig. 6.11 Illustration shows the US Risser grading system. The US system comprises six grades. The US Risser 0 is defined as no ossification. The iliac wing is then divided into quarters, defining the first four grades (1, 2, 3, 4) of ossification of the apophysis (capping). The US Risser 5 begins when the ossified apophysis starts fusing to the wing at its posterior extremity. It continues during the whole process of apophysis fusion, which might take as much as 2 years. Reprinted from Kotwicki [30]

correct the curvature, but rather to prevent progression and to avoid the need for surgical correction.

The most common type of bracing used is the TLSO. The benefit of bracing has been shown to increase with longer hours of wear [31]. Patients should be counseled on the fact that their cosmetic deformity is unlikely to improve with bracing.

Surgical treatment is reserved for patients with curves >45° who are Risser 2 or less, or for curves >50° who are Risser 3 and greater [25]. This consists of fusion of the spine using instrumentation and often bone grafting. The exact details of the fusion will depend on curve magnitude, type, and skeletal maturity level.

Considerations for the Dancer with Scoliosis: Risk of Injury and Prevention Strategies

After identifying the dancer with scoliosis it is important to consider how this may affect their ability to dance and how it may impact their risk of injury. Joint hypermobility is seen most commonly in adolescents with scoliosis, in both males and females, with rates of up to 51% noted compared to just 19% in nondancers [32]. Given that joint hypermobility is a beneficial attribute for the dancer, this may explain some of the increases in prevalence of scoliosis seen in this population.

Scoliosis may predispose the dancer to an increased risk of dance-related injuries. While this risk seems to decrease with age, even by age 16 a dancer with scoliosis is still 1.2× more likely to have an injury than a dancer without scoliosis [26]. In particular, dancers with scoliosis are more likely to present with back injuries than their nonscoliotic peers [26]. Regarding the presence of other anatomic variations, knee varum, knee hyperextension, long-plantar planus foot type, and hallux valgus have been found to be significantly more common in a population of young female dancers with scoliosis than in dancers without this condition [26]. These underlying anatomic variations may increase the risk of lower extremity injuries or pain.

The term "functional scoliosis" is used to describe a curvature without an underlying structural or neurologic anomaly, and is therefore more easily correctable and important to identify. An example of this is the case of a limb length discrepancy. Limb length discrepancies of up to 1 cm are noted in 3–15% of the population [33]. It is important to detect this condition, as correction of the discrepancy results in partial or total regression of the spinal curvature in as little as two weeks [33].

Treating underlying muscle imbalances in the scoliotic dancer can help to improve posture, minimize deformity, and reduce pain. Preventative strategies for low back pain include concentrating on the lower abdominal and transverse abdominus muscles. After evaluation of the curvature in the scoliotic dancer, asymmetric strengthening of the obliques may be helpful, and the significance of scapular winging can be minimized with posterior shoulder strengthening.

Modalities such as gyrotonics and Pilates can be useful adjuncts when targeting these areas.

Conclusions

The causes of back pain in the young adolescent dancer are varied, but a careful history, physical examination, and evaluation of technique are often sufficient to determine the underlying diagnosis. Imaging is helpful to confirm the diagnosis and rule out other causes of pain. Treatment should be targeted to the principal cause, but in all cases technique must be evaluated and any deficiencies corrected in order to ensure full recover and minimize the risk of future injury. A broad range of modalities, including medications, physical therapy, and Pilates, are beneficial when treating the young dancer with back pain.

References

1. Rodriguez D, Pouissant T. Imaging of back pain in children. Am J Neuroradiol. 2010;31(5):787–802.
2. Yin AX, Sugimoto D, Martin DJ, Stracciolini A. Pediatric dance injuries: a cross-sectional epidemiological study. PM R. 2015;8(4):348–55.
3. Gamboa JM, Roberts L, Maring J, Fergus A. Injury patterns in elite preprofessional ballet dancers and the utility of screening programs to identify risk characteristics. J Orthop Sports Phys Ther. 2008;38(3):126–36.
4. Garrick JG, Requa RK. An analysis of epidemiological and financial outcome. Am J Sports Med. 1993;21(4):586–90.
5. Stracciolini A, Yin AX, Sugimoto D. Etiology and body area of injuries in young female dancers presenting to sports medicine clinic: a comparison by age group. Phys Sportmed. 2015;43(4):342–7.
6. Gelabert R. Dancers'spinal syndromes. J Orthop Sports Phys Ther. 1986;7(4):180–91.
7. Gottschlich LM, Young CC. Spine injuries in dancers. Curr Sports Med Rep. 2011;10(1):40–4.
8. Syrmou E, Tsitsopoulos PP, Marinopoulos D, Tsonidis C, Anagnostopoulos I, Tsitsopoulos PD. Spondylolysis: a review and reappraisal. Hippokratia. 2010;14(1):17–21.
9. Amato M, Totty WG, Gilula LA. Spondylolysis of the lumbar spine: demonstration of defects and laminal fragmentation. Radiology. 1984;153(3):627–9.
10. Shrader K. Biomechanical evaluation of the dancer. Orthop Phys Ther Clin North Am. 1996;5(4):455–75.
11. D'Hemercourt PA, Gould LE, Bottino NM. The young female athlete, spondylolysis, Contemporary pediatric and adolescent sports medicine series. Berlin: Springer; 2016. p. 87–99.
12. Tsirikos AI, Garrido EG. Spondylolysis and spondylolisthesis in children and adolescents. J Bone Joint Surg Br. 2010;92(6):751–9.
13. Omey ML, Micheli LJ, Gerbino PG. Idiopathic scoliosis and spondylolysis in the female athlete. Tips for treatment. Clin Orthop Relat Res. 2000;372:74–84.
14. Standaert CJ, Herring SA. Spondylolysis: a critical review. Br J Sports Med. 2000;34(6):415–22.

15. Dizdarevic I, Bishop M, Sgromolo N, Hammoud S, Atanda A. Approach to the pediatric athlete with back pain: more than just the pars. Phys Sportsmed. 2015;43(4):421–31.
16. Wenger DR, Frick SL. Scheuermann kyphosis. Spine (Phila Pa 1976). 1999;24(24):2630–9.
17. D'Hemecourt PA, Gerbino PG, Micheli LJ. Low back injuries in the young athlete. Sport Med Arthrosc Rev. 1996;4(2):122–31.
18. Richardson CA, Snijders CJ, Hides JA. The relation between the transversus abdominis muscles, sacroiliac joint mechanics, and low back pain. Spine (Phila Pa 1976). 2002;27(4):399–405.
19. Frush TJ, Lindenfeld TN. Peri-epiphyseal and overuse injuries in adolescent athletes. Sports Health. 2009;1(3):201–11.
20. Cortes DH. The intervertebral disc: overview of disc mechanics. Berlin: Springer; 2014.
21. Huxel Bliven KCH, Anderson BE. Core stability training for injury prevention. Sports Health. 2013;5(6):514–22.
22. Konieczny MR, Senyurt H, Krauspe R. Epidemiology of adolescent idiopathic scoliosis. J Child Orthop. 2013;7(1):3–9.
23. Kenanidis EI, Potoupnis ME, Papavasiliou KA, Sayegh FE, Kapetanos GA. Adolescent idiopathic scoliosis in athletes: is there a connection? Phys Sportsmed. 2010;38(2):165–70.
24. Rogala E, Drummond D, Gurr J. Scoliosis: incidence and natural history. A prospective epidemiological study. J Bone Joint Surg Am. 1978;60(2):173–6.
25. El-Hawary R, Chukwunyerenwa C. Update on evaluation and treatment of scoliosis. Pediatr Clin North Am. 2014;61(6):1223–41.
26. Steinberg N, Hershkovitz I, Peleg S, Dar G, Masharawi Y, Zeev A, et al. Morphological characteristics of the young scoliotic dancer. Phys Ther Sport. 2013;14(4):213–20.
27. Warren M, Brooks-Gunn J, Hamilton L, Warren L, Hamilton W. Scoliosis and fractures in young ballet dancers. Relation to delayed menarche and secondary amenorrhea. N Engl J Med. 1986;314(21):1348–53.
28. Longworth B, Fary R, Hopper D. Prevalence and predictors of adolescent idiopathic scoliosis in adolescent ballet dancers. Arch Phys Med Rehabil. 2014;95(9):1725–30.
29. Studer D, Awais A, Williams N, Antoniou G, Eardley-Harris N, Cundy P. Selective fusion in adolescent idiopathic scoliosis: a radiographic evaluation of risk factors for imbalance. J Child Orthop. 2015;9(2):153–60.
30. Kotwicki T. Improved accuracy in Risser sign grading with lateral spine radiography. Eur Spine J. 2008;17(12):1676–85 (With permission of Springer).
31. Weinstein SL, Dolan LA, Wright JG, Dobbs MB. Effects of bracing in adolescents with idiopathic scoliosis. N Engl J Med. 2013;369(16):1512–21.
32. Czaprowski D, Kotwicki T, Pawłowska P, Stoliński L. Joint hypermobility in children with idiopathic scoliosis: SOSORT award 2011 winner. Scoliosis. 2011;6:22.
33. Raczkowski JW, Daniszewska B, Zolynski K. Functional scoliosis caused by leg length discrepancy. Arch Med Sci. 2010;6(3):393–8.

Chapter 7
Hip Injuries in the Young Dancer

Emily Niu, MD and Mininder S. Kocher, MD, MPH

Pertinent Definitions

Abduction: The movement of the limb away from the median plane of the body, for example, a side kick.
Acetabulum: The "socket" of the hip, into which the femoral head fits.
Adduction: The movement of the limb toward the median plane of the body, for example, crossed legs.
Anterior inferior iliac spine (*AIIS*): A bony eminence on the anterior inferior aspect of the ilium.
Apophysis: A growth plate near the insertion of a tendon, making it susceptible to injury due to the high tension of the tendons; unlike a physis, an apophysis does not contribute to the length of the bone.
Cam impingement: Hip impingement caused by excess bone along the upper surface of the femoral head and neck.
Chondral: Articular cartilage.
Coxa valga: An increased angle between the head and neck of the femur (normal 135°).
Extra-articular: Outside of the joint; in this context, pertaining to the capsule, ligaments, muscles and tendons, and bony structures surrounding the hip joint.

E. Niu, MD (✉)
Division of Sports Medicine, Boston Children's Hospital,
319 Longwood Avenue, Boston, MA 02115, USA
e-mail: emily.niu@childrens.harvard.edu; niumeister@gmail.com

M.S. Kocher, MD, MPH
Division of Sports Medicine, Department of Orthopaedic Surgery,
Boston Children's Hospital, 300 Longwood Avenue, Hunnewell 2,
BCH 3220, Boston, MA 02115, USA
e-mail: mininder.kocher@childrens.harvard.edu

R. Solomon et al. (eds.), *Prevention of Injuries in the Young Dancer*,
Contemporary Pediatric and Adolescent Sports Medicine,
DOI 10.1007/978-3-319-55047-3_7

Femoral anteversion: The femoral head and neck are anteriorly directed with respect to the axis of the thigh bone (femur); this manifests as inward twisting of the femur and relative inward turning of the knees and feet ("pigeon-toed" appearance: see Fig. 7.1b).
Femoral head: The "ball" of the hip; the highest portion of the femur.
Femoral retroversion: The femoral head and neck are posteriorly directed with respect to the axis of the femur; this manifests as outward twisting of the femur and relative outward turning of the knees and feet (see Fig. 7.1c).
Femoroacetabular impingement (FAI): Increased coverage of the femoral head by the acetabulum; see pincer and cam impingement.
Hip capsule: A membranous envelope of tissue that surrounds the hip joint, acting as a seal for the joint space.
Hip dysplasia: Inadequate coverage of the femoral head by the acetabulum.

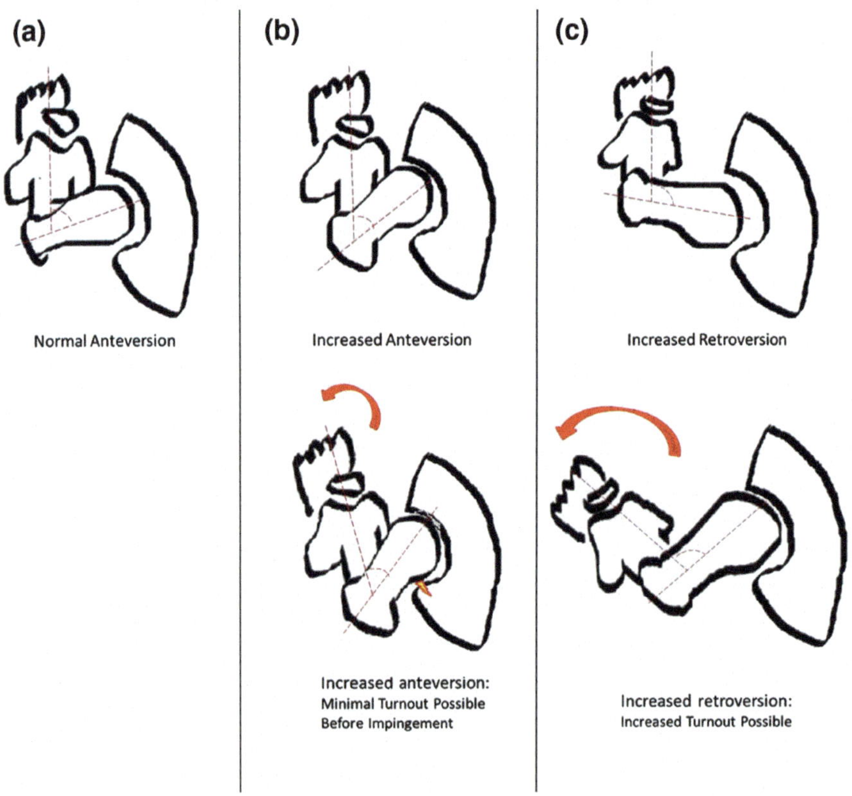

Fig. 7.1 Femoral version as it affects turnout of the feet. **a** Normal anteversion of the femoral neck, demonstrating relationship to the distal femur (knee) with the foot pointed straight ahead. **b** Increased anteversion of the femoral neck with the foot initially pointed straight ahead, demonstrating impingement at the hip as the hip externally rotates. **c** Increased retroversion of the femoral neck with the foot initially pointed straight ahead, demonstrating increased ability to externally rotate at the hip without impingement and thus ability to achieve greater turnout

Intra-articular: Inside the joint; in this context, pertaining to the bony structure of the femoral head and acetabulum and their articulation with each other, cartilage, and labrum of the hip joint.
Labrum: Horseshoe-shaped ring of connective tissue that rims the acetabulum; acts like a rubber seal to increase the stability of the hip joint.
Ligament: A band of fibrous connective tissue that connects two bones, when crossing a joint can contribute to the stability of the joint.
Pincer impingement: Hip impingement caused by excess growth of the upper rim of the acetabulum.
Sub-spine impingement: Occurs when the AIIS contacts the femoral neck during extreme hip flexion.
Tendon: a cord of strong fibrous collagen tissue attaching a muscle to a bone.
Version: The relation of the femoral head and neck with respect to the axis of the femur; see: femoral anteversion, retroversion.

Introduction

It has been said that the feet are the end goal in a dancer; however, the art begins with turn out of the hips. As such, the dancer's hip is unique in the extreme range of motion required of it and the subsequent stresses placed on the hip and its surrounding structures. These stresses can have a particularly pernicious effect on young dancers, due to their ongoing growth and development and the potential for exposure to ill-conceived methods of training. Appropriate prevention, diagnosis, and treatment of common hip injuries are important to help the young dancer return to dance, and more importantly prevent further injury.

Epidemiology

Dance training is often begun at an early age, and time spent in training increases considerably during adolescence, placing increased stress on the developing hip. It is estimated that 35% of adolescent girls participate in some form of dance [1]. Hip injuries have been reported to comprise from 7 to 50% of injuries in dancers [2–4]. This can have long-term consequences, as hip pain is nearly three times more common in retired ballet dancers than in non-dancers [5]. Years of dancing may also contribute to the development of early osteoarthritis in dancers with chronic hip pain [6]. It is clear that hip pain and injuries affect a significant portion of dancers and can persist even after dance activities have ceased.

Risk Factors in Dancers

Not only are dancers required to achieve extremes in range of motion, they must also sustain flexibility and strength within these extremes. The young dancer may lack the neuromuscular control and strength required by such demands. Bennell et al. [7] compared 77 novice dancers ages 8–11 (average age 9.6 years) to similarly aged controls (non-dancers) and found that initially the dancers had significantly less strength in hip flexors, internal and external rotators, and adductors than the control group. At 1-year follow-up of the same two groups [8], the dancers had an interval preferential increase of strength in their hip external rotators, abductors, and adductors; all muscle groups that are targeted in their training. However, the selective strengthening of isolated muscle groups may lead to muscle imbalance and susceptibility to injury [9].

Some dancers may not possess the anatomic makeup required to achieve certain ballet positions, such as "perfect" (180°) turnout. Degree of turnout at the hip is determined by skeletal anatomy, hip capsule laxity, and muscle strength. The skeletal anatomy that dictates hip rotation is version, i.e., the relation of the femoral head and neck with respect to the axis of the femur. Increased retroversion is conducive to greater hip external rotation and ultimately increased turnout (Fig. 7.1). However, this angle is primarily predetermined by genetics and also changes during development [10]. Newborns have an average of 40° of femoral anteversion, which decreases by age 8 to the average adult value of 15° [10].

While some studies have shown that ballet dancers have increased turnout angles and hip external rotation compared to controls [4, 11, 12], these studies were done on advanced dancers and are unlikely to represent the young dancer population. Bennell et al. [7] examined the degree of hip external rotation in novice dancers compared to controls and found that the dancers had on average 5° less external rotation. Increased turnout and external rotation seen in more advanced dancers are likely due to a combination of training and selection.

A common technique used by less experienced dancer to achieve turnout is "screwing the knee." The feet are placed in 180° of turnout with the hips and knees flexed, and the rest of the body is then positioned to accommodate this alignment without moving the feet. This results in compensatory stress seen not only at the hips but also at the knees and lower back, which may predispose the dancer to injury [13].

Hip Anatomy

Skeletal Anatomy

The hip is typically described as a "ball and socket" joint, with the femoral head forming the ball and the acetabulum comprising the socket. The acetabulum is formed by three pelvic bones—the ilium, ischium, and pubis—which join at the triradiate cartilage, a Y-shaped growth plate that fuses at the age of 14–16 years.

The femoral head rotates within the acetabulum, with the tapered femoral neck serving as the connection between the head and the rest of the femur. The congruence of the spherical head within the cuplike acetabulum allows for the extent of range of motion seen in the hip.

Hip Labrum

The labrum is a horseshoe-shaped structure formed of dense connective tissue and fibrocartilage that rims the acetabulum [14]. In addition to increasing the acetabular volume by 33% [15] and acting like a suction cup to resist joint distraction and improve hip stability [16], the labrum is believed to act as a seal to preserve the intra-articular joint fluid [17], which lubricates the joint surfaces and allows for a smooth gliding motion.

Capsular and Ligamentous Structures

The hip joint is reinforced by the capsule and four ligaments. The capsule is composed of circular fibers forming a collar around the femoral neck, called the zona orbicularis, as well as longitudinal fibers traveling parallel to the neck and carrying the blood vessels that supply the intra-articular structures [18]. The ligaments are the iliofemoral, ischiofemoral, and pubofemoral, which are extra-capsular, and the intra-capsular ligamentum teres [19]. Together with the hip capsule, these ligaments facilitate hip range of motion while simultaneously providing additional stability to the joint.

Musculature

The muscles surrounding the hip function along three primary axes of motion: flexion–extension, internal–external rotation, and abduction–adduction. A list of the functional muscle groupings and primary participating muscles is provided in Table 7.1.

Table 7.1 The functional muscle groups and associated muscles of the hip

	Muscles
Flexion	Iliopsoas (Iliacus + Psoas), rectus femoris, sartorius, pectineus
Extension	Hamstrings (semitendinosus, semimembranosus, biceps femoris)
Internal rotation	Adductor magnus, gluteus medius and minimus (anterior fibers)
External rotation	Piriformis, obturator internus and externus, superior and inferior gemellus, quadratus femoris
Abduction	Gluteus maximus, gluteus medius, gluteus minimus, tensor fascia lata
Adduction	Adductor longus, adductor brevis, adductor magnus, gracilis

Intra-articular Causes of Hip Pain

The extremes of motion and force demanded of the dancer's hip can lead to pain and injury even in the presence of normal anatomy. Certain structural variations, such as hip dysplasia or femoroacetabular impingement (FAI), may increase susceptibility to injury.

Hip Dysplasia

Dysplasia refers to inadequate coverage of the femoral head by the acetabulum. This may be due to either a shallow acetabulum, or an increased femoral-head-to-neck angle (coxa valga), effectively creating a femoral head that lacks coverage relative to a normal acetabulum. The degrees of rotation of the acetabulum and femoral head (anteversion or retroversion) relative to each other and to the rest of the lower extremity can also affect the total coverage of the femoral head by the acetabulum [20]. Decreased coverage can lead to instability and increased shearing between the femoral head and the anterolateral rim of the acetabulum [21]. Increased forces caused by this shearing can then lead to labral tears, as well as injury to the adjacent cartilage.

Femoroacetabular Impingement (FAI)

FAI is the opposite scenario to hip dysplasia. Again, the abnormality can originate from either the acetabulum or femoral head, or a combination of both [22]. Acetabular abnormality is dubbed pincer impingement, and refers to excess coverage of the femoral head by the acetabulum. Cam impingement refers to abnormal shape of the femoral head and neck junction, with decreased offset (difference in diameters) between the femoral head and neck. This can lead to abnormal forces and loading between the femoral head/neck junction and the rim of the acetabulum, even when the hip is taken through a normal range of motion [23]. Monazzam et al. [24] performed CT review on 225 patients age 2–19 years and found that (1) the prevalence of cam and pincer morphology is similar in adolescent and adult populations, and (2) this morphology occurs as early as age ten and 12, respectively, in this cohort.

Hip Labral Tears

Labral tears may be a source of hip pain either in isolation or in association with other injuries, such as damage to adjacent cartilage or inflammation of the surrounding muscles and tendons. Multiple types of sensory nerves and free nerve endings have been identified within the labrum, including pain receptors [25]. Therefore, even in the absence of other abnormalities, a labral tear can cause hip pain.

More commonly, the labral tear is seen in conjunction with other insults. Harris et al. [26] noted that chondral wear and labral tears in the hip often occur in the same location. Although there are no definitive studies demonstrating that labral tears result in hip arthritis, there are several basic science studies [16, 27] demonstrating that labral tears lead to increased strain within the articular cartilage. In theory, this could lead to degeneration of the joint and resulting arthritis, but further studies are necessary to demonstrate a true causative relationship.

Labral tears may also lead to micro-instability within the hip. Crawford et al. [28] demonstrated that a labral tear decreased the force required to distract the hip by 60%. The micro-instability resulting from a labral tear may cause the other stabilizing structures around the hip, specifically the surrounding musculature, to overcompensate, resulting in injuries.

Stress Reaction/Fracture

Though a relative rarity, young dancers are at risk for stress reaction and stress fracture of the femoral neck [29]. These injuries occur when the bone is subjected to repeated abnormal stresses, and the risk is increased in females with amenorrhea [30]. Thus, young dancers engaging in intensive dance training, who may also have altered eating habits and poor nutrition, are at particular risk.

Extra-articular Causes of Hip Pain

Capsular/Ligamentous Laxity

The majority of hip joint stability is contributed by its osseous and labral restraints [18, 31]. However, studies have shown that the hip joint may not be perfectly spherical or congruent [32], resulting in rolling and gliding of the joint as well as translation of the rotational center [33]. This motion is compounded by generalized laxity or focal capsular laxity resulting from repetitive micro-trauma. In dancers, repetitive external rotation of the hip pushes the femoral head anteriorly, which over time may lead to focal anterior capsular laxity [34]. Young dancers, in particular, may have generalized ligamentous laxity [35, 36], making them susceptible to instability and injuries about the hip.

In serial studies, Klemp et al. [37, 38] found that dancers who progressed to become company dancers had a significantly lower rate of hypermobility. McCormack et al. [36] also found that as dancers advanced in their careers they had lower rates of hypermobility than younger dancers in training. Though no direct correlation has been demonstrated, it is possible that hypermobility leads to increased susceptibility to injuries about the hip and elsewhere [39, 40], which in turn prevents further progression in dance training and performance.

Extra-articular Impingement

Due to the extremes of motion achieved by dancers, certain extra-articular boney prominences about the hip that might otherwise not contact each other can be a source of impingement and pain. One such occurrence involves the AIIS and distal femoral neck, termed sub-spine impingement [2], which can occur with extreme flexion of the hip, as in a high extension à la seconde.

Tendinopathy

Dancers are susceptible to derangements in the tendons crossing the hip joint, as well as strains in the muscles that control hip motion. Internal or external snapping hip is reported in up to 91% of dancers and produces pain nearly 60% of the time [41]. Internal snapping hip occurs when the iliopsoas tendon snaps over the ilio-pectineal eminence, femoral head, or lesser trochanter [41, 42]. If pain is experienced with this phenomenon, it is located in the anterior groin and is associated with extension and external rotation of the hip from a flexed position. External snapping hip involves the IT band or anterior border of the gluteus maximus muscle snapping over the greater trochanter of the femur. Pain is located over the lateral aspect of the hip and can be associated with trochanteric bursitis [41, 42].

Additionally, injury can occur at any of the muscle groups surrounding the hip. These injuries may present as chronic overuse strains, or be the result of an acute indirect traumatic event leading to an avulsion of the muscle tendon from its bony attachment. Young dancers may be particularly susceptible to apophyseal avulsion injuries due to the inherent weakness of the open growth plate [42, 43]. Avulsions of the ischial tuberosity, the attachment site of the proximal hamstrings, are most common, representing approximately 50% of all avulsion fractures [43]. Other sites include the AIIS (attachment of the rectus femoris), ASIS (attachment of the sartorius), and inferior pubic ramus (attachment of the hip adductors).

Diagnosis

The diagnosis of young dancers with hip pain consists of a focused history, physical examination, and additional tests such as imaging as required. History taking should include questions directed at the location and duration of pain, any preceding injuries related to the onset of pain, exacerbators and alleviators of pain, and the dancer's current functional status. Any interventions or treatments attempted and their efficacy should be recorded. Additionally, the dancer's training program should be explored, including dance styles, level of training, years in training, and hours per week spent in training. Specific symptoms such as snapping and the position of the hip when this occurs can give clues to the source of hip discomfort [2, 44]. A history of pain and/or snap with developpé may be indicative of labral tear, iliopsoas impingement, or both (Fig. 7.2).

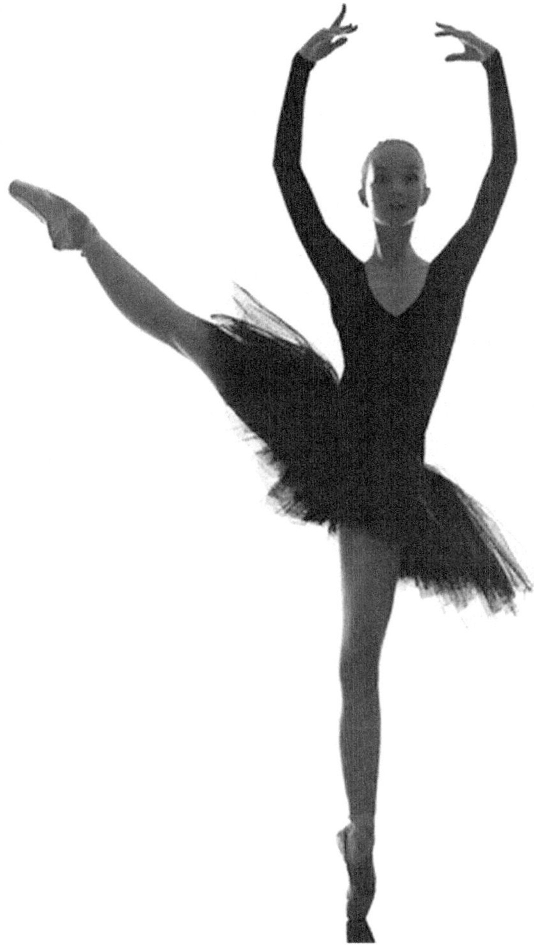

Fig. 7.2 A dancer at the end position of developpé. Symptoms such as pain or snapping of the hip when going through this movement may indicate a labral tear, iliopsoas impingement, or both. The specific positions at which certain symptoms occur can provide important information on the source and nature of the derangement

The physical exam should include the dancer in standing, sitting, supine, lateral, and prone positions; evaluating for overall alignment and range of motion of the hips [45]. Special tests can examine for specific injury patterns. For example, hip pain in flexion, adduction and internal rotation may indicate labral tear or impingement, while pain with extreme flexion may indicate sub-spine impingement. Suspected abductor injury or tendinopathy can be tested for weakness with resisted abduction in the lateral position or with the Trendelenburg test. Subtle instability can be tested with the hip extended and externally rotated, placing a force against the anterior capsuloligamentous complex. Apprehension in this position may indicate laxity or micro-instability. Potential sources of referred pain such as the lumbar spine, sacroiliac joints, and pubic symphysis should also be examined [2, 42]. Finally, the dancer's technique should be evaluated to ensure that no undue strain is being placed on the hip and other structures due to improper training.

Suspected hip injuries on the basis of history and physical exam can be evaluated using imaging modalities including XR, ultrasound, and MRI. Initial XRs, including an AP pelvis and cross-table or Dunn lateral view, can be used to evaluate for bony injuries such as apophyseal avulsions or fractures, in addition to FAI or hip dysplasia. The false profile view can evaluate for anterior acetabular coverage. Ultrasound is useful for evaluating soft tissue structures such as the musculature and tendons surrounding the hip, as well as the labrum. It is particularly efficacious in performing dynamic examination of snapping hip [41, 46, 47] and subtle instability. It can also be used in adjunctive treatment as a guide for injections either intra-articularly or to surrounding structures. MRI, particularly MR arthrogram, can be used to identify labral tears. It is also useful when looking for inflammation within the surrounding muscles and tendons, as well as stress reactions or fractures that do not show up on plain radiographs.

Prevention and Treatment

Defense against injuries in the young dancer begins with a combination of proper technique and a strong, flexible body. Often young dancers are thrust into a demanding pattern of long hours of practice and intensifying physical demands before they have formed a foundation of proper technique. Thus, such habits as the aforementioned "screwing the knee" to achieve turnout are perpetuated, with the compensatory stresses that can cause injuries. Additionally, in spite of (or due to) their youthfulness and high levels of physicality, the exposure to repetitive movements can lead to preferential strengthening of specific muscle groups and imbalance in others [7, 8]. Young dancers should engage in a balanced aerobic and strengthening program outside of classes to prevent this imbalance. Also, stretching of various muscle groups, in particular the hip abductors and hip flexors that are frequently tight in dancers, may help prevent injury and tendinopathies [3]. An individualized regimen of balanced strength and flexibility, targeting the specific needs of the dancer, is the first line of defense and treatment.

There are many secondary contributors to injury that are readily preventable. Reid [48] found in a study of 75 young dancers (average age 13.5) that over one-third had 8 years of training and practiced an average of 14.7 hours per week. This demanding training schedule starting from such a young age places increased stresses on the growing musculoskeletal system. Injury can also result from training on poor surfaces with inadequate footwear [49, 50]. A survey of work incidence report forms filed by dancers performed by Wanke et al. [51] found that dance floor surfaces were the causative factor in 12.8% of all accidents.

Dance combines athletics with aesthetics; therefore, young dancers are susceptible to altered eating habits and poor nutrition. Koutedakis et al. [52] report that female dance students consume below 70% of the recommended daily allowance. This risk factor is not limited to female dancers; Micheli et al. [12] found that percentage of body fat ranges from 13.5 to 16.5% in female professional dancers and from 4.98 to 8.77% in males. In addition to affecting growth and development in the young dancer, poor nutrition can lead to poor bone health due to decreased calcium intake, placing them at risk for stress reactions and fractures, and early fatigability resulting from iron deficiency. These factors in turn lead to higher risk of injury. It is important to recognize these risks and implement early interventions.

When a hip injury does occur in a young dancer the preferred treatment almost invariably begins with a conservative approach utilizing "relative rest" and any number of therapeutic modalities that are commonly practiced by any dance-trained physical therapist. If symptoms persist, treatment options include targeted steroid injections to affected muscles and tendons that can decrease inflammation and help the dancer participate better in rehabilitative exercises. Such injections into the hip joint can be both therapeutic and potentially diagnostic for intra-articular pathology as the source of pain. If non-operative modalities fail, surgery, which is becoming increasingly versatile as arthroscopic techniques continue to improve, can be used to treat labral tears, FAI, chondral lesions and intra-articular loose bodies, and internal and external snapping hip.

Summary

The extreme ranges of motion demanded of the dancer's hip place it at risk for injury. A balance of strength and muscular control along with flexibility is necessary to limit stresses across the hip and surrounding structures. A focused history and physical as well as appropriate imaging aids in diagnosis of apparent injury and can provide keys to counseling the dancer and creating an individualized rehabilitation program. Prevention and physical therapy are the first lines of treatment, but targeted injections and surgical intervention are options in dancers who have failed other treatment modalities. A thorough understanding of the mechanics of dance, the pertinent hip anatomy, and the clinical etiology of injury aids in the design of an effective rehabilitation and treatment program.

References

1. Turner R, O'Sullivan E, Edelstein J. Hip dysplasia and the performing arts: is there a correlation? Curr Rev Musculoskelet Med. 2012;5(1):39–45.
2. Moser BR. Hip pain in dancers. Curr Sports Med Rep. 2014;13(6):383–9.
3. Reid DC. Prevention of hip and knee injuries in ballet dancers. Sports Med. 1988;6(5):295–307.
4. Reid DC, Burnham RS, Saboe LA, Kushner SF. Lower extremity flexibility patterns in classical ballet dancers and their correlation to lateral hip and knee injuries. Am J Sports Med. 1987;15(4):347–52.
5. Ronkko R, Heliovaara M, Malmivaara A, et al. Musculoskeletal pain, disability and quality of life among retired dancers. J Dance Med Sci. 2007;11(4):105–9.

6. Angioi M, Maffulli GD, McCormack M, Morrissey D, Chan O, Maffulli N. Early signs of osteoarthritis in professional ballet dancers: a preliminary study. Clin J Sport Med. 2014;24(5):435–7.
7. Bennell KL, Khan KM, Matthews BL, De Gruyter M, Cook E, Holzer K, Wark JD. Hip and ankle range of motion and hip muscle strength in young novice female ballet dancers and controls. Br J Sports Med. 1999;33(5):340–6.
8. Bennell KL, Khan KM, Matthews BL, Singleton C. Changes in hip and ankle range of motion and muscle strength in 8–11 year old novice female ballet dancers and controls: a 12 month follow up study. Br J Sports Med. 2001;35(1):54–9.
9. Jacobs M, Young R. Snapping hip phenomenon among dancers. Am Correct Ther J. 1978;32(3):92–8.
10. Lincoln TL, Suen PW. Common rotational variations in children. J Am Acad Orthop Surg. 2003;11(5):312–20.
11. Khan K, Roberts P, Nattrass C, Bennell K, Mayes S, Way S, et al. Hip and ankle range of motion in elite classical ballet dancers and controls. Clin J Sport Med. 1997;7(3):174–9.
12. Micheli LJ, Gillespie WJ, Walaszek A. Physiologic profiles of female professional ballerinas. Clin Sports Med. 1984;3(1):199–209.
13. Coplan JA. Ballet dancer's turnout and its relationship to self-reported injury. J Orthop Sports Phys Ther. 2002;32(11):579–84.
14. Safran MR. The acetabular labrum: anatomic and functional characteristics and rationale for surgical intervention. J Am Acad Orthop Surg. 2010;18(6):338–45.
15. Seldes RM, Tan V, Hunt J, Katz M, Winiarsky R, Fitzgerald RH Jr. Anatomy, histologic features, and vascularity of the adult acetabular labrum. Clin Orthop Relat Res. 2001;382:232–40.
16. Terayama K, Takei T, Nakada K. Joint space of the human knee and hip joint under a static load. Eng Med. 1980;9(2):66–74.
17. Ferguson SJ, Bryant JT, Ganz R, Ito K. An in vitro investigation of the acetabular labral seal in hip joint mechanics. J Biomech. 2003;36(2):171–8.
18. Shu B, Safran MR. Hip instability: anatomic and clinical considerations of traumatic and atraumatic instability. Clin Sports Med. 2011;30(2):349–67.
19. Boykin RE, Anz AW, Bushnell BD, Kocher MS, Stubbs AJ, Philippon MJ. Hip instability. J Am Acad Orthop Surg. 2011;19(6):340–9.
20. Hingsammer AM, Bixby S, Zurakowski D, Yen YM, Kim YJ. How do acetabular version and femoral head coverage change with skeletal maturity? Clin Orthop Relat Res. 2015;473(4):1224–33.
21. Shoenecker PL, Clohisy JC, Millis MB, Wenger DR. Surgical management of the problematic hip in adolescent and young adult patients. J Am Acad Orthop Surg. 2011;19(5):275–86.
22. Parvizi J, Leunig M, Ganz R. Femoroacetabular impingement. J Am Acad Orthop Surg. 2007;15(9):561–70.
23. Ganz R, Parvizi J, Beck M, Leunig M, Notzli H, Siebenrock KA. Femoroacetabular impingement: a cause for osteoarthritis of the hip. Clin Orthop Relat Res. 2003;417:112–20.
24. Monazzam S, Bomar JD, Dwek JR, Hosalkar HS, Pennock AT. Development and prevalence of femoroacetabular impingement-associated morphology in a paediatric and adolescent population: a CT study of 225 patients. Bone Joint J. 2013;95-B(5):598–604.
25. Kim YT, Azuma H. The nerve endings of the acetabular labrum. Clin Orthop Relat Res. 1995;320:176–81.
26. Harris WH, Bourne RB, Oh I. Intra-articular acetabular labrum: a possible etiological factor in certain cases of osteoarthritis of the hip. J Bone Joint Surg Am. 1979;61(4):510–4.
27. Ferguson SJ, Bryant JT, Ganz R, Ito K. The influence of the acetabular labrum on hip joint cartilage consolidation: a poroelastic finite element model. J Biomech. 2000;33(8):953–60.
28. Crawford MJ, Dy CJ, Alexander JW, Thompson M, Schroder SJ, Vega CE, Patel RV, Miller AR, McCarthy JC, Lowe WR, Noble PC. The 2007 Frank Stinchfield Award. The biomechanics of the hip labrum and the stability of the hip. Clin Orthop Relat Res. 2007;465:16–22.

29. Mattila VM, Niva M, Kiuru M, Pihlajamaki HK. Risk factors for bone stress injuries: a follow-up study of 102,515 person-years. Med Sci Sports Exerc. 2007;39(7):1061–6.
30. Tibor LM, Sekiya JK. Differential diagnosis of pain around the hip joint. Arthroscopy. 2008;24(12):1407–21.
31. Cereatti A, Margheritini F, Donati M, Cappozzo A. Is the human acetabulofemoral joint spherical? J Bone Joint Surg Br. 2010;92(2):311–4.
32. Afoke NY, Byers PD, Hutton WC. The incongruous hip joint. A casting study. J Bone Joint Surg Br. 1980;62(4):511–4.
33. Gilles B, Christophe FK, Magnenat-Thalmann N, Becker CD, Duc SR, Menetrey J, Hoffmeyer P. MRI-based assessment of hip joint translations. J Biomech. 2009;42(9):1201–5.
34. Martin HD, Savage A, Braly BA, Palmer IJ, Beall DP, Kelly B. The function of the hip capsular ligaments: a quantitative report. Arthroscopy. 2008;24(2):188–95.
35. Grahame R, Jenkins JM. Joint hypermobility—asset or liability? A study of joint mobility in ballet dancers. Ann Rheum Dis. 1972;31(2):109–11.
36. McCormack M, Briggs J, Hakim A, Grahame R. Joint laxity and the benign joint hypermobility syndrome in student and professional ballet dancers. J Rheumatol. 2004;31(1):173–8.
37. Klemp P, Chalton D. Articular mobility in ballet dancers: a follow-up study after four years. Am J Sports Med. 1989;17(1):72–5.
38. Klemp P, Stevens JE, Isaacs S. A hypermobility study in ballet dancers. J Rheumatol. 1984;11(5):692–6.
39. Briggs J, McCormack M, Hakim AJ, Grahame R. Injury and joint hypermobility syndrome in ballet dancers—a 5-year follow-up. Rheumatology. 2009;48(12):1613–4.
40. Scheper MC, deVries JE, deVos R, Verbunt J, Nollet F, Englebert RH. Generalized joint hypermobility in professional dancers: a sign of talent or vulnerability? Rheumatology. 2013;52(4):651–8.
41. Winston P, Awan R, Cassidy JD, Bleakney RK. Clinical examination and ultrasound of self-reported snapping hip syndrome in elite ballet dancers. Am J Sports Med. 2007;35(1):118–26.
42. Frank JS, Gambacorta PL, Eisner EA. Hip pathology in the adolescent athlete. J Am Acad Orthop Surg. 2013;21(11):665–74.
43. Rossi F, Dragoni S. Acute avulsion fractures of the pelvis in adolescent competitive athletes: prevalence, location and sports distribution of 203 cases collected. Skeletal Radiol. 2001;30(3):127–31.
44. Bedi A, Dolan M, Leunig M, Kelly BT. Static and dynamic mechanical causes of hip pain. Arthroscopy. 2011;27(2):235–51.
45. Martin HD, Kelly BT, Leunig M, Philippon MJ, Clohisy JC, Martin RL, et al. The pattern and technique in the clinical evaluation of the adult hip: the common physical examination tests of hip specialists. Arthroscopy. 2010;26(2):161–72.
46. Pelsser V, Cardinal E, Hobden R, Aubin B, Lafortune M. Extraarticular snapping hip: sonographic findings. AJR Am J Roentgenol. 2001;176(1):67–73.
47. Wunderbaldinger P, Bremer C, Matuszewski L, Marten K, Turetschek K, Rand T. Efficient radiological assessment of the internal snapping hip syndrome. Eur Radiol. 2001;11(9):1743–7.
48. Reid DC. Preventing injuries to the young ballet dancer. Physiother Can. 1987;39(4):231–6.
49. Fong YA, Hiller C, Smith R, Vanwanseele B. Effect of footwear on dancers: a systematic review. J Dance Med Sci. 2011;15(2):86–92.
50. Washington EL. Musculoskeletal injuries in theatrical dancers: site, frequency and severity. Am J Sports Med. 1978;6(2):75–98.
51. Wanke EM, Mill H, Wanke A, Davenport J, Koch F, Groneberg DA. Dance floors as injury risk: analysis and evaluation of acute injuries caused by dance floors in professional dance with regard to preventative aspects. Med Probl Perform Artist. 2012;27(3):137–42.
52. Koutedakis Y, Jamurtas A. The dancer as a performing athlete: physiological considerations. Sports Med. 2004;34(10):651–61.

Chapter 8
Knee Problems in the Young Dancer

Peter G. Gerbino, MD, Andrea Stracciolini, MD, FAAP, FACSM and Marina G. Gearhart, BA

Pertinent Definitions

Anterior knee pain: Any pain in the front of the knee resulting from any cause
Patellofemoral pain syndrome (*PFPS*): Anterior knee pain arising in the patella subchondral bone
Plica: A vestigial fold of tissue most commonly on the medial side of the knee that can be painful
Hoffa's fat pad: A large pad of fat behind and adjacent to the patellar tendon thought to provide protection to the joint
Back knee/hyperextension: The condition where a dancer hyperextends her knees
Hyperlaxity: The genetic condition where a dancer has the ability to bend most joints past the normal range of motion
Patella dislocation/subluxation: Translation of the patella (usually laterally) beyond the normal range. Subluxation is a partial dislocation

P.G. Gerbino, MD (✉)
Department of Orthopedic Surgery, Community Hospital of the Monterey Peninsula, 900 Cass St., Suite 200, Monterey, CA 93940, USA
e-mail: peter.gerbino@chomp.org; peter.gerbino@gmail.com

A. Stracciolini, MD, FAAP, FACSM (✉)
Division of Sports Medicine, Department of Orthopaedics, Boston Children's Hospital, 300 Longwood Avenue, Boston, MA 02115, USA
e-mail: andrea.stracciolini@childrens.harvard.edu

M.G. Gearhart, BA
Division of Sports Medicine, Boston Children's Hospital, 319 Longwood Ave., Boston, MA 02115, USA
e-mail: marinagearhart@gmail.com

R. Solomon et al. (eds.), *Prevention of Injuries in the Young Dancer*, Contemporary Pediatric and Adolescent Sports Medicine,
DOI 10.1007/978-3-319-55047-3_8

Osgood–Schlatter syndrome (*OSS*): Tendon injury and traction physeal stress fracture where the patellar tendon connects to the tibia at the tibial tubercle (apophysis)
Sinding–Larsen–Johansson syndrome (*SLJS*): Tendon injury and traction stress injury where the patella tendon connects to the distal pole of the patella (ossific nucleus)
Iliotibial band (ITB) syndrome: An overuse syndrome where there is pain in the iliotibial band at the lateral knee; can lead to bursitis and/or tendinosis
Chondromalacia: Cartilage damage. Typically damage to the retropatellar cartilage
Patellar tendinitis/tendinosis: Inflammation at the patella tendon (tendinitis) or damage to the tendon (tendinosis)

Introduction

Young dancers face unique risk factors for injury related to growth. Combined with less than fully developed experience and skill, they have relatively weak muscles and are skeletally immature, with open growth plates (physes) that are vulnerable to injury during times of growth. Other important extrinsic risk factors include dancing in studios with suboptimal floors that may increase risk for injury [1]. As in any other high-performance athlete, if the performance envelope is pushed too far, injury will occur, either as a result of macrotrauma (from a specific incident), micro-trauma (overuse), or a combination thereof [2]. In the young dancer, these additional factors often combine with the traditional risk factors associated with classic dance, including excessive training, disordered eating, and difficulty distinguishing the pain associated with injury from the routine discomfort resulting from intense dance training [3]. This chapter deals specifically with knee injuries and the need for all healthcare practitioners to understand the injury profile of knee injuries in young dancers, including which injuries occur, why they occur, how to treat them, and how to prevent them from recurring.

Epidemiology

A significant proportion of injuries to young dancers involve the knee. Reid found that 14–20% of ballet dancers' injuries were to the knee and that 50% of those were due to patellofemoral problems [4]. In 2012, Steinberg et al. studied 1336 8- to 16-year-old dancers in Israel. They found that 42.6% had been injured. Early age at onset of dancing, technique problems, and time spent en pointe were specifically associated with knee injuries, and not body structure or anatomic abnormalities [5]. A recent epidemiological study in pediatric dancers showed that 28% of injuries to young dancers presenting to a sports and dance medicine clinic were of the knee [6]. In a similar study of young Irish step dancers, 19.7% of injuries were knee related [7], the major knee problem being patellofemoral pain syndrome [8].

In elite pre-professional dancers aged 15–19 years, the clinical risk of injury was found to be 1.42 injuries per dancer, and 76% risk of recordable injury over the past year [9]. Among professional ballet dancers, knee injury patterns have been shown to differ by sex, with males suffering mostly acute knee injuries and females mostly overuse knee injuries [10]. Teitz found that most knee injuries in adult dancers were patellofemoral, plica-related, or meniscal [11]. Also in professional level dancers, Wanke et al. found that 10.9% of male and 17.5% of female revue dancers' injuries were knee related [12].

Growth and Development as a Risk Factor for Knee Injury

A basic understanding of child and adolescent development as it relates to injury profile is critical when caring for or training pediatric dancers. Currently, there is a trend toward an earlier age of menarche for girls across the United States, with the average age of 12.6 years [13], and girls tend to reach their peak height and body mass at approximately 15 years of age [14]. The onset of puberty in the child dancer may be delayed, extending both the dancer's growth period and duration of increased vulnerability to injury [15]. Overall body mass and height may increase at a dramatic rate in the pre-adolescent and adolescent years. Steinberg et al. report that joint hypermobility is common among young non-professional female dancers compared with control subjects [16]. It is hypothesized that increased joint laxity combined with the physiological changes that occur during growth (i.e., neuromuscular control) may affect the type, severity, and incidence of injuries in the maturing female adolescent population [17, 18]. It has also been suggested that cyclic changes in the hormonal development of females may play a role in injury patterns. As a result, young dancers in the process of growth and maturation may be at higher risk of knee injuries [19–21].

Maturation, growth, body mass, and lower extremity alignment were measured in adolescent ballet dancers (female = 30, male = 16) from the Australian Ballet School over the course of six months. Lower extremity alignment was assessed using a tondu (single knee bend in external rotation) and temps levé (single leg vertical jump in turnout) while being photographed from different angles. The results of this study indicated that knee angles, pelvic angles, and foot length were associated with increase in injury risk. As the dancer manifests changes in the body, his or her injury risk increases [22]. Additionally, once a young dancer has had a lower extremity injury, he or she is at an increased risk for another injury [23, 24]. Initiating integrative resistance training targeting strength, flexibility, and neuromuscular deficits that develop during the puberty process in the dancer early, before injury onset, is critical [25].

Macrotrauma

Macrotrauma occurs with a fall, twist, collision, or other single violent act. It results in contusions, fractures, and ligament injuries about the knee.

ACL Tear

Landing from a jump incorrectly is the most common way for a dancer to tear the anterior cruciate ligament (ACL). These injuries are uncommon in dancers, but do occur, and can be career-ending [26, 27]. A fall with an audible "pop," rapid effusion, and inability to continue dancing is suspicious for ACL tear. Instability and giving way is the typical complaint.

Examination shows a large effusion and increased anterior translation of the tibia. Radiographs are typically normal, other than soft-tissue swelling. MRI will document the tear and other associated injuries (Fig. 8.1). Treatment is usually ACL reconstruction with autograft [26].

Rehabilitation can take more than a year, and some dancers will never regain their previous level of achievement [27]. There is good science showing that ACL injuries can be decreased by incorporating certain exercises into an athlete's training. The PEP program is the best known of these exercises [28]. While PEP is geared toward young female soccer players, it may be helpful in young dancers as well. ACL injury prevention in the dancer may need to be modified given the inherent training of the dancer that incorporates balance and coordination and is less focused on building strength. Perhaps most importantly, a recent meta-analysis of 14 ACL injury-prevention studies concluded that greater success in knee injury

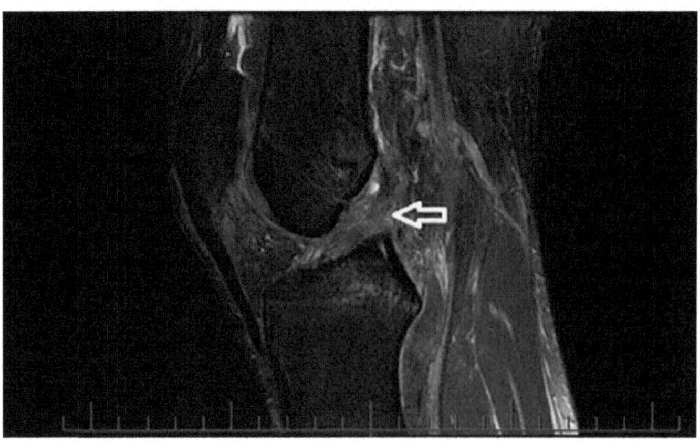

Fig. 8.1 MRI showing torn ACL. Anterior translation of the tibia creates the "question mark sign" in the PCL that is now under less tension

reduction in female athletes was achieved when preventive neuromuscular training commenced before the onset of neuromuscular deficits and peak knee injury incidence, optimally during early adolescence [29].

PCL Tear

Posterior cruciate ligament (PCL) tear is even less common in dancers. It typically occurs when the dancer falls on a flexed knee, striking the proximal tibia on the floor. The tibia is driven back, rupturing the PCL. Exam shows increased posterior translation of the tibia on the femur. MRI is the imaging study of choice.

Unlike the ACL, isolated PCL tears may not need reconstruction [30]. If rehabilitation results in a stable knee that does not give way, the dancer can go back to full activity without surgery or restriction. Persistent instability warrants reconstruction [31]. Prevention of falls through concentration on balance and achievement of center would be a good way to decrease these injuries.

MCL/LCL Tears

When the knee is forced medially (valgus) or laterally (varus), the medial collateral ligament (MCL) or lateral collateral ligament (LCL), respectively, can be torn. Pain and instability can prevent the dancer from dancing. Examination demonstrates varus or valgus laxity and pain. MRI will show the injury. Partial to complete MCL tears usually heal without surgery [32]. If the posteromedial corner is also damaged, a medial side repair of both is done [33]. Return to dance can take weeks to months, depending on the severity of the injury. Like the MCL, the LCL will typically heal without surgery in 6–8 weeks. Also like the medial side, if LCL and posterolateral corner are damaged, an open reconstruction is necessary [34]. In other sports, bracing helps decrease these injuries, but in dance, they are already uncommon. No special prevention strategies are known.

Meniscus Tear

When the knee is under load and twists during a landing or forced turnout, the meniscus can be squeezed and sheared, resulting in a tear. Symptoms can range from mild joint line pain to locking, where the knee cannot be fully extended. This is one of the more common injuries in dancers' knees [11, 35].

Examination for meniscus tear involves checking range of motion and palpating the medial and lateral joint lines. Pain along either joint line should prompt the examiner to check for a McMurray sign, which is a painful snap as the knee is extended from a flexed position. In the past, physicians were told that clinical

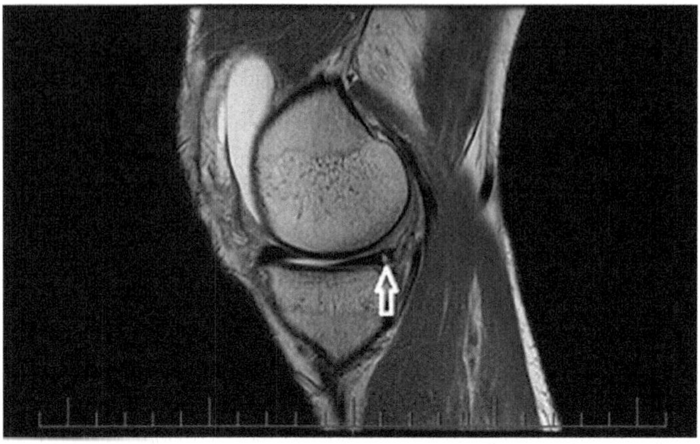

Fig. 8.2 MRI view of a medial meniscus tear

diagnosis was adequate. Unfortunately, a contusion to the femur or tibia can mimic a meniscal tear and result in an unnecessary operation. Confirmation of the diagnosis is made with the MRI (Fig. 8.2).

Treatment of meniscus tear varies. A locked knee must be treated surgically, urgently, to achieve motion and the best chance for repair [36]. Only the smallest tears can be treated non-operatively with rest and rehabilitation [37]. Most meniscus tears are treated with arthroscopic repair or partial resection. Good dance technique is the best prevention here. Knowing when you are fatigued enough to stop dancing is the key to prevention.

Patella Dislocation

A direct blow to the medial side of the patella or a landing where the knee rotates inward can cause the patella to dislocate laterally. This is especially true in dancers with hyperlaxity or a history of patella subluxation. A dislocated patella is hard to miss, as the patella sits on the outside of the knee rather than in its groove (Fig. 8.3). Acutely, the patella is reduced by straightening the knee and pushing the patella medially. Radiographs determine whether a piece of bone was knocked off, requiring surgical repair versus resection. MRI can provide details about articular cartilage damage, location of medial patellofemoral ligament (MPFL) damage, and associated bone bruises [38].

Treatment for first time dislocations is rest, bracing, and rehabilitation. Recurrent dislocation or subluxation calls for MPFL repair or reconstruction [39]. This injury is more common in dancers with hyperlaxity syndrome. They need to know that they have the syndrome and to strengthen their quadriceps, especially the vastus medialus obliquus (VMO), to decrease the likelihood of dislocation.

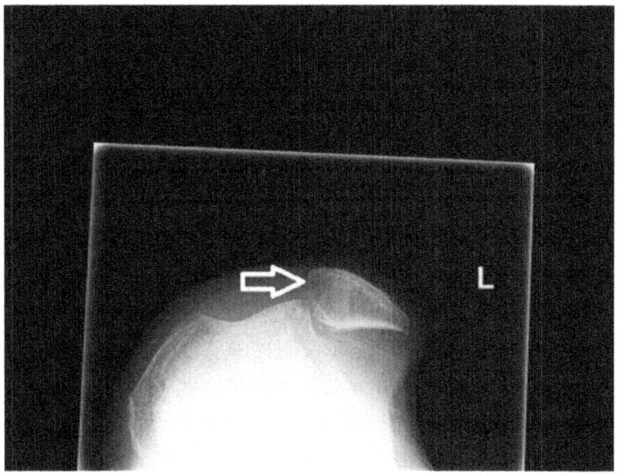

Fig. 8.3 Patella dislocation as seen in MRI axial cut

Fracture

In the knee, the patella, femur, and tibia can break. In the young dancer, the distal femur and proximal tibia physes can be fractured as well. Powerful trauma is required to break bones; hence, fractures are unusual in dancers. Fracture of the patella, femur, or tibia is diagnosed by radiographs. If the fracture is non-displaced, it can be treated by non-weight-bearing in a cast or immobilizer. Repeat radiographs for the first few weeks are needed to ensure the fracture remains non-displaced. Displaced fractures require open reduction and internal fixation with hardware. Fractures typically heal in 6–10 weeks.

Most injuries that result in a broken bone cannot be prevented. Bone strength can be improved, and dancers often have low bone density due to poor diet, abnormal menstrual periods, and/or an eating disorder. Teaching proper calcium, vitamin D, and protein intake should be part of every young dancer's education. Avoiding smoking [40] and correcting disordered eating will optimize bone strength.

Micro-trauma/Overuse

With repetitive, strenuous use of a structure, breakdown occurs, leading to micro-injuries. These can be very painful and destructive over time. Most of the knee injuries sustained by young dancers are from overuse [5]. In general, overuse means too much, too soon. This can include advancing too rapidly for age, training level, conditioning, strength, or balance. It can also mean advancing too rapidly for a given environment, including studio temperature, quality of the dance floor, skill of the dance partner, or teacher's expectations.

Overuse Knee Injuries Unique to Dancers with Open Growth Plates

Osgood–Schlatter Syndrome

Excessive traction forces on the patella tendon in dancers in their early teens can lead to stress fracture of the tibial tubercle physis (growth plate) and small tears in the tendon's attachment fibers on the tibia. The physis can separate a bit, causing a bump at the tibial tubercle. Acute aggravation can cause additional swelling of the area. Examination demonstrates a bump at the tibial tubercle that is tender to palpation. Radiographs show widening of the tibial tubercle physis and frequently fragmentation of the apophysis.

The excess traction leading to physeal stress fracture is treated with rest. Relative rest allowing the tissues to heal should be effective. Such pain-free rest is difficult to achieve, and the pain and injury can persist. In the past, casting was employed to facilitate adequate rest [41]. Now this is rarely done; instead, a knee brace and physical therapy are prescribed. The goal is to restore knee strength and decrease traction at the tubercle through the use of strengthening and flexibility exercises. Unless the lesion becomes completely pain-free to palpation, it usually recurs. For prevention, avoid too much jumping in the immature dancer. Ensure that young dancers have excellent hamstring and quadriceps flexibility.

Sinding–Larsen–Johannson Syndrome

This problem is the same as Osgood–Schlatter, except it occurs in 10- and 11-year olds and at the patella distal pole rather than the tibial tubercle. Treatment is similar.

Common Overuse Knee Injuries in Young Dancers

Patellofemoral Pain Syndrome (PFPS)

This is the most common cause of knee pain in dancers, young and old [1–5, 7, 10]. The pain is thought to arise from the subchondral bone nerves in the patella. The cartilage has no nerves and does not contribute to the patella pain [42]. Asymmetrical overloading of the patella may cause patella deformation and pain [43]. Stairs, jumping, and grand plié are the main culprits (Fig. 8.4).

The dancer will complain of pain with any activity requiring a bent knee. This is when compressive loads on the patella are greatest. The damage can result after a single jump but more often occurs from cumulative jumps and grand pliés when the patella bone fatigues and deforms to a greater extent.

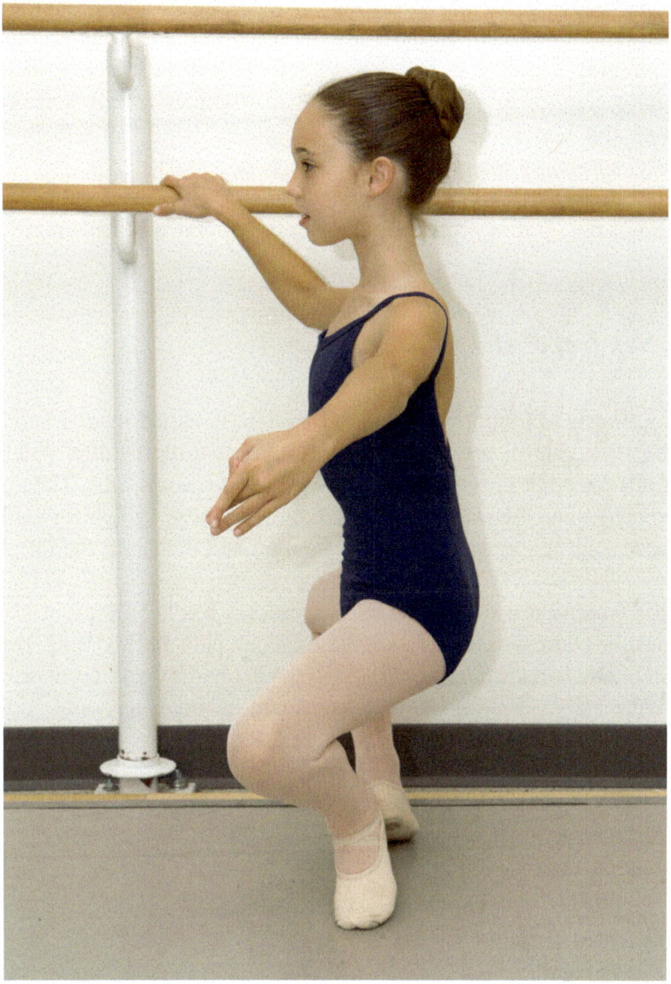

Fig. 8.4 Grand plié with deep knee flexion leads to overload and injury to the patellofemoral joint. Photo courtesy of James Koepfler

Examination consists of evaluating the patella for pain with loading. This can be done by pressing the patella into the trochlea and assessing for pain. Patella tracking is explored to determine whether changing the tracking can be used to modify forces on the damaged parts of the patella. Medial–lateral translation indicates whether hypermobility is a factor. Radiographs can determine patella tilt, patella alta or infera, and whether there is bone damage to the patella or trochlea is hypoplastic. Documenting the subtle subchondral micro-trauma has proven to be more difficult. Bone scan has been shown to indicate subchondral trauma in some patients with PFPS [44], and MRI has documented patella bone changes related to PFPS [45].

The goal of treatment of an isolated patellofemoral problem is force reduction. Depending on whether the force overload is symmetric or asymmetric, different strategies can be employed. If the force is uniform on a well-tracking patella, decreased jumping, grand plié, and overall activity will be effective. If the patella tracks laterally, a brace or taping that medializes the patella may help. Over time, strengthening the VMO and stretching the iliotibial band can relieve pain [46]. Occasionally, surgically realigning the patella is necessary.

Excellent quadriceps [47], hip external rotator, and abductor strength [48], and avoiding grand plié, aid in protecting the patellofemoral mechanism.

Fat Pad Syndrome (FPS)

FPS is also known as Hoffa's syndrome. Swollen, enlarged medial and lateral fat pads can be very painful [49]. This condition tends to occur after patellofemoral pain syndrome, or other knee pathology has existed for some time. The diagnosis is under-appreciated and frequently missed. Examination is straightforward, looking at fat pad size with the knee flexed and extended and palpating the fat pads under stress.

Since this condition occurs after another process has been present, the primary problem must be addressed first. To decrease fat pad pain and swelling, rest and oral NSAIDs are started. If ineffective, injecting the fat pad(s) with corticosteroids can be tried. Ultimately, if non-operative treatment is not successful, arthroscopic removal of the hypertrophic tissue is warranted (Fig. 8.5). As previously noted, the condition typically occurs after a long period of patellofemoral pain syndrome, so preventing PFPS is probably the best prevention for FPS.

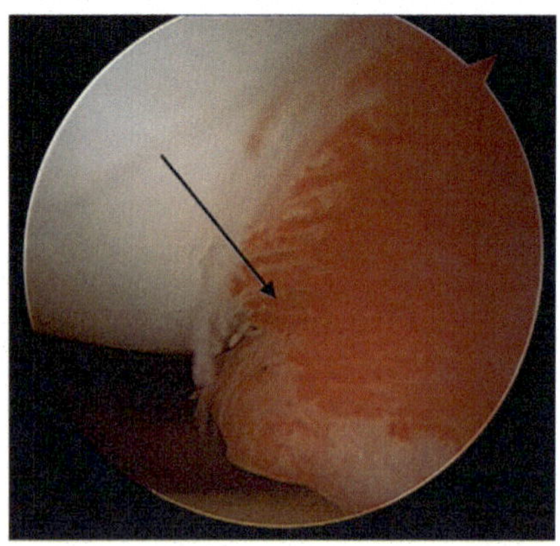

Fig. 8.5 Fat pads can encroach anteriorly in the knee causing impingement

Plica Syndrome

The medial plica is present in most knees. These plicae can become thickened and rub against the medial femoral condyle during flexion. This is a common cause of knee pain in dancers [11]. Whether the plica or the medial femoral condyle synovium is the source of the pain is unknown. Why some plicae rub and others do not is also unknown. Some clinicians believe the rubbing results from the patella tracking laterally, pulling all medial structures laterally with it. Palpation of the plica and medial femoral condyle synovium demonstrates tenderness, making the diagnosis. An enlarged plica can be seen on MRI axial cuts and at arthroscopy (Fig. 8.6).

The goal of initial treatment is to stop the plica from rubbing against the medial femoral condyle. This may be done by medializing the patella with taping, bracing, and strengthening the VMO. In addition, the plica can be injected with corticosteroid under ultrasound guidance. If these efforts are unsuccessful, the plica can be arthroscopically excised, and if necessary, the patella can be surgically medialized. Prophylactic VMO strengthening might prevent the problem from arising.

Synovitis

Synovitis occurs when microscopic cartilage wear particles or other irritants cause the synovium to secrete macrophages and fluid to remove the irritants. The knee is symmetrically enlarged and boggy. Range of motion is limited by capsule distention.

Since synovitis occurs when something irritates the synovium, the source of irritation must be addressed. After ruling out gout, infection, and internal derangement, consider particulate debris from chondral degeneration. Determine the cause of abnormal cartilage wear, such as patella malalignment, patella overload, excessive valgus, or excessive varus. Treat the mechanical deformity causing the wear. The patella can be realigned by taping, bracing, VMO strengthening, or, as a last resort, surgical modification. Varus and valgus can be modified by bracing and possibly by technique changes. Treat underlying degenerative and inflammatory conditions to minimize knee synovitis.

Fig. 8.6 Arthroscopic view of a medial plica

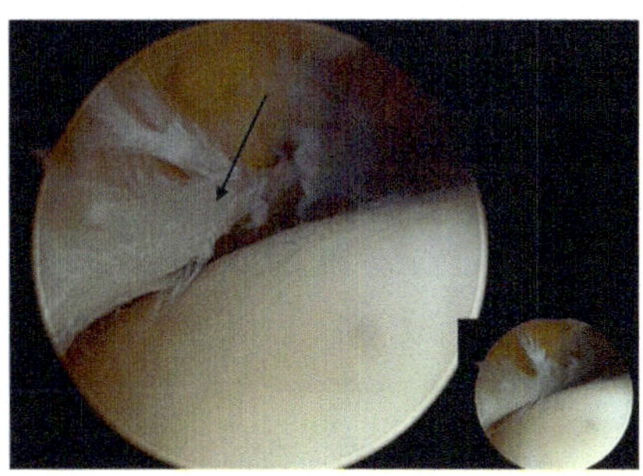

Patella Subluxation and Back Knee

Young dancers have a higher incidence of hyperlaxity syndrome [16] which predisposes them to unique injury patterns. Patellar subluxation occurs when there is hyperlaxity, abnormal tracking, patellofemoral hypoplasia, or a previous dislocation. It is almost always lateral subluxation. On exam, multiple signs of hyperlaxity are present, or the patella is hypermobile from prior dislocation. The apprehension test is positive when the patella is manually translated laterally and the dancer becomes apprehensive. Sources of pain from subluxation are not well understood but may arise from abnormal patellofemoral forces when the patella is in a suboptimal tracking position.

Treatment requires determining the cause of the subluxation. It could be hyperlaxity, patella alta, severe lateral tracking, genu valgum, prior dislocation, patella and/or trochlear hypoplasia, or a combination of these. In all cases begin with taping, bracing, and VMO strengthening. If these interventions are not effective, additional measures can be employed.

The medial patellofemoral ligament can be shortened or augmented surgically [39]. In patella alta, the tibial tubercle can be surgically advanced [50]. Hypoplasia has been treated with patella and/or trochlear osteotomy to create a better capture [51]. Genu valgum can be treated with distal femoral opening-wedge osteotomy [52]. Prevention here is the same as for patella dislocation. VMO strength is critical. Preventive taping or bracing can be employed.

Back knee is the lay term for genu recurvatum, a knee that hyperextends beyond neutral (Fig. 8.7). Dancers with hyperlaxity are more prone to hyperextend. Attempts to get more turnout or a better fifth position can lead some dancers to hyperextend their knees. Back knee can lead to a stretched posterior knee capsule, pain, and a predisposition to ACL injury.

When formulating an injury-prevention strategy, first determine whether hyperlaxity is present by evaluating for hyperextension of the wrist, fingers, and elbows. If the dancer has hyperlaxity, only technique improvement, resisting knee "locking" into a hyperextended position, and use of a brace to limit extension can prevent the problem. If hyperlaxity is present, a generalized strengthening program will be helpful.

If there is not hyperlaxity, the dancer has been forcing the knee backward to achieve a position not attainable without the abnormal knee position. Evaluate and correct technique. Otherwise, look for restricted range of motion in the ankles and hips that force the knee to have extra motion.

Patellar Tendinitis/Tendinosis

Inflammation (tendinitis) or tendon micro-tears (tendinosis) result from too much jumping. A sudden increase in amount of jumping due to a demanding production

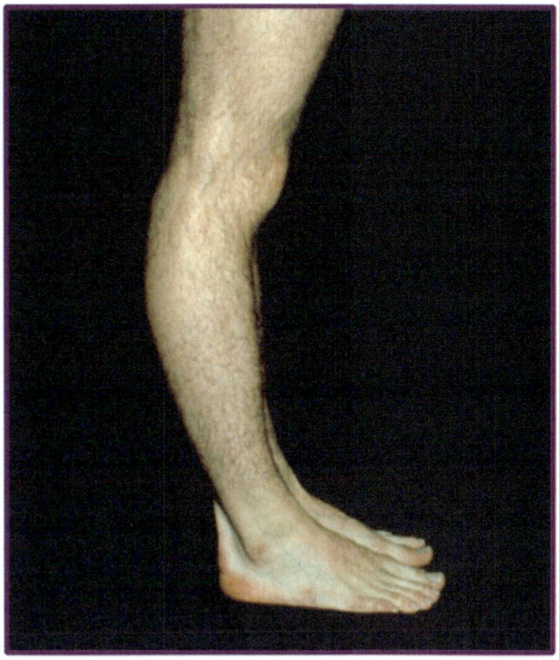

Fig. 8.7 "Back knee" hyperextension in a ballet dancer

or after a period away from dancing can cause these injuries. Palpation at the tendon origin at the distal pole of the patella will demonstrate tenderness. In the very young dancer, this could indicate Sinding–Larsen–Johansson syndrome. In the older teen, patellar tendon injury is possible. MRI will show increased fluid and edema at the site. A partial tear of the patellar tendon is possible.

When this type of injury occurs, jumping is stopped completely. If necessary, running is also stopped and only barre is allowed. Oral or topical anti-inflammatory medicines can help. Gentle, progressive eccentric quadriceps strengthening exercises have been shown to be the optimal intervention [53]. Prevent by increasing jumping gradually; no more than 10% increase per week has been shown to be safe in other athletes.

Iliotibial Band (ITB) Syndrome

Pain on the lateral knee along the iliotibial band (ITB) results from excessive tension on the ITB. This can occur from tight ITB or overuse of the ITB's muscle, the gluteus maximus. ITB excessive tightness has been documented in older dancers, and it is believed that concentrating more on abduction, rather than adduction, is responsible [54]. The gluteus maximus can be overused if it is weak, if hip strength is weak, if core strength is weak, or if there is improper technique [55].

If the ITB is tight as determined by the Ober test, stretching and strengthening will help. If the ITBs are being overused, the gluteus maximus must be assessed. If it is weak, it can be strengthened. If it is fatigued, it must be rested. This can be done with simple rest, but sometimes strengthening the core muscles and other hip muscles is necessary to give the gluteus maximus a rest. If the gluteus maximus is being overused as a brake when landing jumps, technique should be assessed. Emphasize core strength and proper technique. Ensure good ITB flexibility.

Stress Fracture

Stress fractures in dancers occur from overuse of normal bone or from appropriate training in weak bone. Young dancers can have weak bones due to poor diet, disordered eating, low vitamin D, low calcium, or metabolic disorders. Pain with activity that persists at rest, especially at night, is suspicious for stress fracture. Point tenderness at the bone in question will be present. These days, MRI is used to make a definitive diagnosis.

When a stress fracture is found in a dancer, the quality of the bone is assessed. Menstrual history is obtained. The dancer's diet is documented. Calcium and protein intake is noted. Vitamin D3 level is checked. An Israeli study found 73% of athletes and dancers were vitamin D deficient [56].

Recommended levels for calcium and vitamin D intake are controversial. The United States government guidelines are 1000 and 1300 mg calcium and 800 I.U. vitamin D daily [57]. The best current recommendation for athletes is to take in enough vitamin D to achieve >40 ng/mL blood levels [58].

Consuming adequate calories and protein is necessary for strong bone and can be a problem for young dancers. In one study, 80% of ballet dancers with stress fractures had body weights less than 75% of ideal for height [59]; 1.2–1.8 gm/kg body weight of protein is thought to be optimal for teen and adult aerobic athletes [60]. Disordered eating, irregular menses, and osteopenia are the three elements of the Female Athlete Triad, which is certainly seen in adolescent dancers [61]. Disordered eating requires professional counseling.

If the dancer is felt to be at risk for insufficient bone strength, a bone density study (DEXA) is ordered. If bone density is normal, technique and training intensity are assessed. Poor technique and excessive training both require better teaching. Insufficient bone density can be improved by correcting the deficiencies found above.

Summary

Knee injuries in dancers are similar to knee injuries in other athletes, with a few exceptions. Patellofemoral pain and patella tendinitis/tendinosis occur more often due to the jumping demands placed upon dancers. Back knee, patella subluxation, and patella dislocation occur more frequently due to the increased incidence of hyperlaxity syndrome in dancers. Smoking, low vitamin D, abnormal menses, and disordered eating lead to a higher incidence of stress fractures.

References

1. Hackney J, Brummel S, Newman M, Scott S, Reinagel M, Smith J. Effect of reduced stiffness dance flooring on lower extremity joint angular trajectories during a ballet jump. J Dance Med Sci. 2015;19(3):110–7.
2. Micheli LJ. Overuse injuries in children's sports: the growth factor. Orthop Clin North Am. 1983;14(2):337–60.
3. Anderson R, Hanrahan SJ. Dancing in pain. J Dance Med Sci. 2008;12(1):9–16.
4. Reid DC. Prevention of hip and knee injuries in ballet dancers. Sports Med. 1988;6(5):295–307.
5. Steinberg N, Siev-ner I, Peleg S, Dar G, Masharawi Y, Zeev A, Hershkovitz I. Extrinsic and intrinsic risk factors associated with injuries in young dancers aged 8–16 years. J Sports Sci. 2012;30(5):485–95.
6. Yin AX, Sugimoto D, Martin DJ, Stracciolini A. Pediatric dance injuries: a cross-sectional epidemiological study. PM R. 2016;18(4):348–55.
7. Stein CJ, Tyson KD, Johnson VM, Popoli DM, D'Hemecourt P, Micheli LJ. Injuries in Irish dance. J Dance Med Sci. 2013;17(4):159–64.
8. Beasley MA, Stracciolini A, Tyson KD, Stein CJ. Knee injury patterns in young Irish dancers. Med Probl Perform Art. 2014;29(2):70–3.
9. Ekegren CL, Quested R, Brodrick A. Injuries in pre-professional ballet dancers: incidence, characteristics and consequences. J Sci Med Sport. 2014;17(3):271–5.
10. Nilsson C, Leanderson J, Wykman A, Strender LE. The injury panorama in a Swedish professional ballet company. Knee Surg Sports Traumatol Arthrosc. 2001;9(4):242–6.
11. Teitz CC. Hip and knee injuries in dancers. J Dance Med Sci. 2000;4(1):23–9.
12. Wanke EM, Arendt M, Helmgard Mill H, Koch F, Wanke A, Groneberg DA. Traumatic injuries in revue dancers. J Dance Med Sci. 2014;18(1):22–8.
13. Euling SY, Herman-Giddens ME, Lee PA, Selevan SG, Juul A, Sørensen TI, et al. Examination of US puberty-timing data from 1940 to 1994 for secular trends: panel findings. Pediatrics. 2008;121(Suppl 3):S172–91.
14. Malina R, Bouchard C, Bar-Or O. Growth, maturation and physical activity. 2nd ed. Champaign, IL: Human Kinetics; 2005.
15. Brooks-Gunn J, Warren MP. The effects of delayed menarche in different contexts: dance and nondance students. J Youth Adolesc. 1985;14(4):285–300.
16. Steinberg N, Hershkovitz I, Zeev A, Rothschild B, Siev-Ner I. Joint hypermobility and joint range of motion in young dancers. J Clin Rheumatol. 2016;22(4):171–8.
17. Quatman CE, Ford KR, Myer GD, Paterno MV, Hewett TE. The effects of gender and pubertal status on generalized joint laxity in young athletes. J Sci Med Sport. 2008;11(3):257–63.
18. Myer GD, Ford KR, Paterno MV, Nick TG, Hewett TE. The effects of generalized joint laxity on risk of anterior cruciate ligament injury in young female athletes. Am J Sports Med. 2008;36(6):1073–80.
19. Heitz NA, Eisenman PA, Beck CL, Walker JA. Hormonal changes throughout the menstrual cycle and increased anterior cruciate ligament laxity in females. J Athl Train. 1999;34(2):144–9.
20. Wojtys EM, Huston LJ, Lindenfeld TN, Hewett TE, Greenfield ML. Association between the menstrual cycle and anterior cruciate ligament injuries in female athletes. Am J Sports Med. 1998;26(5):614–9.

21. Slauterbeck JR, Fuzie SF, Smith MP, Clark RJ, Xu K, Starch DW, et al. The menstrual cycle, sex hormones, and anterior cruciate ligament injury. J Athl Train. 2002;37(3):275–8.
22. Bowerman E, Whatman C, Harris N, Bradshaw E, Karin J. Are maturation, growth and lower extremity alignment associated with overuse injury in elite adolescent ballet dancers? Phys Ther Sport. 2014;15(4):234–41.
23. Murphy DF, Connolly DA, Beynnon BD. Risk factors for lower extremity injury: a review of the literature. Br J Sports Med. 2003;37(1):13–29.
24. Bowerman EA, Whatman C, Harris N, Bradshaw E. A review of the risk factors for lower extremity overuse injuries in young elite female ballet dancers. J Dance Med Sci. 2015;19(2): 51–6.
25. Stracciolini A, Hanson E, Kiefer AW, Myer GD, Faigenbaum AD. Resistance training for pediatric female dancers. J Dance Med Sci. 2016;20(2):64–71.
26. Meuffels DE, Verhaar JAN. Anterior cruciate ligament injury in professional dancers. Acta Orthop. 2008;79(4):515–8.
27. Liederbach M, Dilgen FE, Rose DJ. Incidence of anterior cruciate ligament injuries among elite ballet and modern dancers: a 5-year prospective study. Am J Sports Med. 2008;36(9): 1779–88.
28. Mandelbaum BR, Silvers HJ, Watanabe DS, Knarr JF, Thomas SD, Griffin LY, et al. Effectiveness of a neuromuscular and proprioceptive training program in preventing anterior cruciate ligament injuries in female athletes. 2-year follow-up. Am J Sports Med. 2005;33(7): 1003–10.
29. Myer GD, Sugimoto D, Thomas S, Hewett TE. The influence of age on the effectiveness of neuromuscular training to reduce anterior cruciate ligament injury in female athletes: a meta-analysis. Am J Sports Med. 2013;41(1):203–15.
30. Keller PM, Shelbourne KD, McCarroll JR, Rettig AC. Nonoperatively treated isolated posterior cruciate ligament injuries. Am J Sports Med. 1993;21(1):132–6.
31. Fanelli GC, Bradley MD, Giannotti F, Edson CJ. The posterior cruciate ligament arthroscopic evaluation and treatment. Arthrosc J Arthrosc Relat Surg. 1994;10(6):673–88.
32. Indelicato PA, Hermansdorfer J, Huegel M. Nonoperative management of complete tears of the medial collateral ligament of the knee in intercollegiate football players. Clin Orthop Rel Res. 1990;256:174–7.
33. Lind M, Jakobsen BW, Lund B, Hansen MS, Abdallah O, Christiansen SE. Anatomical reconstruction of the medial collateral ligament and posteromedial corner of the knee in patients with chronic medial collateral ligament instability. Am J Sports Med. 2009;37(6): 1116–22.
34. Cooper JM, McAndrews PT, LaPrade RF. Posterolateral corner injuries of the knee: anatomy, diagnosis, and treatment. Sports Med Arthrosc. 2006;14(4):213–20.
35. Chang G, Diamond M, Nevsky G, Regatte RR, Weiss DS. Early knee changes in dancers identified by ultra high field 7 T MRI. Scand J Med Sci Sports. 2014;24(4):678–82.
36. Allum RL, Jones JR. The locked knee. Injury. 1986;17(4):256–8.
37. Weiss CB, Lundberg M, Hamberg P, DeHaven KE, Gillquist J. Non-operative treatment of meniscal tears. J Bone Joint Surg Am. 1989;71(6):811–22.
38. Guerrero P, Li X, Patel K, Brown M, Busconi B. Medial patellofemoral ligament injury patterns and associated pathology in lateral patella dislocation: an MRI study. Sports Med Arthrosc Rehabil Ther Technol. 2009;1(1):17.
39. Reagan J, Kullar R, Burks R. MPFL reconstruction: technique and results. Orthop Clin North Am. 2015;46(1):159–69.
40. Castillo RC, Bosse MJ, MacKenzie EJ, Patterson BM, The LEAP Study Group. Impact of smoking on fracture healing and risk of complications in limb-threatening open tibia fractures. J Orthop Trauma. 2005;19(3):151–7.
41. Antich TJ, Brewster CE. Osgood-schlatter disease: review of literature and physical therapy management. J Orthop Sports Phys Ther. 1985;7(1):5–10.
42. Biedert RM, Stauffer E, Friederich NF. Occurrence of free nerve endings in the soft tissue of the knee joint. A histologic investigation. Am J Sports Med. 1992;20(4):430–3.

43. Kerr H, Gerbino P, Soto R, Zurakowski D, Muller J. Load-deformation characteristics of the patella: relationship to intraosseous pressure. Med Sci Sports Exerc. 2007;39(Suppl 5):S472.
44. Hejgaard N, Diemer H. Bone scan in the patellofemoral pain syndrome. Int Orthop. 1987;11(1): 29–33.
45. Niva MH, Kiuru MJ, Haataja R, Pihlajamäki HK. Bone stress injuries causing exercise-induced knee pain. Am J Sports Med. 2006;34(1):78–83.
46. Cowan SM, Bennell KL, Hodges PW, Crossley KM, McConnell J. Delayed onset of electromyographic activity of vastus medialis obliquus relative to vastus lateralis in subjects with patellofemoral pain syndrome. Arch Phys Med Rehab. 2001;82(2):183–9.
47. Natri A, Kannus P, Järvinen M. Which factors predict the long-term outcome in chronic patellofemoral pain syndrome? A 7-yr prospective follow-up study. Med Sci Sports Exerc. 1998;30(11):1572–7.
48. Ireland ML, Willson JD, Ballantyne BT, Davis IM. Hip strength in females with and without patellofemoral pain. J Ortho Sports Phys Ther. 2003;33(11):671–6.
49. Dye SF, Vaupel GL, Dye CC. Conscious neurosensory mapping of the internal structures of the human knee without intraarticular anesthesia. Am J Sports Med. 1998;26(6):773–7.
50. Shen HC, Chao KH, Huang GS, Pan RY, Lee CH. Combined proximal and distal realignment procedures to treat the habitual dislocation of the patella in adults. Am J Sports Med. 2007; 35(12):2101–8.
51. Dejour D, Le Coultre B. Osteotomies in patello-femoral instabilities. Sports Med Arthrosc. 2007;15(1):39–46.
52. Marti RK, Beimers L. Open-wedge osteotomy of the lateral femoral condyle for extensor mechanism instability. Oper Orthop Traumatol. 2006;18(3):273–85.
53. Young MA, Cook JL, Purdam CR, Kiss ZS, Alfredson H. Eccentric decline squat protocol offers superior results at 12 months compared with traditional eccentric protocol for patellar tendinopathy in volleyball players. Br J Sports Med. 2005;39(2):102–5.
54. Reid DC, Burnham RS, Saboe LA, Kushner SF. Lower extremity flexibility patterns in classical ballet dancers and their correlation to lateral hip and knee injuries. Am J Sports Med. 1987;15(4):347–52.
55. Fredericson M, Wolf C. Iliotibial band syndrome in runners: innovations in treatment. Sports Med. 2005;35(5):451–9.
56. Contantini NW, Arieli R, Chodick G, Dubnov-Raz G. High prevalence of vitamin D insufficiency in athletes and dancers. Clin J Sport Med. 2010;20(5):368–71.
57. New Recommended Daily Amounts of Calcium and Vitamin D. NIH Medline Plus. https://www.nlm.nih.gov/medlineplus/magazine/issues/winter11/articles/winter11pg12.html. Accessed 27 Apr 2016.
58. Ogan D, Pritchett K. Vitamin D and the athlete: risks, recommendations, and benefits. Nutrients. 2013;5(6):1856–68.
59. Frusztajer NT, Dhuper S, Warren MP, Brooks-Gunn J, Fox RP. Nutrition and the incidence of stress fractures in ballet dancers. Am J Clin Nutr. 1990;51(5):779–83.
60. Lemon PW. Do athletes need more dietary protein and amino acids? Intl J Sport Nutr. 1995;5(Suppl):S39–61.
61. Hoch AZ, Papanek P, Szabo A, Widlansky ME, Schimke JE, Gutterman DD. Association between the female athlete triad and endothelial dysfunction in dancers. Clin J Sport Med. 2011;21(2):119–25.

Chapter 9
Foot and Ankle Injuries in the Adolescent Dancer

Nancy J. Kadel, MD

Pertinent Definitions

Physis: The growth plate, or segment of bone responsible for longitudinal growth.
Apophysis: A site of tendon attachment and a normal bony outgrowth that arises from a secondary ossification center and fuses with the bone in course of time.
Apophysitis: An overuse injury of inflammation, irritation, and microtrauma unique to the skeletally immature athlete at the biomechanically weak apophysis, resulting from repetitive traction stress at the attached musculotendinous unit.
Osteochondritis dessecans: A disorder of the subchondral bone and its overlying articular cartilage (most common in the knee, elbow, and ankle joints). An area of articular cartilage becomes separated from the underlying subchondral bone. The fragment may lose its blood supply and develop into a loose body in the joint, or become a painful flap of cartilage leading to swelling, vague joint pain, catching, or locking.

Introduction

Dance as an art form requires intense training from an early age, which includes periods of rapid skeletal growth, for those who aspire to perform at an elite level. The young dancer's foot and ankle complex are subjected to high forces, often in the extremes of joint range of motion, particularly ankle plantar flexion [1–3]. The foot and ankle complex functions as a base of support, a lever to propel the dancer

N.J. Kadel, MD (✉)
Seattle Dance and Performing Arts Medicine (SeaPAM), Seattle, Washington, USA
e-mail: nancykadelmd@gmail.com

R. Solomon et al. (eds.), *Prevention of Injuries in the Young Dancer*,
Contemporary Pediatric and Adolescent Sports Medicine,
DOI 10.1007/978-3-319-55047-3_9

in dynamic maneuvers, and a shock absorber. Contrary to most other sports, in dance the foot is essential for expressing the artistic (aesthetic) line of the leg, regardless of the style being performed. This chapter will present some common foot and ankle problems found in the young dancer.

Scope of the Problem (Epidemiology)

Epidemiological studies in young dancers have reported injury incidence rates ranging from 0.77 to 1.55 per 1000 dance hours. During adolescence, an important time of growth and maturation, the concurrent rise in training volume and intensity for young dancers appears to increase their risk of injury [4–9]. Over a 2-year period Steinberg et al. found that 40–48% of all dancers aged eight to 18 sustained an injury, and Ekegren found a risk of injury of 76% over one year in pre-professional ballet students [4, 8]. These studies both attributed the high rate of injury in large part to increased training intensity.

The foot and ankle complex is reported in many studies of adolescent dancers to be the most frequently injured body part. The majority of injuries in young dancers are the result of overuse (72–82% is some studies), which is postulated to be due to the highly specific repetitive movements practiced on a day-to-day basis [4–11]. By way of contrast, overuse injuries reported in elite adolescents in other sports account for only (15–63%) of injuries [12]. Training levels in elite young dancers often exceed those in other sports, including technique classes and/or rehearsals 6 days per week.

One retrospective study found a 37% increase in dance related injuries treated in children age 3–19 years at US emergency departments from 1991 to 2007. A total of 113,084 children and adolescents were treated for such injuries, 58% of which involved the lower extremity: 21% ankle and 12% foot [13]. A cross-sectional study of a 5% random sample of dancers (age 5–17 years) treated at a tertiary pediatric sports medicine facility over nine years found the most common diagnosis was tendonitis/tendinopathy, followed by patellofemoral pain syndrome, apophysitis, and ankle impingement [14]. The foot and toes together with the ankle comprised the majority of the injuries reported in those dancers.

Foot

Hallux Valgus/Bunions

Hallux valgus deformity may be seen in young dancers; however, there is conflicting data regarding whether the incidence of hallux valgus in dancers is greater than that in the general population [15–19]. The cause of hallux valgus formation is multifactorial, and likely results from a combination of genetic predisposition, foot shape, and shoe choice. Dancers with bunion-prone feet, those who force their turnout, and those with flexible pes planus may exacerbate an existing or developing bunion deformity. Young dancers with a bunion deformity often have congenital metatarsus primus varus [20]. In dancers who develop bunions, it is recommended to avoid surgical intervention while they are still dancing. Any bunion surgery can lead to loss of dorsiflexion first metatarsophalangeal joint after at the (1 MTPJ), and a minimum of 90° of MTPJ dorsiflexion is required for the demi-pointe position.

Many dancers with mild bunions have few or no symptoms other than angular deformity of the hallux. Some dancers develop pain and swelling of the bursa over the medial 1 MTPJ. Acute inflammation (bursitis) of the 1 MTPJ should be treated with brief icing, non-steroidal anti-inflammatory drugs (NSAIDS), and taping to stabilize the hallux/1 MTPJ. Dancers should be counseled to wear wide toe-box low heeled or athletic type shoes outside of class if bunions are symptomatic. Use of toe spacers between the first and second toes, and in some instances a donut or horseshoe-shaped pad over the medial prominence of the 1 MTPJ worn in the pointe shoes, can help to reduce symptoms while dancing. Intrinsic foot muscle strengthening exercises, including the doming exercise, picking up marbles or pieces of make-up sponge with the toes, and hallux abduction exercises are important for all young dancers, but especially so in dancers with feet prone to hallux valgus. Attention to pointe shoe fit is critical for dancers with hallux valgus, as is emphasis on proper foot and leg alignment during technique class and avoidance of forced turnout. Dancers with bunions may find a pointe shoe with a wider, square-shaped box and/or a higher than normal vamp or wings extending over the hallux MTPJ more supportive and comfortable. Attention to proper alignment during training of young dancers can help to avoid exacerbation of bunion-prone feet [21].

Sesamoid Injuries

The differential diagnosis for pain at the plantar aspect of the 1 MTPJ in a young dancer includes: sesamoiditis, bursitis, osteonecrosis, stress or acute fracture of one or more sesamoid bone(s), and sprain of a bipartite sesamoid. (Of course infection, systemic inflammatory conditions, nerve entrapment, and tumor should be ruled out.) Bipartite sesamoids are present in 10–33% of feet [22–24]. The sesamoid bones are small bones imbedded within the flexor hallucis brevis (FHB) tendons, and articulate with the plantar surface of the first metatarsal head. Their function is to stabilize the 1 MTPJ and improve the power of the FHB tendons, much as the patella assists the quadriceps muscles. The sesamoids are subjected to high stress when the dancer rolls up onto demi-pointe or full pointe, or when taking off and landing a jump.

Presenting symptoms are pain under the first metatarsal head on the plantar forefoot, worst with relevé (rolling up onto the ball of the foot), running, and jumping. The dancer will be tender to palpation of the sesamoid bone, and a swollen and inflamed fluid filled bursa may be palpable. The tibial sesamoid is most frequently involved. The sesamoids are embedded in the FHB tendons; therefore, the tenderness should move distally with dorsiflexion of the great toe on physical exam.

Injecting a small amount of local anesthetic will confirm the diagnosis. Bone scan and MRI may be needed to identify stress fractures or osteonecrosis. Plain radiographs (with sesamoid views) or CT scans can identity fractures. Bipartite sesamoids will have rounded edges on a radiograph compared to the sharply defined edges of an acute sesamoid fracture. Technical errors such as rolling in, pronation, or forcing turnout can result in excessive loading of the sesamoids, and must be corrected for successful resolution of symptoms. Improper jump landings without plié (slight bend in the knees) and the practice of walking with an out-toeing gait can contribute to sesamoid problems.

Treatment includes a trial of padding to off-load the area. Felt dancer (sesamoid) pads with a cut-out for the sesamoids may help, and use of a stiff-soled shoe such as a clog or hiking boot outside of class to limit hallux MTP joint motion may reduce symptoms. A removable cast boot can be used if symptoms are severe. Assessing and correcting alignment and technical problems are important for success. Corticosteroid injections in this area (and in young dancers) should be used rarely, and only after technical errors are addressed. Sesamoid problems may take months to resolve fully, and surgical excision is not recommended in dancers, as potential loss of plantar flexion strength could end a dance career [21–24]. Bone stimulators have been reported to improve healing in sesamoid fractures [25].

Metatarsophalangeal Joints

Metatarsalgia is not particularly common in dancers, so in a dancer with forefoot pain Frieberg's infarction or MTPJ synovitis or instability should be suspected. Frieberg's infarction is an idiopathic osteonecrosis (most often of the second metatarsal head) that is more common in females, and may present in adolescence as metatarsalgia and MTPJ swelling and pain. Clinical symptoms often precede radiographic changes by 6 months, but a bone scan or MRI can provide an earlier diagnosis. Radiographs may reveal a flattening or fragmentation of the metatarsal head. Physical exam will demonstrate tenderness and often an effusion and decreased range of motion of the MTPJ. Conservative treatment including taping the toe, stiff-soled shoes out of class, and avoidance of painful activities should be employed [23].

MTPJ instability can be seen in dancers. The demi-pointe position, with weight bearing on the ball of the foot during relevé, transmits excess loads to the second and third metatarsal heads. Dancers will have plantar MTPJ tenderness on physical exam, yet report dorsal MTPJ pain with relevé. In addition, the painful MTPJ will have increased passive anterior/posterior translation (+MTPJ Lachman or Drawer test) [26]. NSAIDS, padding, and taping the toe (to either the next toe or the plantar foot) can be used to help alleviate symptoms. Referral to an orthopaedic foot and ankle specialist is recommended if symptoms persist.

Fifth Metatarsal Fracture

Fractures of the fifth metatarsal are common in dance. The mechanism for injury is usually a missed jump landing or rolling over the outer border of the foot while on demi-pointe. The dancer will present with lateral foot pain, swelling, and ecchymosis. Physical exam findings include tenderness over the lateral metatarsal. Radiographs are needed for accurate diagnosis, as treatment is based on the location and type of fracture. A spiral shaft fracture, known as a "dancer's fracture," can be treated without surgery, regardless of displacement [27]. A removable cast boot, with weight bearing as tolerated, is used until pain-free walking is possible, usually within 6 weeks. As soon as comfort allows, pool exercises and gentle active range of motion exercises are begun out of the boot. Return to dance is progressed slowly, first with barre work and pain-free exercises, and progression to center, turns, and jumps as symptoms resolve. Physical therapy focusing on proprioception, core, and foot intrinsic strength training is recommended. The clinician should evaluate the ankle for associated instability or ligament sprain, as both injuries may occur with this mechanism.

Avulsion fractures of the proximal fifth metatarsal are associated with the above mechanism of an ankle inversion injury. Typically extra-articular, the fracture line is through the tuberosity. Treatment with a stiff-soled shoe or removable cast boot to control symptoms is sufficient. Surgical treatment is reserved for the rare case of significant displacement or articular involvement. In skeletally immature dancers, pain on the lateral border of the foot at the proximal end of the fifth metatarsal is more likely to be apophysitis (see Iselin's disease), whether insidious or traumatic in onset [24, 28, 29].

Jones fractures occur at the metaphyseal–diaphyseal junction of the fifth metatarsal in more mature young dancers. Because of poor blood supply in this area, these transverse fractures have a propensity for nonunion. Most common in modern and barefoot dancers, Jones fractures can be treated in a short-leg cast for 6–8 weeks with non-weight bearing. However, elite dancers and athletes typically are treated with bone stimulators or surgical intervention to avoid prolonged immobilization and reduce risk of nonunion.

Stress fractures of the proximal fifth metatarsal metaphyseal-diaphyseal area can be seen in dancers, who often report chronic lateral foot pain followed by an acute event. Radiographs demonstrate cortical thickening, periosteal reaction, and a wider fracture line than seen in the acute Jones fracture. These fractures may require operative treatment, often with bone grafting and bone stimulator, due to poor healing potential similar to the acute Jones fracture [22, 27].

Apophysitis Fifth Metatarsal (Iselin's Disease)

Iselin's disease is the term for traction apophysitis at the base of the fifth metatarsal. The apophysis of the proximal fifth metatarsal can be seen on radiographs at about age 10 in girls and age 12 in boys, and fuses approximately two years later. The fibularis brevis and fibularis tertius muscles insert proximally on the fifth metatarsal near the attachment of the metatarsal ligaments as well as the plantar fascia. The secondary ossification center is within the insertion site of the fibularis brevis on the dorsolateral aspect of the tuberosity of the fifth metatarsal. This problem is most typically seen in young dancers undergoing rapid growth, or following an inversion injury to the foot in a skeletally immature dancer. Apophysitis must be differentiated radiographically from an avulsion fracture of the base of the fifth metatarsal, as tenderness would be in a similar location (Fig. 9.1). Treatment includes avoidance of painful activities, removable boot if needed for pain-free walking for three weeks, and gentle fibularis stretching and strengthening after symptoms have improved. Graduated return to dance activities may resume once the foot is no longer tender on physical exam [24, 28, 29].

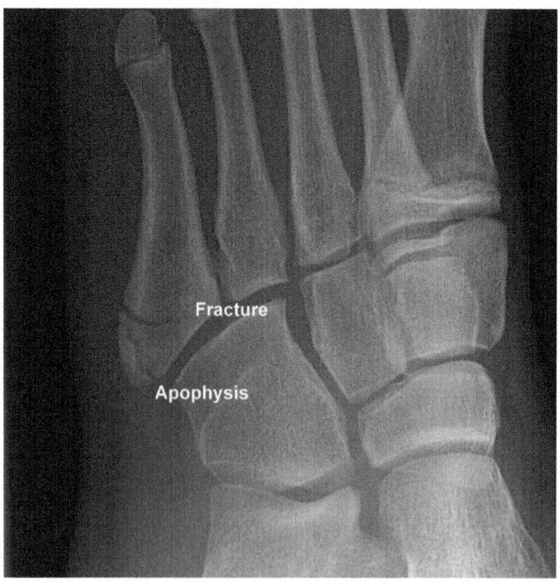

Fig. 9.1 Normal apophysis (more parallel to the shaft) is shown along with an avulsion fracture, which is more transverse at the base of the fifth metatarsal in a skeletally immature foot. Apophysis plus fracture: case courtesy of Dr. Alexandra Stanislavsky

Stress Fractures

Whenever loading is increased too rapidly, or there is repeated microtrauma of physiological loads that exceed the bones reparative capacity, a stress fracture can occur. Increased training intensity, hard floors, nutritional and hormonal factors, menstrual irregularities, low body mass index, and low energy availability have all been implicated in stress fractures. Dancing more than 5 h per day and having amenorrhea greater than 90 days have been demonstrated as risk factors for stress fractures in female dancers [30]. Metatarsal stress fractures are the most common stress fracture reported in dancers [30, 31]. The fibula, tibia, spine, and hip are other potential sites.

The dancer with a stress fracture will report a dull, achy pain in the injured area. Initially pain will typically occur near the end of class or with jumps. A marked increase in training intensity (such as a summer dance program) often precedes the symptoms. As symptoms progress pain becomes more constant, and may occur with walking and at night. Rarely is swelling present, and often pain is not well localized. Bony tenderness may be present. Initial radiographs are often normal. Radionuclide bone scans can be positive only a few days after the injury, but MRI is recommended to make the diagnosis (Fig. 9.2a, b).

(a) (b)

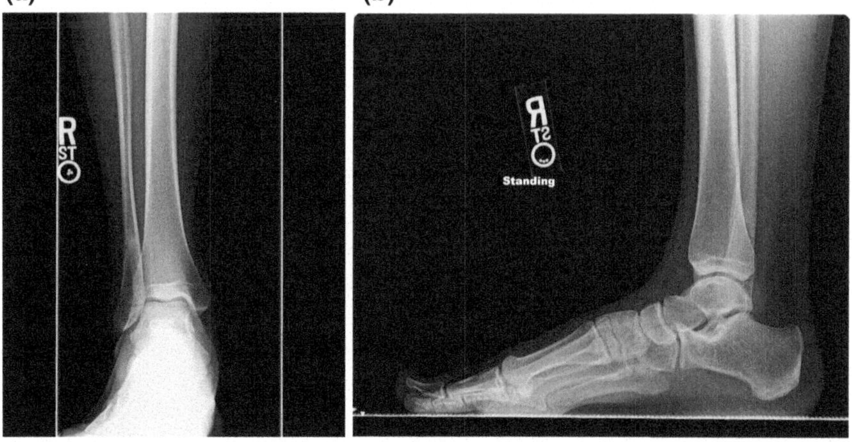

Fig. 9.2 **a** Anteroposterior radiograph of healing right fibula stress fracture in 14-year-old female elite ballet dancer who developed ankle pain week 5 of a 6-week summer dance intensive program. **b** Lateral radiograph of the same healing right fibula stress fracture. The dancer was able to walk without pain after a total of 3 weeks in a removable boot and was allowed to weight-bear in sneakers and start pool, Pilates, and elliptical trainer exercises. Graduated return to full dance activities was begun after additional 3 weeks when radiographs demonstrated further healing

Dancers are at risk for a stress fracture at the base of the second metatarsal. Running athletes typically will have a stress fracture of the midshaft or more distal aspect of the metatarsal [31, 32]. In the midfoot, the second metatarsal is recessed and the second metatarsal-cuneiform joint is more proximal than the first or third metatarsal-cuneiform joints. The first and second metatarsals bear the majority of a dancers' weight whether on demi-pointe, pointe, or in landing from a jump, and those stresses are transmitted proximally to the midfoot, where the base of the second metatarsal is locked in [33].

Synovitis of Lisfranc's joints (the metatarsal-cuneiform joints) and a proximal second metatarsal stress fracture are difficult to distinguish with physical exam or a bone scan [31, 32, 34–36]. Therefore, MRI has become the preferred test in a dancer with midfoot pain, a suspected stress fracture, and negative radiographs. Healing time is prolonged for the stress fracture (6–8 weeks) compared to synovitis (3 weeks); hence, accurate diagnosis is important for managing these injuries [34]. Treatment for foot and ankle stress fractures does not usually require casting, but some dancers need a removable cast boot for pain-free walking outside of class. Bone stimulators are often used to aid healing. Attention to energy availability, calcium and vitamin D levels, and correction of any deficits is important. Conditioning can be maintained with floor barre, Pilates, pool exercises, and exercise bicycle or elliptical trainer barring pain at the fracture site with those activities. Rehabilitation includes gradual return to class with avoidance of painful activities such as pointe work, jumps, turns, and demi-pointe until healing is completed and pain resolved.

Lisfranc Sprain/Fractures

Midfoot sprains/fractures in young dancers are not common, but the physician treating dancers should have a high index of suspicion because if this injury is not recognized and treated it can be career ending. The ligaments of the tarso-metatarsal joints act to support the medial and longitudinal arches of the foot. These injuries can be easily missed as radiographic findings may be subtle, and the midfoot pain can be mistaken for possible stress fracture or synovitis. Usually, these injuries have more swelling when compared to a stress fracture or isolated synovitis. Tenderness over the dorsal midfoot (especially the first and second metatarsal-cuneiform joints) is present. In acute cases plantar midfoot ecchymosis may be seen, increasing the likelihood of a Lisfranc injury diagnosis. *Weight bearing* AP radiographs may show a small diastasis between the first and second metatarsal bases (comparison views of the opposite foot aid in making the diagnosis). Lisfranc's ligament is located between the medial cuneiform and the base of the second metatarsal. An avulsed fragment of bone between the first and second metatarsal bases may be seen if the ligament is injured.

The mechanism of injury to Lisfranc's joints in dancers has been described to include a fall off pointe position, missed jump landings, take-off for a jump, and a foot catching a seam or irregularity in the floor. These injuries occur in ankle plantar flexion, with or without rotation, often with the metatarsal-phalangeal joints in maximal dorsiflexion (demi-pointe) [29, 37–39]. Most Lisfranc injuries require surgical treatment, and only a simple sprain with no instability should be treated non-surgically. Any suspected Lisfranc injury should be referred to an orthopaedic surgeon for evaluation. Recovery is prolonged, and immobilization with avoidance of weight bearing activities for 6–12 weeks is required. Rehabilitation of the entire kinetic chain will be needed to return the dancer to full performance level.

Plantar Fasciitis

The plantar aponeurosis is a strong band of fascia extending from the calcaneal tuberosity to attach at the plantar aspect of the proximal phalanges. In young dancers plantar fasciitis usually coincides with calcaneal apophysitis, but in older adolescent dancers with closed physes it can exist by itself and presents as plantar-medial arch or heel pain [40]. The literature suggests that this is not a true inflammatory condition, but rather the result of repetitive microtrauma after increased training intensity [41]. Dancers will usually have pain with their first few steps in the morning, which improves quickly and then worsens later with increased activity. Diagnosis is based on history and physical exam findings of tenderness over the anteromedial aspect of the heel, worst with the foot and toes in dorsiflexion and less tender with plantar flexion of the toes. This, like Sever's disease, is a clinical diagnosis, because radiographs are often not helpful. However, tenderness of the calcaneal wall should alert the clinician to a possible calcaneal stress fracture (or Sever's disease in a skeletally immature dancer), and further imaging is needed.

Treatment should include relative rest (including avoidance of painful activities), dorsiflexion night splint for sleeping, and gastrocnemius, soleus, and plantar arch stretches. Use of a stiff-soled shoe for walking, such as hiking boots or clogs, can help to avoid stressing the plantar fascia by limiting flexion of the MTP joints [41]. Use of the night splint and stiff-soled shoes is often needed for 4–6 weeks minimum. Taping the foot arch can improve symptoms in many dancers.

Apophysitis of the Os Calcis (Sever's Disease)

Sever's disease (calcaneal apophysitis) is a traction apophysitis and should be considered in any young dancer with open physes (growth plates) who complains of heel pain. The calcaneal apophysis is located in the posterior calcaneus, oriented perpendicular to the long axis of the tuberosity. It first appears on radiographs at ages 4–7 years in females and 4–10 years in males; it does not fuse until an average age of 16 years. The Achilles tendon inserts along the posterior calcaneal tuberosity, and the plantar fascia on the plantar medial tuberosity [28, 29]. The diagnosis is particularly common in Irish step dancers, and seen in both males and females [40]. The dancer may complain of heel pain in the morning, pain with jumping, on heel strike when walking, and with percussive movements. Radiographs are often negative, but fragmentation or widening of the growth plate may be present. Physical exam findings include tenderness to palpation over the apophyseal calcaneal growth plate and posterior heel, pain with medial and lateral squeeze test of the calcaneus, weakness of ankle dorsiflexion, and contracture of the Achilles tendon [24].

Treatment includes avoidance of painful activities, and in most cases use of a removable walking boot cast for three weeks, plantar fascia night splint for sleeping, and gentle Achilles stretches along with ankle dorsiflexion resistance band strengthening. The young dancer may need to continue use of the night splint for sleep and wearing a cushioned supportive shoe outside of class for an additional 4–6 weeks as symptoms subside. Return to dance includes relative rest, such as avoidance of jumps and other painful maneuvers, until symptoms are resolved.

Ankle

Ankle Sprain

Ankle sprain is the most frequent traumatic injury in dancers, and may be related to the increased time dancers spend weight bearing in ankle plantar flexion, a highly unstable position for the ankle joint. Rolling over the lateral border of the foot while on pointes or demi-pointe, or landing poorly from a jump, is the usual mechanism of injury. In most ankle sprains, the lateral ligaments are injured, especially the anterior talofibular ligament (ATFL). The ATFL is injured when the ankle is in plantarflexion; the calcaneofibular ligament (CFL) is injured when the inversion occurs with the ankle (foot) in dorsiflexion (or neutral) position. It is important to note that in younger dancers with open growth plates there is a higher risk of physeal injury or fracture rather than ligamentous disruption. Any tenderness of the distal fibula should be assessed for possible distal fibula fracture or physeal (growth plate) injury. It is well recognized that the greatest risk factor for an ankle sprain is a previous inversion injury, and those dancers with a cavus foot type and varus heel also have higher inversion injury risk [42–46].

Findings on examination include tenderness to palpation over the anterolateral ankle ligaments, swelling, and ecchymosis. Laxity on ankle drawer testing may be present, but must be compared to the contralateral ankle. Any tenderness over the fibula, sinus tarsi, or fifth metatarsal should alert the clinician to obtain foot and ankle radiographs. A computed tomography (CT) scan or magnetic resonance imaging (MRI) scan should be obtained to identify possible osteochondral injury to the talus or occult fracture if symptoms have not started to improve in one week. In cases of recurrent sprains, AP stress views of both ankles can help quantitate the degree of instability, with 5° difference between sides considered significant.

The majority of sprains resolve with conservative management. Early functional treatment of ankle sprains is recommended. Compression bandage, brief icing, ankle air-stirrup brace in athletic shoes outside of class, and limited class participation are instituted as pain allows. Severe sprains may require use of a removable walking boot cast for 3 weeks. The boot should be removed for icing and range-of-motion exercises, and worn for walking and sleeping until pain resolves (not more than 3 weeks). McCormack et al. observed that dancers with generalized hypermobility have a more prolonged recovery from soft tissue injuries than non-hypermobile dancers [47, 48].

Attention to strengthening, edema control, and range of motion and proprioception exercises are needed for rehabilitation from an ankle sprain. Ballet dancers require full mobility of their hindfoot, midfoot, and ankle joints to dance en pointe. Failure to restore posterior talar glide and full ankle dorsiflexion following ankle sprain may lead to posterior ankle impingement [49]. The insufficient ATFL allows the talus to translate forward in the ankle mortise in the plantar flexed position, resulting in impingement of bone and/or soft tissues in the posterior ankle joint. It is important in dancers to encourage work on attaining full dorsiflexion at the tibiotalar joint following an ankle sprain; therapists should be encouraged to assist the dancer in achieving posterior talar glide and restoration of subtalar joint mobility with manual therapy.

Dancers often have a very flexible ankle and a moderately or highly arched (cavus) foot. Subtle hindfoot varus may be present, increasing the prospect of re-injury. Studies have found dancers and athletes with previous ankle sprain have impaired dynamic postural control (more postural sway than controls or uninjured dancers). Even after return to full professional dance or sport participation, and without complaints of instability, measurable differences in postural sway can be demonstrated [42–46].

Work on the entire kinetic chain is crucial for full recovery. Core strengthening, proprioception, and proximal hip strengthening exercises should be included in any dancer's rehabilitation from ankle sprain, in addition to fibularis longus and brevis muscle strengthening. Work on unstable surfaces and balance tasks with eyes closed will assist return of proprioception and full function. Practicing relevés in parallel position with a tennis ball held between the malleoli can help the injured dancer retrain ankle strength and motion in a neutral ankle joint position, avoiding sickling during relevé [21].

Osteochondritis Dessecans

Osteochondritis dessecans of the talus is an injury or abnormality of the articular cartilage and subchondral bone of the talar dome. In the ankle, an osteochondral lesion on the talus is an area of subchondral bone with poor blood supply and inflammation, osteonecrosis, and delamination, with an abnormality of the overlying articular cartilage. Theories regarding the cause include repeated microtrauma, multiple ankle sprains, and genetic factors. A history of trauma is implicated in 75–94% of patients, less often in posteromedial lesions. Lesions may be bilateral in up to 10% of cases. Exact incidence is unknown, but is estimated to occur in 40–70% of cases after ankle sprain. Age at presentation is most commonly the second decade, but ranges from age 10 to 40. Symptoms typically include deep ankle pain with weight bearing activities, stiffness, and limited range of motion. Catching, clicking, locking, and swelling may occur. MRI is the best study for suspected lesions, as they may be difficult to identify on radiographs. These dancers should be referred to an orthopaedic foot and ankle specialist for treatment. Initial treatment in adolescents involves casting in removable boot, crutches, and non-weight bearing in an attempt to heal the lesion if not displaced [50–52].

Ankle Impingement Syndromes

Posterior Ankle Impingement

The term "posterior ankle impingement" is used to describe any painful condition due to compression of soft tissues or bone between the posterior edge of the tibia and the calcaneus, typically when the ankle is in plantar flexion. A normal ossification center is located at the posterior aspect of the talus. It usually appears at 9–12 years of age and fuses 1 year after its appearance. If it does not fuse with the talus, an ossicle develops, known as the os trigonum [29]. This ossicle or a large posterior lateral process of the talus called a Steida process are the usual sources of bony impingement (Fig. 9.3a, b). While it may be seen at any age, most commonly this problem presents in the adolescent dancer. Flexor hallucis longus (FHL) tenosynovitis secondary to an impinging os trigonum is also reported in dancers, and should be suspected in any dancer with posterior ankle pain [53–63]. An acute fracture of the posterolateral process of the talus can also cause posterior ankle pain [58].

(a) (b)

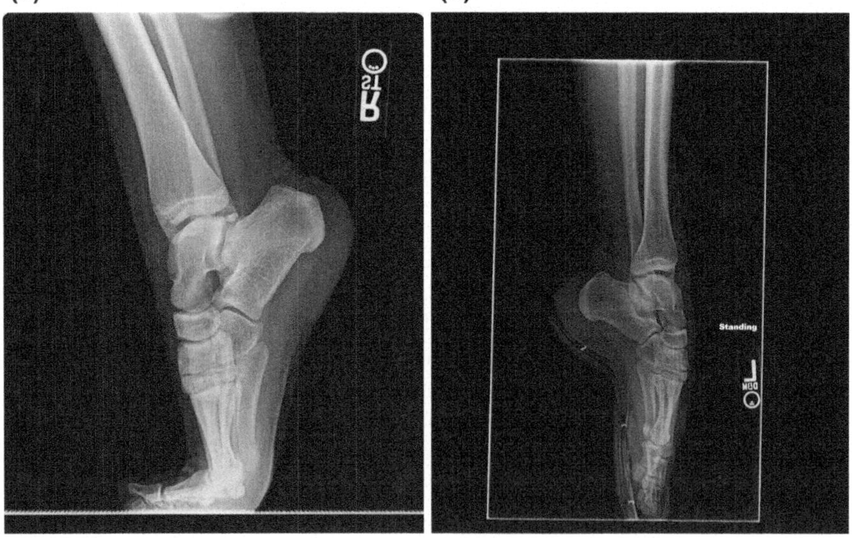

Fig. 9.3 **a** Radiograph of a 13-year-old dancer with posterior impingement and a painful os trigonum. Note that the dancer is unable to achieve full demi-pointe position with weight bearing (i.e., she is unable to align her metatarsals under the tibia or get maximal ankle plantarflexion). **b** Radiograph of a 15-year-old dancer demonstrating the "en pointe" position of the foot. Although this dancer has a prominent Steida process, she had no impingement symptoms at the time of the radiograph, and could easily achieve maximal ankle plantarflexion

Dancers with posterior ankle impingement usually describe pain in the posterolateral ankle behind the fibularis tendons, along with stiffness and limitation in plantar flexion motion. Pain is worse with plantar flexing of the foot, as in tendu and relevé maneuvers. This condition may be mistaken for fibularis or Achilles tendonitis, and may follow an ankle sprain [49]. An affected dancer may have difficulty achieving the full pointe position on the affected side. Swelling and tenderness may be present behind the lateral ankle joint anterior to the Achilles tendon. Dancers with posterior ankle impingement will have a positive *plantar flexion sign*: pain with forced passive ankle plantar flexion with the dancer's knee flexed at 90° will reproduce the symptoms. This test will not be positive in Achilles, fibularis, or isolated FHL tendinitis [53–57, 60–63]. Those with FHL tendonitis and an os trigonum will have posteromedial ankle tenderness and pain with flexion of the great toe against resistance. Palpable crepitus just posterior to the medial malleolus may be found with range of motion of the great toe. Triggering or locking of the great toe may be present [62, 63].

Radiographs in maximal plantar flexion, or with the dancer en pointe, can demonstrate a bony block or os trigonum. MRI is useful to identify bone edema in the posterior talus, os trigonum, and calcaneus, and to demonstrate fluid in the FHL tendon sheath [58, 59]. Relief of pain with an injection of lidocaine posterior to the fibularis tendons can confirm the diagnosis [22, 53, 54]. Treatment consists initially of limitation of painful activities, including pointe work, and physical therapy to encourage strengthening and mobilization of the ankle joint. The dancer should sleep with a night splint to help reduce stiffness and synovitis until symptoms resolve. Intrinsic foot strengthening exercises along with practice pointing the foot with a relaxed calf can reduce symptoms [60]. Surgery to remove the os trigonum and/or release the FHL tendon sheath is reserved for those dancers who fail physical therapy and correction of technical errors. Recovery time after surgery varies, and dancers often have some persistent symptoms for one year, but most return to full participation by 4–6 months. Some dancers find benefit from changing their pointe shoe style and fit.

FHL Tendinitis

Flexor hallucis longus (FHL) tendinitis is common in dancers; hence the term "dancer's tendinitis." While present rarely in other athletes, it is seen most frequently in the female ballet dancer [53, 54, 60–63]. A biomechanical study demonstrated that the muscles crossing the metatarsophalangeal joints work 2.5–3 times harder than those crossing just the ankle joint in dancers rising on to full pointe position, placing these muscles and tendons (FHL, and flexor digitorum longus) at risk for overuse injuries [1]. The repetitive foot transition from full plantar flexion of the en pointe position to plié with the ankle in dorsiflexion can compress the FHL tendon in its fibro-osseous tunnel along the posteromedial talus under the sustentaculum tali, leading to inflammation.

Dancers may complain of posteromedial ankle pain, swelling, or popping. Some dancers develop triggering or locking of the great toe, the result of a nodule forming on the tendon. Crepitus can be palpated at the posteromedial ankle, and pain with resisted flexion of the hallux interphalangeal (IP) joint may be present. Functional hallux rigidus may be present, as demonstrated by a limitation of great toe dorsiflexion with the knee fully extended and the ankle in full dorsiflexion, known as the Thomasen test [63]. FHL inflammation may be present with or without an os trigonum or prominent Steida process; therefore the FHL tendon should be evaluated in any dancer suspected of posterior ankle impingement. Ultrasound and/or MRI are the recommended diagnostic tests.

Conservative treatment including temporary cessation of pointe work and jumps, physical therapy, and anti-inflammatory medication usually resolves the problem. Corticosteroid injection into the FHL tendon sheath may be considered only if done by an experienced ultrasonographer, as a rupture could end a dancer's career. In those dancers with triggering of the hallux or a nodule on the tendon, surgical release of the FHL sheath may be required, as well as in dancers that fail non-operative treatment [62]. Return to full dance participation typically is 3–6 months.

Anterior Ankle Impingement

Anterior impingement in dancers may be a consequence of compression of soft tissues or osteophytes (talar neck and/or distal tibia) in the anterior ankle joint. The osteophytes are proposed to be a consequence of repeated ankle sprains or microtrauma from repetitive impact of loaded dorsiflexion [64–66]. Anterior impingement is more common in male dancers and in dancers with cavus feet. Symptoms of anterior impingement include anterior ankle joint pain with jump landings, plié, and loss of ankle dorsiflexion. Some have pain when descending stairs. Swelling may or may not be present. Tenderness to palpation of the anterior ankle joint is usually found. Pain with passive ankle dorsiflexion can be present, but may be falsely negative in anterior impingement [64, 65].

Radiographs of the ankle and an oblique view of the foot will demonstrate osteophytes. Treatment includes relative activity limitation, including avoidance of jumps and forcing demi-plié, and use of a felt pad under the heel in ballet and street shoes. Physical therapy to correct technical errors such as improper alignment in plié and hindfoot supination, and taping the foot to support the subtalar joint and hindfoot may help to resolve symptoms. A brief trial in a walking boot cast and a night splint for three weeks may help alleviate pain and inflammation. Judicious use of a single intra-articular corticosteroid injection may be tried in select cases, followed by a walking cast for three weeks. If pain persists, surgical treatment with arthroscopic or open debridement of osteophytes and soft tissue may be required [67–69]. Postoperative care, including Pilates, floor barre, and pool exercises (once incisions are healed) should be initiated early, with an increase of dance activity as pain allows. Full pain-free dance participation may take as long as 3–6 months.

Achilles Tendinitis

Achilles problems are commonly seen in adolescent dancers, particularly those who force their turnout, leading to increased pronation in the midfoot and hindfoot, or those with flexible pes planus. Failure of the dancer to land from jumps with his or her heels on the ground also can contribute to contracture of the Achilles tendon and subsequent risk of injury. In young dancers, during periods of rapid growth there is relative tightness and weakness of the gastrocnemius–soleus complex, placing them at increased risk for Achilles tendinitis. Mahieu and colleagues identified plantar flexion weakness and increased dorsiflexion excursion as significant predictors for Achilles tendon overuse injury in one prospective study [70]. Tight ribbons around the ankle in ballet dancers may cause irritation of the tendon; use of elastic ribbons or shoes with elastic sewn into the area over the tendon can reduce pain [21, 22].

Careful stretching and strengthening of the calf muscles and the use of a night splint while sleeping can alleviate most symptoms. Eccentric strengthening exercises, physical therapy with deep tissue massage, or modalities such as Graston technique may be beneficial. For young dancers in a rapid growth phase some reduction in jumps and dance participation may be temporarily required.

Future Directions

Foot and Ankle Injury Prevention for Dancers

Dancers require a balance of overall flexibility and strength, muscular endurance, and control. The adolescent dancer has the added challenge of a growing skeleton, along with complex emotional and hormonal changes. Difficulties experienced by young dancers during periods of active growth include the temporary loss of coordination, flexibility, and strength at a time when skill acquisition is becoming more challenging and training loads are increasing. All of these factors may contribute to foot and ankle injuries in young dancers. As a physician evaluating a young dancer, it is important not only to examine the area of injury but also to look at the entire kinetic chain. Core strength, muscle imbalances, and even leg length discrepancies (not uncommon during periods of rapid growth) may be contributing to a foot or ankle injury. Correction of alignment, technical errors, and muscle imbalances will not only help in rehabilitation from an injury but may prevent future injuries from occurring.

Summary

The young dancer's foot and ankle are subjected to high forces and unusual stresses in training and performance. The foot and ankle are reported to be the most frequently injured areas in adolescent dancers. In addition, the young dancer is at risk for some unique injuries found only in the immature skeleton. Periods of rapid growth are an especially risky time for young dancers, as transient loss of flexibility, coordination, and strength leave them more vulnerable to injury.

Elite adolescent dancers often have a very high performance and rehearsal load, with little time for attention to aerobic fitness and general health. Unlike Little League Baseball, with defined pitch counts by age group, no similar recommended dance load limitations exist [71]. Monitoring practice and performance loads should be considered. Adequate rest, fitness, recovery time, and nutrition are critical to maximize a dancer's healing potential if an injury does occur. Correction of muscle imbalances, attention to proper technique, sequential skill progression, and proper shoe fit may help limit acute injuries to the foot and ankle in a young dancer.

Physicians must not limit their exam to the foot and ankle, but should assess the entire kinetic chain of the dancer. Injury or pain in the foot may predispose the dancer to problems further up the kinetic chain, and these must be addressed for successful return to performance. The physician treating dancers must be sensitive to the fact that even young dancers consider pain and injury a normal part of daily life. In their competitive world, dancers may fear treatments that could result in loss of rehearsal or performance time and possibly dance roles or participation in an upcoming audition. Creativity is needed to build trust with the young dancer, and it is important whenever possible to modify treatment plans to accommodate the dancer's need to maintain strength, flexibility, and fitness during recovery.

References

1. Dozzi P, Winter D. Biomechanical analysis of the foot during rises to full pointe: implications for injuries to the metatarsal–phalangeal joints and shoe redesign. Kinesiology and Medicine for Dance. 1993–1994;16(1):1–11.
2. Galea V, Norman R. Bone-on-bone forces at the ankle joint during a rapid dynamic movement. In: Winter DA, Norman RW, Wells RP, Hayes KC, Patla AE, editors. Biomechanics IX-A: proceedings of the ninth international congress of biomechanics. Champaign, IL; Human Kinetics; 1985. p. 71–6.
3. Russell J, McEwan I, Koutedakis Y, Wyon M. Clinical anatomy and biomechanics of the ankle in dance. J Dance Med Sci. 2008;12(3):75–82.
4. Steinberg N, Aujla I, Zeev A, Redding E. Injuries among talented young dancers: findings from the U.K. centres for advanced training. Int J Sports Med. 2014;35(3):238–44.
5. Steinberg N, Siev-Ner I, Peleg S, Dar G, Masharawi Y, Zeev A, Hershkovitz I. Injury patterns in young non-professional dancers. J Sports Sci. 2011;29(1):47–54.
6. Leanderson C, Leanderson J, Wykman A, Strender LE, Johansson SE, Sundquist K. Musculoskeletal injuries in young ballet dancers. Knee Surg Sports Traumatol Arthrosc. 2011;19(9):1531–5.

7. Gamboa JM, Roberts LA, Maring J, Fergus A. Injury patterns in elite pre-professional ballet dancers and the utility of screening programs to identify risk characteristics. J Orthop Sports Phys Ther. 2008;38(3):126–36.
8. Ekegren CL, Quested R, Brodrick A. Injuries in pre-professional ballet dancers: incidence, characteristics and consequences. J Sci Med Sport. 2014;17(3):271–5.
9. Smith PJ, Gerrie BJ, Varner KE, McCullogh PC, Lintner DM, Harris JD. Incidence and prevalence of musculoskeletal injury in ballet. A systemic review. Orthop J Sports Med. 2015;3(7):2325967115592621.
10. Luke A, Kinney S, D'Hemecourt PA, Baum J, Owen M, Micheli LJ. Determinants of injuries in young dancers. Med Probl Perform Art. 2002;17(3):105–12.
11. Wiesler ER, Hunter DM, Martin DF, Curl WW, Hoen H. Ankle flexibility and injury patterns in dancers. Am J Sports Med. 1996;24(6):754–7.
12. Baxter-Jones A, Maffulli N, Helms P. Low injury rates in elite athletes. Arch Dis Child. 1993;68(1):130–2.
13. Roberts K, Nelson N, McKenzie L. Dance-related injuries in children and adolescents treated in US emergency departments in 1991–2007. J Phys Activity Health. 2013;10(2):143–50.
14. Yin A, Sugimoto D, Martin D, Stracciolini A. Pediatric dance injuries: a cross-sectional epidemiological study. PM R. 2016;18(4):348–55.
15. Davenport K, Simmel L, Kadel N. Hallux valgus in dancers: a closer look at dance technique and its impact on dancers' feet. J Dance Med Sci. 2014;18(2):86–92.
16. Desoille H, Bourguignon A, Chavy AL. Statistical study of the frequency of hallux valgus and of different forms of the foot in classical dancers. Arch Mal Prof. 1960;21:343–9.
17. Einarsdóttir H, Troell S, Wykman A. Hallux valgus in ballet dancers: a myth? Foot Ankle Int. 1995;16(2):92–4.
18. van Dijk CN, Lim LS, Poortman A, Strübbe EH, Marti RK. Degenerative joint disease in female ballet dancers. Am J Sports Med. 1995;23(3):295–300.
19. Kennedy JG, Collumbier JA. Bunions in dancers. Clin Sports Med. 2008;27(2):321–8.
20. Coughlin MJ. Juvenile hallux valgus: etiology and treatment. Foot Ankle Int. 1995;16 (11):682–97.
21. Kadel N. Foot and ankle problems in dancers. Phys Med Rehab Clin N Am. 2014;25(4):829–44.
22. Hamilton WG, Hamilton LH. Foot and ankle injuries in dancers. In: Mann R, Coughlin M, editors. Surgery of the foot and ankle. 7th ed. St. Louis: Mosby Incorporated; 1999. p. 1225–56.
23. Prisk V, O'Loughlin P, Kennedy J. Forefoot injuries in dancers. Clin Sports Med. 2008;27 (2):305–20.
24. Houghton KM. Review for the generalist: evaluation of pediatric foot and ankle pain. Pediatr Rheumatol Online J. 2008;6:6. http://www.ped-rheum.com/content/6/1/6.
25. Bronner S, Novella T, Becica L. Management of a delayed-union sesamoid fracture in a dancer. J Orth Sport Phys Ther. 2007;37(9):529–37.
26. Thompson FM, Hamilton WG. Problems of the second metatarsophalangeal joint. Orthopedics. 1987;10(1):83–9.
27. O'Malley MJ, Hamilton WG, Munyak J. Fractures of the distal shaft of the fifth metatarsal. Dancer's fracture. Am J Sports Med. 1996;24(2):240–3.
28. Frush TJ, Lindenfeld TN. Peri-epiphyseal and overuse injuries in adolescent athletes. Sports Health. 2009;1(3):201–11.
29. Malanga GA, Ramirez-Del Toro JA. Common injuries of the foot and ankle in the child and adolescent athlete. Phy Med Rehabil Clin N Am. 2008;19(2):347–71.
30. Kadel N, Teitz C, Kronmal R. Stress fractures in ballet dancers. Am J Sports Med. 1992;20 (4):445–9.
31. O'Malley MJ, Hamilton WG, Munyak J. Stress fractures at the base of the second metatarsal in ballet dancers. Foot Ankle Int. 1996;17(2):89–94.
32. Micheli L, Sohn R, Solomon J. Stress fractures of the second metatarsal involving Lisfranc's joint in ballet dancers. J Bone Joint Surg Am. 1985;67A(9):1372–5.

33. Kadel N, Boenisch M, Teitz C, Trepman E. Stability of Lisfranc joints in ballet pointe position. Foot Ankle Int. 2005;26(5):394–400.
34. Harrington T, Crichton K, Anderson I. Overuse ballet injury to the base of the second metatarsal a diagnostic problem. Am J Sports Med. 1993;21(4):591–8.
35. Nussbaum AR, Treves ST, Micheli L. Bone stress lesions in ballet dancers: scintigraphic assessment. Am J Roentgenol. 1988;150(4):851–5.
36. Albisetti W, Perugia D, De Bartolomeo O, Tagliabue L, Camerucci E, Calori G. Stress fracture of the base of the metatarsal bones in young trainee ballet dancers. Int Orthop. 2010;34(1):51–5.
37. DellaValle C, Su E, Nihal A, Rosenberg Z, Trepman E. Acute disruption of the tarsometatarsal (Lisfranc's) joints in a ballet dancer. J Dance Med Sci. 2000;4(4):128–31.
38. Kadel N, Donaldson-Fletcher E. Lisfranc's fracture–dislocation in a male ballet dancer during take-off of a jump: a case report. J Dance Med Sci. 2004;8(2):56–8.
39. Gillespie P, Robertson A, George B, Nihal A. Acute Lisfranc joint disruption in a ballet dancer. Foot Ankle Surg. 2005;11(2):105–8.
40. Walls R, Brennan S, Hodnett P, O'Byrne JM, Eustace SJ, Stephens MM. Overuse ankle injuries in professional Irish dancers. Foot Ankle Surg. 2010;16(1):45–9.
41. Schwartz E, Su J. Plantar fasciitis: a concise review. Perm J. 2014;18(1):e105–7.
42. Hiller CE, Refshauge KM, Beard DJ. Sensorimotor control is impaired in dancers with functional ankle instability. Am J Sports Med. 2004;32(1):216–23.
43. Leanderson J, Eriksson E, Nilsson C, Wykman A. Proprioception in classical ballet dancers. A study of the influence of an ankle sprain on proprioception in the ankle joint. Am J Sports Med. 1996;24(3):370–4.
44. Lin C, Lee I, Liao J, Wu W, Su F. Comparison of postural stability between injured and uninjured ballet dancers. Am J Sports Med. 2011;39(6):1324–31.
45. Steib S, Zech A, Hentschke C, Pfeifer K. Fatigue-induced alterations of static and dynamic postural control in athletes with a history of ankle sprain. J Athl Train. 2013;48(2):203–8.
46. Schmitt H, Kuni B, Sabo D. Influence of professional dance training on peak torque and proprioception at the ankle. Clin J Sport Med. 2005;15(5):331–9.
47. McCormack M, Briggs J, Hakim A, Grahame R. A study of joint laxity and the impact of benign joint hypermobility syndrome in student and professional ballet dancers. J Rheumatol. 2001;31(1):173–8.
48. Briggs J, McCormack M, Hakim A, Grahame R. Injury and joint hypermobility syndrome in ballet dancers—a 5 year follow-up. Rheumatology (Oxford). 2009;48(12):1613–4.
49. Moushine E, Crevoisier X, Leyvraz PF, Akiki A, Dutoit M, Garofalo R. Post-traumatic overload or acute syndrome of the os trigonum: a possible cause of posterior ankle impingement. Knee Surg Sports Traumatol Arthrosc. 2004;12(3):250–3.
50. Kennedy JG, Hodgkins CW, Colombier JA, Guyette S, Hamilton WG. Foot and ankle injuries in dancers. Int SportMed J. 2007;8(3):141–65.
51. van Dijk CN, Reilingh ML, Zengerink M, van Bergen CJ. Osteochondral defects in the ankle: why painful? Knee Surg Sports Traumatol Arthrosc. 2010;18(5):570–80.
52. Lynch SA, Renstrom PA. Treatment of acute lateral ankle ligament rupture in the athlete: conservative versus surgical treatment. Sports Med. 1999;27(1):61–71.
53. Hamilton W. Posterior ankle pain in dancers. Clin Sports Med. 2008;27(2):263–77.
54. Hamilton WG, Geppert MJ, Thompson FM. Pain in the posterior aspect of the ankle in dancers: differential diagnosis and operative treatment. J Bone Joint Surg Am. 1996;78A (10):1491–500.
55. Marotta J, Micheli LJ. Os trigonum impingement in dancers. Am J Sports Med. 1992;20 (5):533–6.
56. Kadel N, Micheli L, Solomon R. Os trigonum impingement syndrome in dancers. J Dance Med Sci. 2000;4(3):99–102.
57. Russell J, Kruse D, Koutedakis Y, McEwan I, Wyon M. Pathoanatomy of posterior ankle impingement in ballet dancers. Clin Anat. 2010;23(6):613–21.

58. Robinson P, White LM. Soft tissue and osseous impingement syndromes of the ankle: role of imaging in diagnosis and management. Radiographics. 2002;22(6):1457–71.
59. Peace K, Hillier JC, Hulme A, Healy J. MRI features of posterior ankle impingement syndrome in ballet dancers: a review of 25 cases. Clin Radiol. 2004;59(11):1025–33.
60. Albisetti W, Ometti M, Pascale V, DeBartolomeo O. Clinical evaluation and treatment of posterior impingement in dancers. Am J Phys Med Rehabil. 2009;88(5):349–54.
61. Giannini S, Buda R, Mosca M, Parma A. Di Caprio F osterior ankle impingement. Foot Ank Int. 2013;34(3):459–65.
62. Kolettis GJ, Micheli LJ, Klein JD. Release of the flexor hallucis longus tendon in ballet dancers. J Bone Joint Surg Am. 1996;78A(9):1386–90.
63. Michelson J, Dunn L. Tenosynovitis of the flexor hallucis longus: a clinical study of the spectrum of presentation and treatment. Foot Ankle Int. 2005;26(4):291–303.
64. O'Kane J, Kadel N. Anterior impingement syndrome in dancers. Curr Rev Musculoskelet Med. 2008;1(1):12–6.
65. van Dijk CN. Anterior and posterior ankle impingement. Foot Ankle Clin. 2006;11(3):663–83.
66. Kleiger B. Anterior tibiotalar impingement syndromes in dancers. Foot Ankle. 1982;3(2):69–73.
67. Stretanski MF, Weber GJ. Medical and rehabilitation issues in classical ballet: literature review. Am J Phys Med Rehabil. 2002;81(5):383–91.
68. Nihal A, Rose DJ, Trepman E. Arthroscopic treatment of anterior ankle impingement syndrome in dancers. Foot Ankle Int. 2005;26(11):908–12.
69. van Dijk C, Bergen C. Advancements in ankle arthroscopy. J Am Acad Orthop Surg. 2008;16 (11):635–46.
70. Mahieu N, Witvrouw E, Stevens V, Van Tiggelen D, Roget P. Intrinsic risk factors for the development of Achilles tendon overuse injury: a prospective study. Am J Sports Med. 2006;34(2):226–35.
71. American Sports Medicine Institute. Position statement for youth baseball pitchers updated Apr 2013; http://www.asmi.org/research.php?page=research&section=positionStatement.

Chapter 10
The Use of Diagnostic and Interventional Ultrasound in Treating and Preventing Injuries in the Young Dancer

Sarah Jackson, MD, CSCS and Pierre d'Hemecourt, MD

Pertinent Definitions

Linear high-frequency probe: A higher frequency transducer or probe (10–12 MHz) that provides the best image resolution for superficial structures. It has a limited depth of penetration (<3–4 cm deep).
Curvilinear low-frequency probe: A lower frequency transducer (<7 MHz) that is required to image deeper structures.
Sagittal: A sagittal plane divides the body into right and left.
Axial: An axial plane divides the body top to bottom.
Oblique: An oblique position of the probe is a slanting configuration, or any variation from the perpendicular or horizontal.
In-plane: A term used to describe the position of the needle in relation to the ultrasound probe. The needle enters the skin alongside the probe. It then traverses the plane of the ultrasound, and the whole shaft is visualized as it progresses toward the target.
Out-of-plane: A term used to describe the position of the needle in relation to the ultrasound probe. The needle enters the skin perpendicular to the probe and is aimed at the plane of sound, which is a thin line projected straight out of the center of the probe. With this approach, only the needle tip is visualized and the remainder of the needle is off the screen.
Eccentric muscle contraction: Active contraction of a muscle occurring simultaneously with lengthening of the muscle and increasing joint angle. Eccentric exercises are frequently a part of post-procedure rehab protocols.

S. Jackson, MD, CSCS (✉) · P. d'Hemecourt, MD
Division of Sports Medicine, Department of Orthopedics,
Boston Children's Hospital, 319 Longwood Ave., Boston, MA 02115, USA
e-mail: Sarah.Jackson@childrens.harvard.edu

P. d'Hemecourt, MD
e-mail: pierre.dhemecourt@childrens.harvard.edu

R. Solomon et al. (eds.), *Prevention of Injuries in the Young Dancer*,
Contemporary Pediatric and Adolescent Sports Medicine,
DOI 10.1007/978-3-319-55047-3_10

Hypoechoic: A region in an ultrasound image in which the echoes are weaker or fewer than normal or in the surrounding regions. This shows up as black on the image.
Hyperechoic: Pertaining to material that produces echoes of higher amplitude or density than the surrounding medium. This shows up as white on the image.
Hydrodissection: A technique employing a pressurized fine stream of solution (typically saline, lidocaine, cortisone, or a mixture of these), used to develop tissue planes or to divide certain tissues.

Introduction

The injury incidence rate of young dancers is 0.77–1.55 per 1000 dance hours [1–3]. Many young dancers put in hours of work to take their technique to the highest level achievable, and some are talented and hardworking enough to pursue careers as professionals. Because of this, our job as sports medicine physicians is to push the envelope and remain on the cutting edge of both diagnostic and treatment options to help them maintain their health and longevity throughout their dance careers and beyond. Musculoskeletal ultrasound has been gaining popularity in the field of sports medicine over the past decade [4]. Ultrasound has a wide range of utility and can often be used in settings where other diagnostics cannot due to its ease of portability. Ultrasound can also be used as a modality by physical therapists; however, this type of ultrasound differs greatly from the use of diagnostic ultrasound. Both utilize acoustic or sound waves, though the frequency of the therapeutic ultrasound used to enhance healing is typically between 1.0 and 3.0 MHz, while the frequency used in diagnostic ultrasound ranges between 2.0 and 15.0 MHz. The higher frequencies correlate with a shorter wavelength and are absorbed more easily and therefore do not penetrate through tissues. For this reason high frequencies are used for more superficial structures, and lower frequencies for deeper structures. In this chapter we will discuss the use of ultrasound in both static and dynamic diagnostics as well as to guide a myriad of different treatment options. We will also discuss the use of diagnostic ultrasound in pre-participation examination and how this can help prevent future injuries.

Utilizing Ultrasound for Interventional Assistance in the Dancer

Ultrasound is a convenient and low-risk tool that can be used to aid in the diagnosis of common injuries seen in the adolescent dancer and as imaging guidance for diagnostic and therapeutic injections. In this section we will discuss specific injuries that can benefit from interventions with ultrasound, such as autologous growth factors.

Spine

Back pain and spinal injuries are a common complaint seen in young dancers presenting to sports medicine and orthopedic clinics. Yin et al. [5] showed that 14.5% of injuries in a group of dancers 5–17 years of age occurred in the spine. However, some of these young dancers do not have structural abnormalities after having undergone extensive evaluations, physical therapy, and strength training in an attempt to improve their pain and support the spine. Once conservative measures have failed an ultrasound-guided steroid/anesthetic injection may be useful. This can help to decrease pain and inflammation, as well as localizing the etiology of their pain. The anesthetic response immediately after the injection helps to localize the source of pain. The steroid component is intended to allow the dancer to increase the physical therapy exercises.

One area that responds particularly well to diagnostic and therapeutic injection is the facet joint. These injections should only be attempted by the trained and experienced physician. Facet joint injuries may produce findings on imaging, but often the associated pain is only elicited on physical examination. Ultrasound is used in this case to guide the injection, using a curvilinear (low-frequency) probe placed in the axial plane in the midline of the back over the central spinous process. In this view the central spinous process is seen as the midline with the lamina on either side, in what some refer to as the "pagoda roof." The facet joints lie on the lateral edge of the lamina, as do the transverse processes (Fig. 10.1). Sliding the probe slightly inferior to the lower edge of the facets will bring the transverse processes into view. Using a lateral to medial approach, in the same plane as the probe, a spinal needle can be inserted into the facet joint and anesthetic and steroid

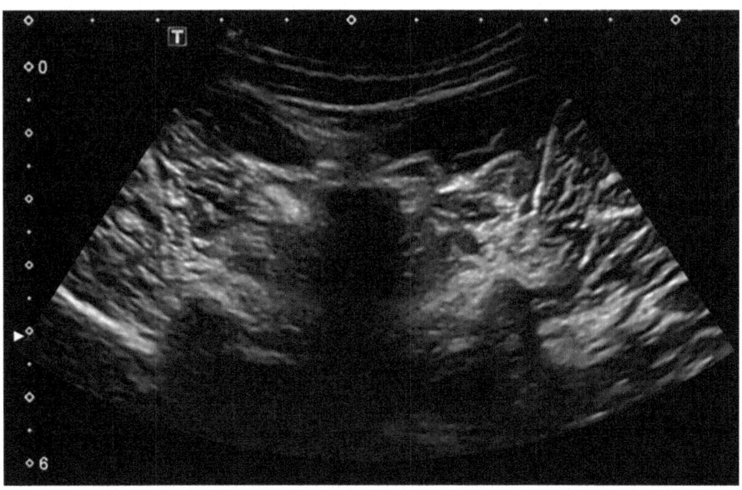

Fig. 10.1 "Pagoda roof" of L5 spinous process with transverse processes and facet joints on either side of the spine

can be injected. Immediately after the procedure facet joint loading with spinal extension and rotation can be performed to assess for pain response to the anesthetic portion of the solution. If complete pain relief is achieved, the physician has confirmation of the specific source of pain and can use this information when making physical therapy recommendations. The steroid portion of the injection can take up to 2 weeks to begin to give relief and will last anywhere from 3 to 6 weeks, allowing the dancer to pursue focused physical therapy.

Similarly, the dancer with interspinous ligament sprain or interspinous bursitis may benefit from a diagnostic and therapeutic injection. Typically, the point of maximal discomfort can be localized by palpating the spinous processes and interspinous spaces to identify the level of the spine at which the dancer is experiencing pain. This injection can be done with the patient prone while lying on a pillow such that the spine is arched into flexion. This will separate the spinous processes, allowing for good visualization under ultrasound. The probe can be placed in the sagittal plane over the midline of the spine, exposing the spinous processes and the interspinous ligaments. For this injection an out-of-plane approach can typically be used to inject anesthetic and steroid just deep to the interspinous ligament. Again, immediately after the procedure, provocative maneuvers such as flexion or extension of the spine can be done to assess for anesthetic response to the injection.

The sacroiliac joint (SIJ) is not an uncommon cause of pain in the young dancer for several reasons. The young female often has more ligamentous laxity than males, and therefore potential instability in the SIJ. Furthermore, the sacrum is more vertical in the female than in the male, which also renders it more vulnerable to instability. Finally, dancers often sustain injuries to the spine, such as spondylolysis. In conditions of this kind the erector spinae, which are the primary stabilizers of the sacrum to pull it forward into a flexed and stable position [6], are inhibited and become weak.

Usually, rehabilitation of the stabilizing muscles is adequate to diminish pain. In some circumstances, however, it is useful from a diagnostic and therapeutic standpoint to perform a diagnostic injection. At times, pain may inhibit proper strengthening, and the corticosteroid may enhance the ability to perform physical therapy. The lower end of the SIJ is most suitable for injection. This is performed with the dancer prone. The posterior superior iliac spine is identified. In the thin dancer a high-frequency linear probe with virtual convexity demonstrates this nicely. The probe is held in an axial plane at the posterior superior iliac spine (PSIS) and slid caudally until the lowest end of the SIJ is seen. Then, from medial to lateral, the area is entered with a 22 spinal needle with an in-plane approach. Visualization of the inferior sacroiliac joint (ISIJ) allows for confirmation of proper placement once the entry has been accomplished. A combination of anesthetic and corticosteroid is used. Provocation maneuvers are performed before and after to assist in confirming the diagnosis of SIJ involvement.

Hip

Hip injuries account for 13.1% of all injuries in the young dancer and can be complex and difficult to treat [5]. Once preliminary diagnostics have been completed, which may include physical examination, plain radiographs, and MRI, ultrasound can be used to examine the hip in both a static and dynamic manner (refer to the hip section in "Diagnostic Ultrasound Examination: Static/Dynamic" for further information on how to perform a static and dynamic examination of the hip). Ultrasound is also used to guide diagnostic and therapeutic injections.

It may be daunting to differentiate between intra-articular and extra-articular causes of the dancer's hip pain. Micheli et al. [7] described three provocative maneuvers for isolating iliopsoas causes of pain. These include pain with passive hip flexion, resisted flexion/abduction/external rotation (FABER) of the hip, and hip extension/internal rotation. Additionally, a Ludloff's test involves pain with resisted straight leg raise with the patient sitting at the edge of the bed and the hip flexed at 90°. Pain with this maneuver is felt to be specifically attributable to the psoas. During these maneuvers a pain score can be obtained from the patient pre- and post-injection. The comparison of "pre-" and "post-injection" scores can be used to identify the etiology of the dancer's pain.

The two main injections used in the hip for both diagnostic and therapeutic value are an intra-articular injection and a psoas bursa injection. Past studies have discussed the use of fluoroscopic guidance of psoas injections [7]; however, more recently ultrasound has been shown to serve this purpose effectively [8, 9]. The psoas bursa injection can be performed in several different ways. Here we will discuss the two most commonly used in our clinical practice. The first method is to have the patient lying supine and placing the probe in the sagittal oblique plane over the hip to visualize the femoral head, neck, and acetabulum (Fig. 10.2). In this plane one can visualize the overlying hip capsule or synovial lining and just superficial to the capsule the psoas muscle/tendon. If the patient has psoas bursitis a hypoechoic, or black layer, will be seen just between the capsule of the hip and the psoas muscle/tendon, representing bursal fluid within the psoas bursa. The injection can then be performed in this plane with an in-plane approach, from distal to proximal, using a spinal needle to inject cortisone and anesthetic into the psoas bursa and the peritendon. The needle tip usually enters the bursa just above the femoral head (see Fig. 10.2). Fluid can be visualized both filling the bursa and washing up through the peritendinous layer. The other approach used for this injection involves obtaining a short axis or axial view of the psoas tendon, which can be done by placing the probe in the direct axial plane of the acetabulum and femoral head with the psoas tendon seen as a hyperechoic or round white structure typically lying in the gutter formed by the acetabulum and the femoral head. Again using an in-plane approach from lateral to medial, the spinal needle can be directed to just beneath the psoas tendon and cortisone and anesthetic can be injected into the pertendinous region as well as the bursa lying below the tendon.

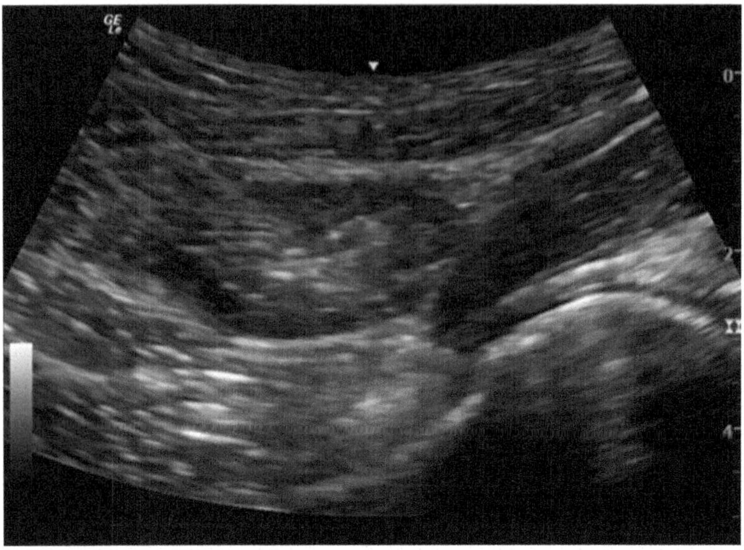

Fig. 10.2 Psoas bursa injection, with probe held in the sagittal oblique plane to visualize the acetabulum, femoral head-neck junction, and overlying psoas tendon. In this image, needle tip is at the level of the psoas bursa just beneath the tendon

The other commonly performed diagnostic and therapeutic procedure performed in the young dancer with hip pain is an intra-articular injection. This injection is typically used prior to surgery for either femoral acetabular impingement (FAI) or labral repair. Many dancers will have labral tears or other pathologic findings on MRI. However, this may not be the source of pain in all cases. One study showed that elite female ballet dancers with pathologic findings on MRI were symptomatic in less than two thirds of the cases [10]. Another study demonstrated that in a group of professional ballet dancers 51% had labral pathology on MRI that was asymptomatic [11]. A diagnostic and therapeutic intra-articular injection can be used to determine whether the dancer may benefit from surgical repair or if the etiology of their pain is due to other extra-articular sources.

The intra-articular injection is performed in a similar fashion to the psoas bursa injection described above with a sagittal oblique view. In this plane one can visualize the femoral head-neck junction, the overlying hip capsule, and the synovial lining. The probe is then slid back and forth medial to lateral to find the midpoint of the femoral head-neck junction. The injection can then be performed in this plane, using an in-plane approach, from distal to proximal. However, the needle is aimed at the femoral head-neck juncture in this case. (Fig. 10.3). Prior to injection of solution confirmation of intra-articular location can be achieved by turning the probe 90° into the axial plane to visualize the needle at the femoral head-neck junction beneath the capsule, or synovial lining. Once confirmation of intra-articular location is established the probe is turned back to the sagittal oblique

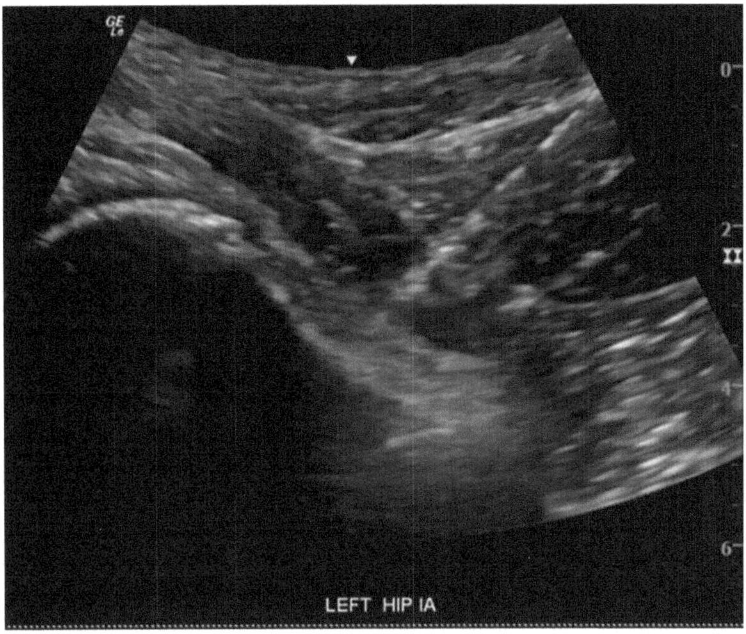

Fig. 10.3 Intra-articular hip injection with probe over the left hip in a sagittal oblique view to visualize the femoral head-neck junction and overlying hip capsule

plane and solution can be injected, watching for the fluid to fill the intra-articular space as the capsule fills.

After any of the above procedures are performed "post-injection" scores should be obtained to determine whether the injection did in fact target the etiology of the dancer's pain. This information can then be used to guide further management.

Knee

Even more common than hip and spine injuries are knee injuries in the adolescent dancer, with a reported rate of 28.8% [5]. The use of ultrasound to both diagnose and treat certain etiologies of knee pain in dancers has been slowly becoming more evidence based. In the section "Diagnostic Ultrasound Examination: Static/Dynamic," we will discuss how to perform the static and dynamic knee examination. In this section we will discuss the interventional uses of ultrasound in the knee.

One source of knee pain commonly seen in the young dancer is medial plica syndrome. This is an area where injection under ultrasound guidance can be used to confirm the diagnosis and to treat the inflammation and improve pain. This injection is performed with the patient lying supine with the knee slightly bent to about 20°

and the leg externally rotated to allow for the medial aspect of the knee to be easily accessed. The high-frequency, or linear, probe is placed in the axial plane, with the patella visualized on one side of the screen and the medial femoral condyle on the opposite side of the screen (Fig. 10.4). Using palpation to locate the plica and area of maximal pain, the probe can be slid distal and proximal until the plica is well visualized between the medial patellar facet and the medial femoral condyle. Then, using an out-of-plane approach, a needle can be dropped directly down adjacent to the plica and cortisone and anesthetic agent can be injected. Immediately after the injection the patient should perform previously determined provocative movements to assess for resolution of pain from the anesthetic portion of the injection.

Similarly, young dancers may have medial knee pain due to Hoffa's fat pad impingement. In this case injection can be performed with the patient supine with the knee flexed to 90° and the foot planted on the table. Then, placing the probe in the axial plane over the patellar tendon, the fat pad can be well visualized below the tendon. Depending on whether the dancer's pain is more medial or lateral, a corresponding approach can be used to concentrate more of the injection at the area of increased discomfort. For medial sided pain a needle can be inserted using an in-plane approach, from medial to lateral, just deep to the patellar tendon, being careful to avoid injecting too closely to the tendon itself. Cortisone and anesthetic can then be injected directly into the fat pad. In some cases the dynamic examination of the patellar tendon's relation to the fat pad is performed by flexing and extending the knee while directly observing the fat pad. It would be abnormal for the fat pad to adhere to the patellar tendon. When it does, a hydrodissection to loosen the fat pad from the tendon is required. This procedure can be performed with the patient in the same position as that used for the fat pad injection; however,

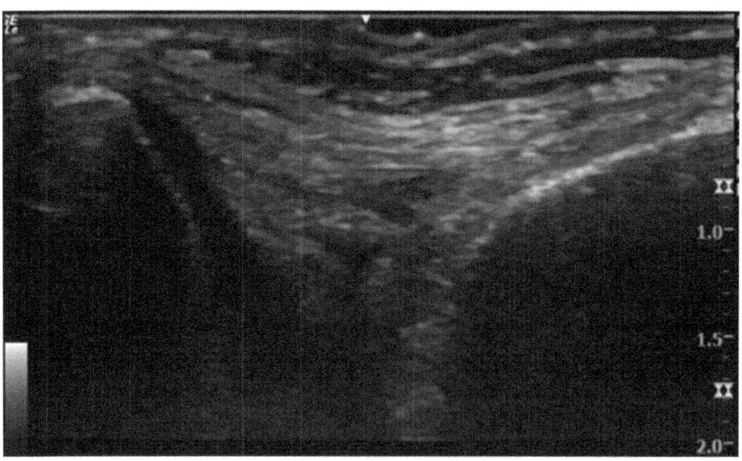

Fig. 10.4 Medial plica seen here with medial facet of the patella on the *left* and medial femoral condyle on the *right*, with hyperechoic area between representing plica

this time as the tendon is visualized in the axial plane the probe is moved obliquely in a diagonal plane, pointing medial to lateral, from distal to proximal. Then, using an in-plane approach, the needle is placed just beneath the patellar tendon and superficial to Hoffa's fat pad. Saline, anesthetic, or a combination of the two can be injected to hydrodissect the fat pad away from the tendon. (Cortisone is never used for this injection site.) This allows the tendon to glide more smoothly without impinging on the fat pad.

Given the amount of rotational force placed on the knee of the young dancer, meniscus injuries can occur. Typically, in young dancers with a moderate to large tear, surgical meniscal repair is recommended, given their age and ability to heal well after a repair. Minor tears or small areas of degeneration seen on either MRI or ultrasound examination, on the other hand, have recently been found to respond well to ultrasound-guided needle fenestration of the meniscus followed by injection with autologous growth factors such as platelet-rich plasma (PRP) or whole blood. Our early experience with this has been encouraging. Further studies in this area are needed. The procedure is performed with the patient in the supine and slightly decubitus position. The high-frequency linear probe is placed in the coronal plane to visualize images of the affected meniscus (medial or lateral). The probe is slid from posterior to anterior to visualize the meniscus between the femoral condyle superiorly and the tibial plateau inferiorly. Using an out-of-plane approach, a 22 to 25-gauge needle is used to make 8–10 fenestrations into the meniscus, injecting small amounts of PRP with each fenestration. The needle is then inserted just between the meniscus and the meniscofemoral ligament if that area is affected, and PRP can be injected between these layers. The patient is then placed in a hinged knee brace with specific limitation in flexion and extension, depending on which horn of the meniscus was fenestrated. Typically, we use a long-hinged knee brace for 2 weeks locked from 0 to 30° of flexion, then 2 weeks at 0–60°, and then progress to full ROM. During this time the patient is also started on physical therapy, consisting of mostly isometric exercises for the first 2 weeks and progressing through increased range of motion as the brace range is increased.

Patellar tendinopathy can be very difficult to resolve, especially once degenerative changes have occurred. When a hypoechoic area has been identified and all conservative management has been exhausted, needle tenotomy with whole blood injection can be performed. This is done with the dancer lying in the supine position, the knee bent to between 45 and 90° of flexion, and the foot placed on the table. A high-frequency linear probe is placed in the axial view to visualize the hypoechoic area of tendon degeneration, typically seen near the proximal insertion at the distal pole of the patella (Fig. 10.5a, b). Using an out-of-plane approach, a 22-gauge needle is inserted through the tendon into the area of degeneration (Fig. 10.5c). Depending on the extent of injury, a number of fenestrations are made to include the entire width and depth of the affected area. Typically, small aliquots of whole blood or PRP are injected with each fenestration. After the procedure is performed the dancer is placed in a knee immobilizer for a few days to control pain, but then mobilized using isometrics and biking for the next 2 weeks. During the third and fourth weeks dynamic exercises, both open and closed chain, and added resistance on the stationary bike can be initiated. Eccentrics are added gradually.

Ankle

Dance is often performed in the plantar flexed position and can lead to impingement of both soft tissue and bony structures, particularly in the posterior ankle between the tibia and calcaneus. Some dancers will have a prominent Stieda process of the posterior talus, while others will have a discrete os trigonum. These conditions are reported to occur in up to 14% of the general population, and when present they are bilateral in 50% of patients [12]. We have a clinical impression that the incidence of os trigonum in dancers is much greater than that of the general population. Diagnosis can be made with a plain lateral radiograph with the dancer in full plantar flexion (en pointe). Ultrasound can be used in this case to perform guided diagnostic injection to confirm the source of pain and help with surgical planning. For this injection the patient is normally lying prone with the foot hanging just off the end of the table. The high-frequency, or linear, probe is placed in the sagittal plane in line with the Achilles tendon and slid out to the lateral ankle. As the Achilles

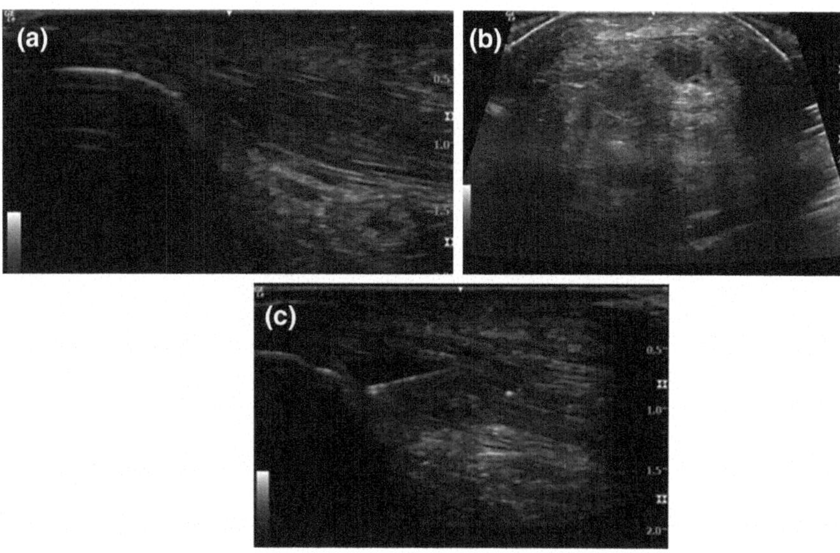

Fig. 10.5 **a** Long axis view of patellar tendon (probe held in direct sagittal plane) with hypoechoic area of degenerative tendon on insertion into patella. **b** Short axis view of patellar tendon (probe held in direct axial plane) with hypoechoic area of degeneration, which correlates with area as shown in Fig. 10.5a. **c** Long axis view with needle in degenerative area during needle tenotomy

goes out of view, the stedia process or os trigonum comes into view, with the calcaneus distal to that. It is sometimes difficult to differentiate between a prominent stieda process and os trigonum with ultrasound, as the bone has acoustic shadowing that may make it difficult to identify. A needle can then be inserted in the in-plane or out-of-plane approach down to the level of the stieda process/os trigonum, and cortisone and anesthetic solution can be injected to encompass the object in question and any surrounding soft tissue while avoiding any vascular or tendon structures. Immediately after this injection is performed provocative movements can be initiated, typically forced plantar flexion, to assess for resolution of pain.

Another typical etiology of ankle region pain in a dancer is subtalar joint pain. There are three facets of the subtalar joint: anterior, middle, and posterior. The largest and most commonly associated with pain in the dancer is the posterior facet [12]. This area can be injected for both diagnostic and therapeutic value, using three different approaches: anterolateral, posterolateral, and posteromedial [13]. In our current practice we normally use the anterolateral approach, which will be described here. The patient is placed in the lateral decubitus position with the lateral aspect of the affected ankle facing up and the leg propped on a towel roll, allowing the foot to invert slightly. Using the linear, or high-frequency, probe placed in the sagittal plane in line with the distal end of the fibula to visualize the calcaneus, the probe is then moved slightly anterior to visualize the lateral aspect of the posterior subtalar joint. Using an out-of-plane approach, the needle is inserted into the subtalar joint and a combination of cortisone and anesthetic is injected. One can confirm that fluid has reached the facet by placing the probe posteriorly. Provocative maneuvers can be performed before and after injection of the anesthetic as the diagnostic portion of the examination.

In terms of tendinitis, such as flexor hallucis longus, tibialis posterior, Achilles, or peroneal tendinitis, ultrasound is used as a diagnostic imaging technique and sometimes for guidance of injections. Due to the risk of tendon rupture with steroid, these injections are reserved as a last resort and would be followed by a period of restricted activity and slow return to dance. The dancer puts great stress and relies on these important tendons for support throughout a majority of movements in dance, and therefore cortisone injections around these structures, especially in the younger/adolescent age group, should be avoided (see the ankle and foot sections in "Diagnostic Ultrasound Examination: Static/Dynamic" for further information regarding diagnostic ultrasound of the ankle and foot).

One particular diagnosis that can be improved with cortisone injection with hydrodissection is crossover syndrome. Crossover syndrome is described as stricture that occurs as the flexor hallucis longus (FHL) crosses the flexor digitorum longus (FDL) and passes through a retinacular structure at the plantar midfoot, known as the Knot of Henry. This occurs in dancers due to repetitive forefoot push off and forced plantar flexion performed in most forms of dance, especially classical ballet. This injury is best visualized with the dancer lying in the lateral decubitus position with the medial side of the affected foot exposed. A high-frequency linear probe can first be placed in an axial plane just posterior to the medial malleolus to visualize its edge, and then moved from anterior to posterior to visualize the tibialis posterior, the FDL, and the FHL tendons. Focusing on the FHL, the probe can be turned 90° to visualize the FHL tendon in a long axis view and then slid distally to follow the FHL as it dives deep to cross the FDL at approximately the level of the navicular bone. Once a good view is obtained of this crossover of the FHL and FDL, the 1st toe can be passively flexed and extended, looking for movement of the two tendons along each other. If there is a stricture or inflammation in this area the tendons may appear to be stuck down and will not have easy motion with this movement. It is in this view that a 22-gauge needle can be inserted between the FHL and FDL to hydrodissect the transition point with a mixed solution of cortisone and anesthetic, while being careful not to inject directly into either tendon. After the hydrodissection is complete, this dynamic examination can be repeated.

Another common cause of ankle pain in the young dancer is a ganglion off the FHL in the posterior ankle. Occasionally, persistence of symptoms will require the need to aspirate the ganglion and inject a small volume of corticosteroid. The FHL sheath can also become stenotic, causing a "trigger"-type sensation in the posterior ankle, similar to a trigger finger. This can be treated with a hydrodissection of the FHL from the sheath. This should be done in the off season to avoid tendon injury. A further concern about this injection is the neurovascular structures on the medial side of the ankle. Attention to these is mandatory during injection.

Similar to patellar tendinopathy, Achilles tendinopathy can be recalcitrant to conservative management. If a hypoechoic area of degeneration is seen (Fig. 10.6a, b), whole blood needle tenotomy can be performed in a similar fashion to that described above for the patellar tendon (refer to the ankle section in "Diagnostic Ultrasound Examination: Static/Dynamic" for diagnostic ultrasound of the Achilles tendon). This can be performed with the dancer lying in the prone position with the feet hanging just off the edge of the examination table. Prior to the tenotomy and whole blood injection, a sural nerve block can be performed, also under ultrasound guidance, to help with anesthesia, in addition to local anesthetic, which is used with

(a) (b)

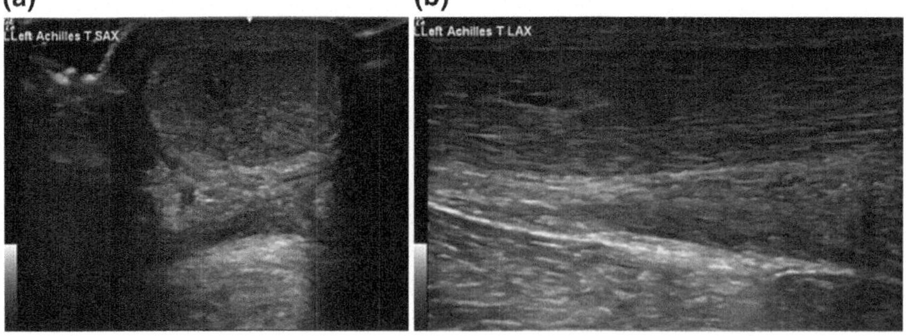

Fig. 10.6 **a** Short axis view with the probe placed in a direct axial plane over the Achilles tendon. Small hypoechoic area represents area of degenerative tendon. **b** Long axis view with the probe placed over the Achilles in the direct sagittal plane, again visualizing hypoechoic area of degeneration

all procedures. The linear, high-frequency probe is placed in the axial view to visualize the hypoechoic area of tendon degeneration. Using a 22-gauge needle in an out-of-plane approach, the needle is inserted through the tendon into the area of degeneration. Adequate fenestrations are made to cover the width and depth of the hypoechoic areas while constantly injecting small aliquots of blood. During these fenestrations the probe can be repetitively turned 90° into the sagittal plane to confirm placement. After the procedure is performed the dancer is placed in a walking boot for the first 2 weeks. During that time the patient starts physical therapy, focusing mostly on isometric exercises, passive range of motion, and stationary biking with no resistance. In the second week active range of motion can be added. During the third and fourth weeks dynamic exercises, both open and closed chain, and added resistance on the bike can be initiated. The fifth and sixth weeks include eccentric strengthening exercises and gradual addition of plyometric exercises.

Foot

Morton's neuroma is a common cause of foot pain in dancers. Typically, MRI has been used to diagnose these injuries, and many clinicians will do blind cortisone injections in attempting to help with relief of pain and inflammation. However, one recent study has shown that ultrasound can diagnose a Morton's neuroma in 85% of cases [14]. While other studies show that MRI does have higher sensitivity, it does have a false negative of 17%, and ultrasound can be used to confirm the diagnosis [15]. To evaluate for a Morton's neuroma the patient is commonly placed in the prone position with the plantar surface of the foot facing the examiner. The linear, or high-frequency, probe is placed in the axial plane to visualize the intermetatarsal space at which the patient is experiencing symptoms. The metatarsals are identified and then scanned proximally and distally. The normal appearance of the interdigital space is homogenous hyperechoic tissue, representing fatty tissue. Morton's neuroma is identified when a hypoechoic or anechoic mass is seen within that space. The probe can then be turned 90° to visualize the neuroma in the sagittal plane, allowing for measurements to be taken in two dimensions. Not only can ultrasound be used to aid in the diagnosis, but it can also help guide more accurate injections of cortisone to help decrease inflammation and pain. When performing a cortisone injection to this area the probe is typically held in the axial plane, and then, using the out-of-plane approach, the needle is placed between the digits deep into the fat pad which overlies the metatarsal head and cortisone and anesthetic agent can be injected to surround the neuroma while being careful not to inject the fat pad with steroid to avoid fat necrosis.

Given the amount of time a dancer is placing the foot in demi-pointe with forced extension of the 1st metatarsal phalangeal (MTP) joint or bearing a significant amount of body weight through the 1st toe while on pointe, the amount of inflammation and degenerative changes that can take place even in the young dancer is not surprising. In this age group we frequently see capsulitis of the joint, but tend not to see arthritic or degenerative changes until dancers are into their 20s. For the dancer with recalcitrant pain and inflammation in the 1st MTP joint, we can perform ultrasound-guided cortisone injections. With the dancer lying in the supine position with knee bent and the foot placed flat on the bed, the linear, high-frequency probe is placed in the sagittal plane, in line with the 1st MTP joint. Sliding the probe distally, the 1st MTP joint will come into view. Then, using an out-of-plane approach, the needle can be dropped into the joint space and a solution of anesthetic and cortisone can be injected into the joint. Normally, a total of 1–2 cc can be injected; however, this space is small and may only be able to accommodate about 1 cc of fluid total.

In the more advanced degenerative joint in the slightly older dancer we have also been using PRP to inject into the joint. If PRP is used, this is usually done at least twice, about 2 weeks apart. Both injections are followed by 5–7 days of relative rest without dancing and gradual return to physical therapy.

Diagnostic Ultrasound Examination: Static/Dynamic

Hip

As described above, hip injuries in dancers are quite common and can be difficult to diagnose. Ultrasound has recently provided a way to help improve the diagnosis of hip injuries by allowing the clinician to perform both a static examination and a dynamic examination of the hip joint and surrounding soft tissue structures. Ultrasound examination allows for assessment to be performed actively in the position of pain and at the point of tenderness [16, 17]. Ultrasound can also be used in a pre-participation physical examination to assess for possible predisposing factors such as instability or structural variants that may lead to injuries. This information can then be used either to modify a dancer's movement or to provide information to physical therapists or instructors to guide rehab and strength training to prevent injury or further damage.

First, the static examination of the anterior hip is performed with the patient lying supine with the hip exposed. Either a high- or low-frequency probe may be used, depending on the thinness of the dancer. The probe is placed in the direct sagittal plane, laterally of the hip, to visualize the anterior inferior iliac spine (AIIS) and the attachment of the rectus femoris tendon as well as the acetabulum. In this view the morphology of the AIIS can be graded, which has been shown to correlate with hip range of motion [18]. Three variants of AIIS have been described, based on the relationship between the AIIS and the acetabular rim. With Type I there is a smooth ilium wall without bony prominence between the AIIS and the acetabular rim. Type II has bony prominences on the ilium wall extending to the acetabular rim but not below, and appears as a "rooflike" prominence over the hip. A type III AIIS extends below the anterior–superior acetabular rim. Type II and III variants have been shown to be associated with decreased hip flexion and internal rotation [18].

Next, the probe is moved to the sagittal oblique plane to visualize the femoral head-neck junction and the acetabulum superiorly. Maintaining this view, the dancer's leg is then internally rotated to 20°. In this view the femoral head-neck offset is evaluated for a possible CAM lesion, which often lies on the superior lateral femoral neck. One study has shown better reliability of ultrasound as a modality to diagnose CAM impingement when compared to both MRI and plain radiographs [19].

Then, the probe is placed in the direct axial plane to visualize the psoas tendon lying in the gutter between the femoral head and the acetabulum. While maintaining this view, the dancer's hip is brought up into flexion, as close to 90° as possible, and internally rotated by the examiner to assess for impingement of either the femoral head-neck junction on the acetabulum, or soft tissue or labrum becoming impinged between the femoral head and the acetabulum. Also, while maintaining this view one can evaluate for snapping psoas tendon. The dancer actively flexes at the hip, abducts, and then extends the leg back down in one smooth motion. During this motion the psoas tendon can be seen moving laterally into the belly of the iliopsoas muscle, and then, as the leg is extended back down and into neutral, the tendon snaps back into place. This is typically also felt, and possibly heard, by the dancer and/or examiner.

Stability of the hip joint can also be assessed from this anterior view. Hip instability can be a factor contributing to pain or predisposing to injury [20]. Dancers tend to be quite flexible from years of stretching and training but also due to natural selection; those at high levels tend to have exceptional ligamentous laxity. Anterior instability is usually experienced in extended and externally rotated positions, such as in développé. To assess for anterior hip stability the probe is first placed over the hip in the sagittal oblique plane to visualize the femoral head and the acetabulum. Scanning from medial to lateral the highest point of the femoral head is determined, and at that point an image is taken and a horizontal line from the tip of the acetabulum is drawn across the femoral head. This is used as the neutral position. Typically, the line will be at the level of the femoral head; however, if it is not, the distance above or below that line can be measured. Next, the dancer is moved to the edge of the table, allowing the leg to be brought into extension and external rotation by the examiner. Concurrently, the dancer is asked to hold the contralateral leg in a flexed position, thereby neutralizing the pelvis. This is commonly referred to as the "apprehension position" (Fig. 10.7a, b). In this position another still image is taken of the acetabulum and the femoral head at the high point. A line is again drawn horizontally out from the rim of the acetabulum, and the amount of anterior excursion of the femoral head above the acetabular rim can be measured using the neutral image as a reference point.

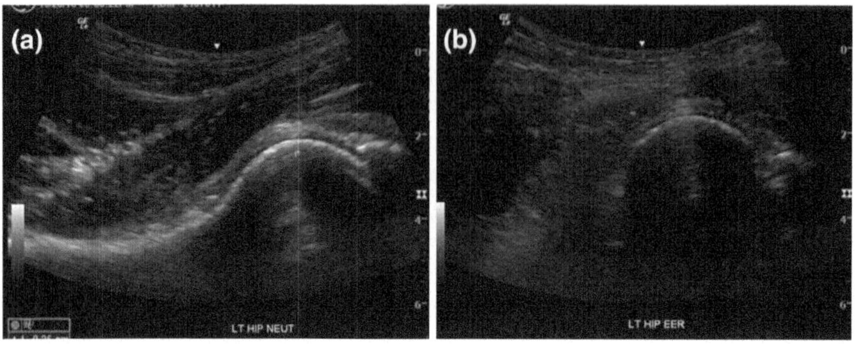

Fig. 10.7 Hip instability examination. **a** A hip in the neutral position (patient lying supine with legs extended on the table) with the femoral head lying just above the rim of the acetabulum. **b** A hip with instability and anterior excursion of the femoral head >2 mm above the level of the acetabulum (patient lying at the edge of the bed with the leg brought into extension and external rotation by the examiner)

Knee

Similar to the hip ultrasound examination portions of the knee examination can be done statically, while others are performed in a more dynamic way to evaluate for movement or adhesion of certain structures. One structure that is well visualized with ultrasound is the meniscus; in one recent study ultrasound was two times more likely than MRI to correctly diagnose presence or absence of meniscal pathology seen arthroscopically [21]. A high-frequency linear probe is first placed in the coronal plane along the medial joint line starting at the posterior portion of the joint to visualize the tibial plateau and medial femoral condyle, with the posterior horn of the medial meniscus lying between. The probe is then moved anteriorly in a radial manner along the joint line. The meniscus is evaluated for irregularities or hypoechoic areas that are evidence of tears. Then, turning the probe 90° into the axial plane, the meniscus can be visualized. The probe can be slid proximally to visualize the femoral condyle and distally to visualize the tibial plateau, confirming visualization of the meniscus. Scanning posterior to anterior the entire medial meniscus can be visualized, again assessing for irregularities or hypoechoic areas, taking axial radial images. The same two views can then be performed for the lateral meniscus. However, for the lateral meniscus the distal border will be the fibular head for a portion of the examination.

Next, the patellar tendon can be evaluated in cases of anterior knee pain consistent with patellar tendinitis, or "jumper's knee". With the dancer lying supine, the knee is placed in flexion, ranging from 30 to 45°, with a towel roll supporting the leg [22, 23]. First, the linear, high-frequency probe is placed over the patellar tendon in the sagittal plane to visualize the attachment of the tendon to the distal pole of the patella, scanning medial and lateral to view the broad attachment site. Measurements can be taken of the thickness or depth of the patellar tendon at its insertion. The probe is then slid distally to visualize the entire length of the patellar tendon as it inserts onto the tibial tubercle. During this maneuver the examiner is also looking for hypoechoic areas consistent with tendon degeneration, or tendonopathy. A normal patellar tendon should have a fibrillar echoic appearance. Next, the probe is turned 90° into the axial plane, and the patellar tendon is scanned starting proximal at the distal pole of the patella down to its insertion, again looking for hypoechoic areas.

While evaluating the patellar tendon in the sagittal plane, Hoffa's fat pad is seen just deep to the tendon. The examiner can flex and extend the dancer's knee while visualizing the proximal end of the patellar tendon and Hoffa's fat pad below, and assess for possible adhesion of the fat pad to the tendon. There is currently no published data on this; however, in our clinical experience we have noticed that this adhesion may be contributing to anterior knee pain seen with fat pad impingement, and hydrodissection of the fat pad from the tendon, as described above, has helped to improve outcomes.

Ankle

Refer to the ankle section of "Utilizing Ultrasound for Interventional Assistance in the Dancer" for a description of static and dynamic examination of the posterior ankle, including Achilles examination and posterior impingement, as well as medial ankle examination, including tibialis posterior, FDL, and FHL tendons as they course behind the medial malleolus and through the medial plantar aspect of the foot. In addition to the views of the medial ankle described above, one can follow the FHL tendon in the long axis view all the way to its distal insertion at the base of the 1st MTP between the two sesamoids. At this level dynamic examination can also be performed by passively flexing and extending the 1st toe at the MTP joint to visualize possible strictures or adhesion of the FHL tendon to the sesamoids or surrounding soft tissue.

Static ultrasound examination of the lateral ankle can also be performed to help with diagnosis of inversion ankle injuries. To assess lateral ankle sprains of the anterior talofibular ligament (ATFL), calcaneofibular ligament (CFL), and then posterior talofibular ligament (PTFL), first the linear, high-frequency probe is placed over the lateral ankle, in line with the fibula. While visualizing the fibular proximally and the calcaneus distally the CFL can be seen as a hyperechoic structure between the two bony structures. Injury to this ligament can be seen as hypoechoic areas, thickening of the ligament, or surrounding hypoechoic fluid. Then, sliding the lower end of the probe into the slightly oblique perspective as the talus comes into view, the ATFL can be seen just above the fibula and attaching onto the talus. Next, the probe is slid directly back into the sagittal plane over the CFL, and then, again, the lower end of the probe is obliqued posteriorly to visualize the posterior aspect of the talus, and the PTFL is seen between the fibula and the talus.

The peroneal tendons can be assessed by placing the probe in the sagittal plane just posterior to the lateral malleolus or distal fibula, and the peroneus brevis and peroneus longus are seen. The peroneus brevis is closest to the fibula, with the perometatarsal and then theneus longus just posterior to it. Following these two tendons in the long axis view the peroneus brevis can be followed to its attachment at the base of the fifth metatarsal, and then peroneus longus as it crosses the cuboid on the lateral foot and then under the plantar surface of the foot to its attachment at the proximal head of the first metatarsal and the medial cuneiform. The course of each of these two tendons can also be visualized starting at the lateral malleolus in the axial view and followed in the short axis view. While scanning these two tendons one will assess for abnormalities such as hypoechoic areas of tendon degeneration or more commonly surrounding hypoechoic fluid indicative of tendinitis.

A dynamic examination of the peroneal tendons can be performed to assess for possible subluxation. With the probe in the axial plane to visualize the distal fibula and the peroneal tendons posterior to the fibula, the dancer is asked to dorsiflex actively and evert the ankle against resistance, while the examiner watches for movement of the tendons anteriorly out of the groove. Peroneal subluxation can be associated with previous injury to the lateral ankle causing weakness or injury to the superior peroneal retinaculum and/or a shallow groove. In a dancer with recurrent subluxation of the peroneal tendon tears within the tendons should be considered, which can be seen during the above-described ultrasound examination.

Foot

Static ultrasound examination can be useful in the diagnosis of plantar fascia abnormalities as well. With the dancer lying prone with the knee bent at 90° and the plantar aspect of the foot fully visualized, the linear, high-frequency probe is placed in the sagittal plane over the calcaneus and slid distally to visualize the insertion of the plantar fascia at the distal end of the calcaneus. In this long axis view of the plantar fascia one can assess for bony irregularities of the calcaneus at the attachment site and hypoechoic areas within the fascia as signs of degenerative changes. The thickness of the fascia can also be measured in this plane, with measurements of greater than 5 mm indicating abnormal thickening of the fascia. Next, the probe is turned 90° to the axial plane to again assess for degenerative changes and measure thickness of the fascia.

Pre-Participation Ultrasound Examination

Several pre-participation ultrasound examinations of the dancer may help to predict injury and focus pre-habilitation in the following areas. Further studies are being performed to assess the utility of these examinations.

Hip: Instability and CAM Impingement

The hip stability examination that is described in the section "Diagnostic Ultrasound Examination: Static/Dynamic," as a portion of the dynamic hip ultrasound examination, can be done during the pre-participation physical. If a dancer is found to have significant laxity or anterior excursion of the femoral head >2 mm (see Fig. 10.7a, b), then that dancer can be given focused strengthening, posterior chain, and core stabilizer exercises to support the hip, while focusing on obtaining a neutrally aligned pelvis.

A CAM deformity may also be detected with the anterolateral sagittal oblique view of the hip, as noted in the spine section of "Utilizing Ultrasound for Interventional Assistance in the Dancer." It is not known whether this deformity will predispose to injury, but its detection may be useful information in the dancer with hip pain.

Patellar Tendinopathy

As part of the pre-participation physical an ultrasound examination of the patellar tendon can be performed (described in the knee section of "Diagnostic Ultrasound Examination: Static/Dynamic"). In one study of asymptomatic athletes 21.7% had positive findings of tendinosis on ultrasound examination [23]. These findings should alert the physician to the risk of tendinosis. Additional follow-up, including specific exercises and injury prevention strengthening programs, can be initiated.

References

1. Ekegren CL, Quested R, Brodrick A. Injuries in pre-professional ballet dancers: incidence, characteristics and consequences. J Sci Med Sport. 2014;17(3):271–5.
2. Gamboa JM, Roberts L, Maring J, Fergus A. Injury patterns in elite pre-professional ballet dancers and the utility of screening programs to identify risk characteristics. J Orthop Sports Phys Ther. 2008;38(3):126–36.
3. Leanderson C, Leanderson J, Wykman A, Strender L, Johansson S, Sundquist K. Musculoskeletal injuries in young ballet dancers. Knee Surg Sports Traumatol Arthrosc. 2011;19(9):1531–5.
4. Sharpe RE, Nazarian LN, Parker L, Rao VM, Levin DC. Dramatically increased musculoskeletal ultrasound utilization from 2000 to 2009, especially by podiatrists in private offices. J Am Coll Radiol. 2012;9(2):141–6.
5. Yin AX, Sugimoto D, Martin DJ, Stracciolini A. Pediatric dance injuries: a cross-sectional epidemiological study. PM R. 2016;8(4):348–55.
6. DeRosa C, Porterfield V. Anatomical linkages and muscle slings of the lumbopelvic region. In: Vleeming A, Mooney V, Rob Stoeckart R, editors. Movement, stability and lumbopelvic pain: integration and research. Edinburgh: Churchill Livingstone; 2007: pp. 47–62.
7. Micheli LJ, Solomon R. Treatment of recalcitrant iliopsoas tendonitis in athletes and dancers with corticosteroid injection under fluoroscopy. J Dance Med Sci. 1997;1(1):7–12.

8. Nazarian LN. Musculoskeletal ultrasound: applications in the hip. J Dance Med Sci. 2011;15 (4):173–6.
9. Adler RS, Buly R, Ambrose R, Sculco T. Diagnostic and therapeutic use of sonography-guided iliopsoas peritendinous injections. Am J Roentgenol. 2005;185(4):940–3.
10. Duthon VB, Charbonnier C, Kolo FC, Magnenat-Thalmann N, Becker CD, Bouvet C, et al. Correlation of clinical and magnetic resonance imaging findings in hips of elite female ballet dancers. Arthroscopy. 2013;29(3):411–9.
11. Mayes S, Ferris A-R, Smith P, Garnham A, Cook J. Similar prevalence of acetabular labral tear in professional ballet dancers and sporting participants: Clin J Sport Med. 2016;26 (4):307–13.
12. Rathur S, Clifford PD, Chapman CB. Posterior ankle impingement: os trigonum syndrome. Am J Orthop (Belle Mead NJ). 2009;38(5):252–3.
13. Smith J, Finnoff JT, Henning PT, Turner NS. Accuracy of sonographically guided posterior subtalar joint injections: comparison of 3 techniques. J Ultrasound Med. 2009;28(11):1549–57.
14. Quinn TJ, Jacobson JA, Craig JG, van Holsbeeck MT. Sonography of Morton's neuromas. Am J Roentgenol. 2000;174(6):1723–8.
15. Torres-Claramunt R, Gines A, Pidemunt G, Puig L, de Zabala S. MRI and ultrasonography in Morton's neuroma: diagnostic accuracy and correlation. Indian J Orthopaedics. 2012;46 (3):321.
16. Chow AHL, Morrison WB. Imaging of hip injuries in dancers. J Dance Med Sci. 2011;15 (4):160–72.
17. Jacobson JA. Ultrasound in sports medicine. Radiol Clin North Am. 2002;40(2):363–86.
18. Hetsroni I, Poultsides L, Bedi A, Larson CM, Kelly BT. Anterior inferior iliac spine morphology correlates with hip range of motion: a classification system and dynamic model. Clin Orthop Relat Res. 2013;471(8):2497–503.
19. Lerch S, Kasperczyk A, Berndt T, Rühmann O. Ultrasound is as reliable as plain radiographs in the diagnosis of cam-type femoroacetabular impingement. Arch Orthop Trauma Surg. 2016;136(10):1437–43.
20. Kalisvaart MM, Safran MR. Microinstability of the hip-it does exist: etiology, diagnosis and treatment. J Hip Preserv Surg. 2015;2(2):123–35.
21. Cook JL, Cook CR, Stannard JP, Vaughn G, Wilson N, Roller BL, et al. MRI versus ultrasonography to assess meniscal abnormalities in acute knees. J Knee Surg. 2014;27 (4):319–24.
22. Cassel M, Baur H, Hirschmüller A, Carlsohn A, Fröhlich K, Mayer F. Prevalence of Achilles and patellar tendinopathy and their association to intratendinous changes in adolescent athletes. Scand J Med Sci Sports. 2015;25(3):e310–8.
23. Toprak U, Ustüner E, Uyanık S, Aktaş G, Kınıklı GI, Baltacı G, et al. Comparison of ultrasonographic patellar tendon evaluation methods in elite junior female volleyball players: thickness versus cross-sectional area. Diagn Interv Radiol Ank Turk. 2012;18(2):200–7.

Chapter 11
Nutrition, Bone Health, and the Young Dancer

Derrick D. Brown, MSc

Pertinent Definitions

Epiphysis: The articular end of a long bone, which during growth is separated from the bone shaft by an area of cartilage.
Macronutrients: Carbohydrate, protein, and fat are the three macro (large) nutrients that the body needs from food in order to function.
Micronutrients: Vitamins and minerals are the micro (small) nutrients that the body relies on for multiple functions. Examples of micronutrients include vitamins, like folate and beta-carotene, and minerals, such as calcium and iron.
Osteogenic: The process that occurs during bone remodelling that allows for the production of new bone.
Periosteum: A fibrous sheath that covers bones, usually thicker in children than in adults.

Introduction

Dance is a beneficial activity for children and adolescents. Similar to sport, it can provide growing bodies with many physiological benefits. For example, targeted exercises such as hops and skips in non-dancing children seem to improve bone growth over a prolonged period [1]. Dance affords additional opportunities for

D.D. Brown, MSc (✉)
Institute of Sport Science/Dance Science, University Bern,
Bremgartenstrasse 145, 3012 Bern, Switzerland
e-mail: derrickdutch@gmail.com

D.D. Brown, MSc
National Centre Performing Arts Onderlangs 9, 6812 CE Arnhem, The Netherlands

R. Solomon et al. (eds.), *Prevention of Injuries in the Young Dancer*,
Contemporary Pediatric and Adolescent Sports Medicine,
DOI 10.1007/978-3-319-55047-3_11

aesthetic development: urban, contemporary styles, classical ballet, and many other genres offer diverse forms of artistic and cultural expression. There are, however, negative consequences that can occur as a result of intense training and performance demands. Extensive studies across a range of dance styles report a high incidence of injuries among adolescent recreational and professional dancers in the spinal region and lower extremities [2–5]. Narratives regarding desirable body types, driven by artistic and fashionable trends, often cause young dancers to attempt to emulate extreme dietary and lifestyle trends, leading to a host of health issues.

Musculoskeletal development and maturation are dynamic interdependent processes encompassing a myriad of factors, not just diet [6]. As shown in Fig. 11.1, physiological, hormonal, mechanical, and genetic factors are contributing influences. Nutrition in particular forms a crucial link to successful growth and maturation. For example, there is consistent and convincing evidence describing the positive effect of calcium and vitamin D on bone accretion during youth [7, 8]. Total bone health, however, is complex, encompassing a diverse spectrum of nutrients, hormonal development, and injury history. Nutritional imbalance coupled with severe long-term restriction of nutrients can lead to lifelong health complications.

Growth, and subsequently maturation, can be seen in three subtly connected phases: infancy, childhood, and puberty [9]. While all three are equally important, dance training generally begins during late childhood into puberty; thus, information regarding the latter two phases will form the core content of this chapter. Firstly, the chapter presents an evaluation of the distribution and determinants of injury in dancers. Next, a topical view of bone growth and maturation is discussed. Finally, the interface between bone health and nutrition will be addressed, concluding with a consideration of hormones and bone health.

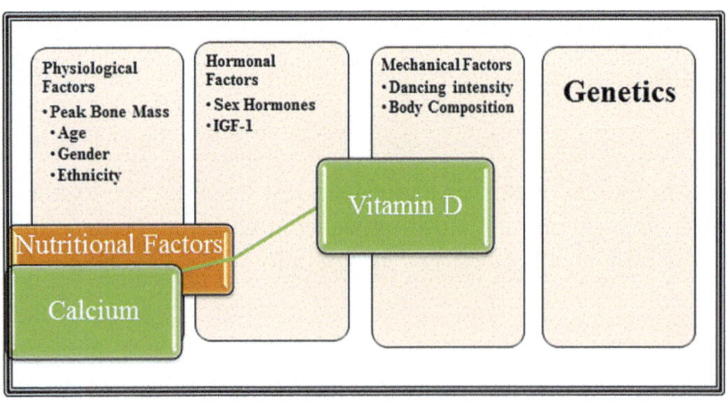

Fig. 11.1 Factors that influence bone health

Epidemiology/Scope of the Problem

Physical and artistic demands are often at odds in the dance profession. When analyzing trends and patterns seen in dancers, most studies observe the distribution and determinants of varying rates and types of injuries. Research reveals a surprising comparison of injury rates; 4.4 injuries per 1000 h in dancers [3] versus 4.1/1000 h in contact sports [10]. Cheerleading is an example of an aesthetic sporting activity, which contains a great deal of dancing. An estimated 208,800 children from 5 to 18 years of age were treated in US hospital emergency departments for cheerleading-related injuries between 1990 and 2002 [11]. Similarly, in a recent retrospective study spanning 17 years, researchers reported that more than 113,084 children with dance-related injuries were treated in US emergency departments [12]. The data revealed that 55% of dance-related injuries occurred in "classical dance" genres (ballet, tap, jazz, and modern). Adolescent dancers (15–19 years) constituted 40% of the injuries, and research in adult dance populations is comparable [13, 14], extending the observation that dance is not without physical risk.

Physical activity enhances skeletal formation and bone mineral density (BMD) [15], yet in professional dancers and other artistic athletes an open question is whether dance activities retard skeletal growth and maturation [16–18]. Physical examination via anthropometry and physiological assessments via specialized scans are established methods of measuring skeletal development and maturation. Israeli researchers determined the body structure and adipose tissue distribution of 1482 female dancers aged 8–16 years compared with a control group of 226 non-dancer girls [19]. Fourteen anthropometric measurements across 15 indices recorded significant difference related to the extent and distribution of adipose tissue. At age 8, both groups showed similar weight, while at age 13, non-dancers were significantly heavier than dancers (48.4 ± 9.8 and 40.6 ± 8.7 kg, respectively). At age 15, weight differences between the two groups decreased to only 2 kg. Moreover, adipose tissue distribution at menarche was 13 years among dancers and 12 years in non-dancers. The researchers concluded that any concerns about dance retarding growth and maturation were negligible, as the differences could be a consequence of "teacher selection".

Anthropometry provides physicians and health care professionals with a macroscopic view of the body. However, physiological changes that occur in dancers are due in part to the intensity of their training combined with negative energy balance. Low BMD is a chronic condition often seen in both genders, which is modifiable via balanced nutritional intake. Dual energy X-ray absorptiometry (DXA) techniques offer an effective means of evaluating the influence of diet and the consequence of intense dance activity by measuring changes in lean tissue, bone mineral content, and fat across key body areas. DXA is generally considered a suitable method for examining and studying children because this technique contains low irradiation and negligible time needed to perform the scans [20].

Several observational studies have utilized DXA to ascertain bone health in adolescent dance populations. In one of the most comprehensive studies to date,

Burckhardt and colleagues, during an internationally renowned ballet competition for pre-professional dancers, examined 127 female participants with average age of seventeen [21]. Using DXA scans, they conducted assessments for body mass index (BMI), bone mineral content (BMC), and bone mineral apparent density (BMAD) at the lumbar spine and femoral neck. Additionally, pubertal stage (Tanner score), psychometric data gathered via the EAT-40 questionnaire, and a self-reported three-day dietary record were collected. The results revealed that BMI for age was on average normal in only 43% of the dancers, while 16% had a more or less severe degree of thinness (12.6% Grade 2 and 3.1% Grade 3 thinness via Tanner scores). For 117 participants, the average age for menarche was late, 13.9 years, with 10 participants found to have primary amenorrhoea, and one secondary amenorrhoea. In terms of diet, the results revealed that food intake, evaluated by the number of consumed food portions, was below the recommendations for a normally active population in all food groups except animal proteins, where the intake was more than twice the recommended amount. Most of the population was in the final stages of their pre-professional education. Thus, their daily activity would qualify as high intensity, intermittent training [22]. In this group, with low BMI and intense dancing, BMC was low and associated with nutritional factors; dairy products having a positive and non-dairy proteins a negative influence, highlighting the adaptable influence of nutrition.

While DXA to date has been the gold standard by which bone health is assessed, it should be interpreted with some caution. The areal or surface density measured is the quantity of BMC per cm^2, which means that bigger bones have greater surface bone density with a comparable real volumetric BMD (g/cm^{-3}). Larger differences are seen in African Americans than in Caucasian American populations [23]. This difference in measurement can be avoided by combining areal BMD with bone and body size-corrected BMC [24]. A recent systematic review of bone health in dancers demonstrated that large discrepancies in methodology complicate ascertaining how large the low BMD problem is in female dancers [25]. Thus, more consistency across studies is needed. Clinical studies have begun to explore the use of computed tomography together with high-resolution magnetic resonance imaging, which offers a three-dimensional depiction of the microarchitecture of both cortical and cancellous bone compartments [26].

Bone Growth and Maturation

During the first 18 months of life, a child will develop approximately 25% of peak bone mass, and by the age of 18, approximately 90% of total peak bone mass has been gained. The last 10% occurs in the final phases of maturation, leading to a fully ossified skeleton, which can happen at any time in the subsequent 10 years, depending on the gender and genetics of the individual [27]. The addition of weight-bearing exercise during puberty confers maximum bone accretion, interconnecting with hormonal development as the child matures. Growth hormone

(GH), insulin-like growth factor-1 (IGF-1), and sex hormones all have effects on bone accretion [28]. Another hormone, leptin, via leptin receptors found in bone, has been suggested as a good biomarker to assess pubertal delay in a young ballet dance population [16]. Adolescence is a period of rapid development towards building adult skeletal strength and thus becomes the key growth phase when discussing physical activity. In girls, the years before menarche provide advantageous osteogenic benefits resulting from weight-bearing physical activity, particularly with regard to bone modelling.

In childhood and throughout adolescence, bones are sculpted by a process called modelling, which allows for the growth of new bone at one site and the removal of old bone from another site within the same bone. Three key principles determine bone remodelling: cellular responses that are mutually dependent on strain, load, and frequency of stimulus—i.e., dynamic (not static) loading—which exerts the strongest bone adaptation response, and as bone cells tend to favour routine movement, variation of stimulus is important to elicit a consistent level of response [29]. Hence, regular weight-bearing physical activity is a modifiable behavior that enhances bone health during growth, and possibly reduces risk of fracture in later life [15]. Research into classical dancers who perform a myriad of repetitive dance steps of short duration has pointed to an osteogenic effect on weight-bearing sites of the skeleton [30], which might help dancers who started ballet early avoid bone problems later in life [31].

When discussing bone maturation in children, two additional concepts are important: plasticity and elasticity. Bones in children allow for a greater degree of deformation than do adult bones before they break. Plastic deformation characterizes bone that deforms but does not fracture [32]. Thus, low modulus of elasticity in growing bones means the bone can be angled beyond its elastic limit without producing a fracture. The periosteum, a fibrous sheath that covers bones, is much thicker in children than in adults and acts as a restraint to displacement. The thick periosteal sleeve is important for paediatric skeletal remodelling. Because of it angular deformation of a child's bone may cause a fracture of the cortices without displacement.

The epiphysis, the rounded end of a long bone, is a secondary ossification site in the growing skeleton, making it sensitive to trauma. Epiphysis development is of crucial concern in all young dancers but particularly in female dance students who wish to pursue a career in classical dance, where they will be called upon to transfer their body weight and balance on the tips of their toes in pointe shoes. This manoeuvre can lead to overuse injuries seen frequently in classical dancers [4]. The fusion of the epiphyses generally occurs earlier in the foot than the leg. From age five through age 12 the average girl's foot grows 0.9 cm (0.35 in.) per year, reaching an average foot length of 23.2 cm (9 in.) at age 12. Hence, the recommendation from physicians to dancers and their support team is to start pointe training around that age, with the caveat that all bodies develop at different rates [33]. During the dynamic growth spurts bones generally lengthen more rapidly than the musculotendinous junctions. Restriction of the muscle tendon units equates to more traction stress on the growing tissue at the insertion point. When coupled with the demands of dance technique proficiency, repetition of many dance steps can cause inflammation and microavulsions at the bone–cartilage junction [34]. Dancers are susceptible to working long hours rehearsing similar movement patterns across dance choreographies. Insufficient time to recover, nutrient deficient diets, and inadequate caloric intake when compared to energy expenditure can ultimately lead to avoidable overuse injuries [35].

During maturation in adolescence bone continue to grow in length and width, as well as to increase in cortical thickness. There is a substantial increase in bone mass and bone density during this period. These processes are interdependent and are influenced by internal factors both genetic and hormonal, and external factors such as nutrient intake and physical demands placed on the system. Gender differentiation, for example, has traditionally been seen as a non-modifiable factor, as males typically have a longer pre-pubertal growth period and in puberty their growth spurt occurs up to 18 months later than in girls, which translates to different skeletal proportions in the lower extremities [36]. Children with intersex disorders, or those who opt for gender reassignment, may be an exception.

Regardless, a convincing factor crucial to successful bone maturation is nutrition. The remodelling of bone is a coordinated relationship between endocrine and nutritional physiology via cell signalling proteins, cytokines, as well as circulating hormones, parathyroid hormone (PTH), insulin-like growth factor 1 (IGF-1), and calcitonin, a naturally occurring hormone that helps to regulate calcium [8]. Additionally, vitamin D is ultimately converted to its biologically active form 1,25-dihydroxyvitamin D (1,25-OH2-D), which stimulates calcium absorption in the intestine. Both calcium and vitamin D are continually emphasized for their role in growth and maturation in children and will be covered later in more detail. While physical activity does confer positive gains in skeletal health, dance as a specific form of exercise is not without its challenges, as discussed below.

Nutrition and Bone Development in Young Dancers

It should be clear that a balanced diet is important for growth, achieving good health, and providing for the basic energy needs in developing youth [37, 38]. Performance nutrition in the context of dancing enhances physical and artistic performance by decreasing fatigue and the risk of disease and injury [39]. Balancing energy intake with energy expenditure is crucial for preventing an energy deficit or excess. Energy deficits may cause delayed puberty, menstrual dysfunction, decreased muscle mass, and increased susceptibility for fatigue or injury [40], while energy excess can result in needless weight gain [41]. We classify the foods we eat into two broad categories: macronutrients and micronutrients. Macronutrients include carbohydrates founds predominately in foods such as vegetables, baked goods and fruit, fats from foods such as butter and olive oil, and protein from foods such as meat, eggs, and/or plant-based sources. Micronutrients are the vitamins and minerals in our food.

Macronutrients

Dietary fats, carbohydrates, and proteins are the basic building blocks from our food that are converted into substances needed for energy, growth, and repair and maintenance of bodily structures. Fats are naturally found in animal and plant foods and provide an abundant source of fuel for energy, which we use mainly when the body is inactive. Carbohydrates, converted into simple and complex sugars, also contain a rich source of energy and are quickly broken down in the body to provide a rapid energy source to the muscles [22]. Proteins, both animal- and plant-based, contain amino acids which form the building blocks of most cells and tissues in the body: hair, muscle, organs, nails, and even tears. A balance in protein ingestion is important to bone health, as imbalance can affect urinary calcium retention or excretion [42]. A classification of macronutrients can be seen in Table 11.1.

Micronutrients

An entire spectrum of micronutrients is important for maturation. Successful bone health requires adequate intake of these micronutrients and the metabolic bioavailability of calcium and vitamin D [8], which is detailed below.

Table 11.1 Classification of macronutrients

	Carbohydrates		Fats	Proteins
Forms	Complex	Simple	Fats, triglycerides, three fatty acid chains, the alcohol glycerol	Amino acids
	Polysaccharides (starches)			
	Disaccharides (sucrose, lactose)	Monosaccharides (glucose, fructose)		
Use in the body	Easily available, preferred energy for physical activity Energy 17 kJ/g (4 kcal/g)		Key form of storage Provides insulation of body tissue and nerve fibres. Maintains cellular structure, hormones Energy 39 kJ/g (9 kcal/g)	Tissue growth and repair. Production of antibodies, enzymes, haemoglobin Energy 17 kJ/g (4 kcal/g) more utilised in the absence of sufficient carbohydrates and/or fats
Food sources	Fruits, vegetables, tubers and starchy edible roots, sugar based foods, refined foods		Plant based (avocado, nuts, vegetables oils) Animal based (dairy, butter, meats)	Plant based (peas, legumes, pulses) Animal based (meats, seafood, eggs, dairy)

Calcium

During the first year of life, calcium intake predominately comes from human milk, or if that is not available an infant-based formula alternative. After year one, the major source of dietary calcium in the USA is derived from dairy-based products. Table 11.2 provides an overview of calcium sources from animal, vegetarian, and vegan sources [43]. Calcium is a key to bone remineralization. The adult human body contains about 1000–1500 g of calcium, and depending on gender, race, and general body size up to 99% is found in bone as hydroxyapatite, a naturally occurring mineral form of calcium apatite. Studies in children and adolescents have shown that ingestion of calcium-enriched foods enhances the rate of bone mineral acquisition and peak bone mass [44, 45]. In a study that assessed calcium balance across 34 studies pooled by age group, Matkovic and Heaney [46] determined an optimal threshold intake of 1500 mg/d for children, adolescents, and young adults.

Vitamin D

Vitamin D is a key micronutrient involved in bone health. The distinctiveness of vitamin D is that it is one of the few known nutrients dependent on sunlight for synthesis in the human body. Approximately 85–90% of vitamin D is formed in the skin following sunlight exposure; the remaining amount is obtained from the diet. The skeletal and endocrine systems are inexorably linked. The skeleton functions to protect vital organs and support movement, and it also, via the endocrine system, plays a role in regulating energy metabolism. Vitamin D exerts considerable influence on the metabolism of micronutrients Ca and phosphorus, as well as key bodily organs: intestine, bone, and kidney. The active metabolite, 1,25(OH)2vitamin D3 (calcitriol), facilitates active Ca absorption in the intestine. Moreover, vitamin D is central to bone turnover, and a suboptimal intake of this nutrient during childhood and adolescence can contribute to BMD decrement.

It is a generally accepted premise that vitamin D is a key micronutrient involved in the regulation of many skeletal and extra-skeletal cellular processes of importance in physical performance. Athletic performers, however, may be subject to vitamin D concentrations below 50 nmol/L [47], and research in adolescent and adult dance populations reveals similar areas for improvement. Wolman et al. [48] studied a group of nineteen UK-based elite classical ballet dancers over a six month period for 25-hydroxyvitamin D. During the winter all 19 dancers were either insufficient (n = 14) or deficient (n = 5) in serum 25(OH)D, and in the summer months only three dancers had normal serum 25(OH)D. In a pilot study of young male dancers in Australia aged 10–19, Ducher and colleagues [49] found similar results, with a group mean of 50.5 nmol/L. While these studies with small cohorts are not generalizable, they do provide a glimpse of the challenges young dancers may face. Notable in both dance studies mentioned is that similar findings were made across genders and,

Table 11.2 Calcium found in foods

Food	Standard portion size	Calories in standard portion	Calcium in standard portion (mg)[a]
Liquids			
Low-fat milk (1%)	1 cup	102	305
Skim milk (non-fat)	1 cup	83	299
Reduced fat milk (2%)	1 cup	122	293
Low-fat chocolate milk (1%)	1 cup	178	290
Reduced fat chocolate milk (2%)	1 cup	190	273
Whole buttermilk	1 cup	152	282
Whole chocolate milk	1 cup	208	280
Whole milk	1 cup	149	276
Evaporated milk	½ cup	170	329
Orange juice, calcium fortified[b]	1 cup	117	349
Soymilk (all flavours)[b]	1 cup	109	340
Almond milk (all flavours)[b]	1 cup	91–120	451
Rice drink	1 cup	113	283
Yoghurt and soft cheeses including dairy alternatives			
Plain yogurt, non-fat	8 oz	127	452
Plain yogurt, low-fat	8 oz	143	415
Vanilla yogurt, low-fat	8 oz	193	388
Fruit yogurt, low-fat	8 oz	238	383
Ricotta cheese, whole milk	½ cup	216	257
Mozzarella cheese, part-skim	1.5 oz	128	304
Hard cheese			
Cheddar cheese	1.5 oz	173	287
Provolone cheese	1.5 oz	149	321
Monterey cheese	1.5 oz	159	317
Muenster cheese	1.5 oz	156	305
Plant-based-calcium rich foods			
Collards, cooked, boiled, drained, without salt	1 cup chopped	62	268
Mustard spinach (tender greens), raw	1 cup	33	315
Tempeh, Raw	½ cup	159	92
Beans, baked, canned, no salt added	1 cup	265	127
Tofu, raw, regular, prepared with calcium sulphate	½ cup	94	434
Seafood			
Sardines, canned in oil, drained	3 oz	177	325

[a]U.S. Department of Agriculture, Agricultural Research Service, Nutrient Data Laboratory. 2014. USDA National Nutrient Database for Standard Reference, Release 27. Available at: http://www.ars.usda.gov/nutrientdata

[b]Calcium fortified

importantly, in different geographic locations. There are several possible reasons for vitamin D deficiency in young dancers, the foremost being that when studying at elite and pre-professional academies most dancers spend considerable time in the dance studio, upwards of 5–6 h a day, and so receive little exposure to sunlight, particularly in the northern latitudes during winter months.

Dietary choice plays a crucial role in micronutrient availability, vitamin D, and Ca, in particular. While a lacto-ovo vegetarian diet appears to offer negligible concerns for vitamin D and Ca deficiency, vegan diets may be more problematic [50]. In particular, risk from fractures in adult vegans appears to be a consequence of lowered calcium intake [51]. Table 11.3 provides an overview of dietary vitamin D from standard and vegetarian diet sources [43]. As dietary patterns fluctuate, particularly in traditionally dairy-rich countries of the West, so do the dietary recommendations from experts in the field [52, 53]. Supplementation is often touted in popular media as a viable choice for vegetarian and vegan diets. There are

Table 11.3 Vitamin D found in foods

Food	Standard portion size	Calories in standard portion	Vitamin D in standard portion (IU)[a]
Liquids/fat			
Milk, low-fat, fluid, 1% milk fat, protein[b, c]	1 cup	119	98
Whole buttermilk	1 cup	152	127
Milk, chocolate, fluid, commercial, whole[b, c]	1 cup	149	276
Milk, evaporated, 2% fat[b, c]	1 cup	270	403
Margarine, regular, 80% fat, composite, stick, with salt[b]	1 tablespoon	100	60
Yoghurt and soft cheeses including dairy alternatives			
Yogurt, fruit, low fat, 9 grams protein per 8 oz[b]	6 oz	169	89
Plant-based—vitamin D rich foods			
Mushrooms, portabella, grilled[d]	1 cup sliced	35	634
Mushrooms, brown, Italian or Crimini, raw[d]	1 cup whole	19	1110
Seafood			
Fish, sardine, Atlantic, canned in oil, drained solids with bone	1 cup	310	287
Swordfish	3 oz	146	566

[a]*Source* U.S. Department of Agriculture, Agricultural Research Service, Nutrient Data Laboratory. 2014. USDA National Nutrient Database for Standard Reference, Release 27. Available at: http://www.ars.usda.gov/nutrientdata
[b]Vitamin D fortified
[c]Vitamin A fortified
[d]Exposed to ultraviolet light

multiple randomized controlled trials purporting to show the benefits of calcium supplementation in otherwise healthy children. Unfortunately, many studies are industry funded, and thus require caution when applying their recommendations [54]. Scant randomized controlled trials have been conducted in large populations of vegetarians and in particular vegans. A recent dietary self-reported study of vegans in Denmark revealed significant deficiencies in vitamin D, Ca, vitamin B12, and iron. Parents of vegetarian and vegan children wishing to provide calcium supplementation should first consult with their primary physicians to discuss the options available.

A complexity with nutrition is that the deleterious effects are often recognized once the problem has become chronic. Figure 11.2 provides an overview of benefits and challenges to bone health. For nutrition to be beneficial, particularly in injury prevention, the body must meet its daily energy needs consistently over time, instead of yo-yo cycles of caloric and nutrient imbalance via extreme dietary restriction. Continuous caloric restriction will limit carbohydrate stored in skeletal muscle and liver as glycogen, which could create problems for physically active individuals [55]. Finally, in children who are picky eaters, lack of financial resources or poor dietary choices can lead to the deficits resulting in chronic conditions.

Nutrition and Hormones

As a close to this chapter, one further subject should be considered, namely the effect of hormones and their connection to nutrition and bone health. Hormones with regard to bone growth were briefly discussed above. Furthermore, a consistent pattern has emerged regarding the negative consequences for skeletal and hormonal health resultant from chronic dietary restriction, amenorrhoea, and disordered eating behavior [30, 56]. Less discussed but equally important are the challenges to

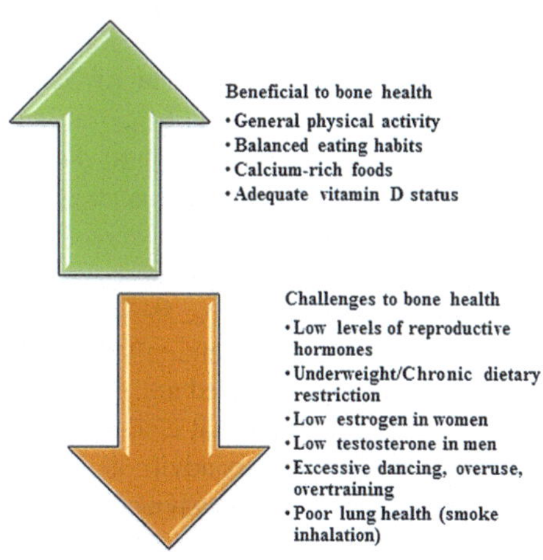

Fig. 11.2 Benefits and challenges to bone health

skeletal health confronting children who, with their parents consent, opt for gender reassignment. Puberty suppression involves the use of gonadotropin-releasing hormone analogues to suppress puberty in adolescents with gender dysphoria [57]. The role of androgens and estrogens in bone metabolism, pubertal bone development, and maintenance of bone mass is well established [40]. Consequently, the surgical and hormonal treatment of male-to-female transsexual adolescents (transsexual girls) could have adverse effects on bone health. Transsexual girls (mean age 14) and boys (mean age 15) have been minimally researched [58]. Key findings in this cohort reveal that from the start of hormone treatment to the age of 22, the lumbar areal BMD z score (for natal sex) in transwomen decreased significantly, and in transmen there was a trend towards decrease, which would suggest that the BMD was below their pre-treatment potential. Gender reassignment challenges are also exacerbated when accompanied by disordered eating challenges [59, 60]. Currently, there are transgender young adults who have entered dance companies and dance academies; we know of them via those who have sought the press to reveal their stories. While there is scant clinical research published on dancers who have completed gender reassignment, there is sufficient anecdotal evidence of reassigned dancers working as professionals to warrant addressing the challenges these future dancers may face with regard to skeletal and hormonal health. Anonymity and gender identity protection are paramount in this vulnerable age group; hence, research has not revealed how many transgender children also dance or the extent of medical and psychosocial support they receive. Thus, for paediatricians, sport physicians, and those involved in primary care a continuous monitoring of bone mass development as well as dietary balance is warranted in this niche group, particularly given the physical and mental demands of these potential dance professionals.

Summary

Adolescence represents a critical stage in a young dancer's life. Many will start dancing at the precarious phase when their bodies acquire more skeletal bone mass. While genetic influences predetermine bone mass to a large extent, external modifiable factors allow for optimized bone mass in childhood. Dance schools that promote a healthy environment for young students via curricula that protect growing bodies are the key. A regular variety of high impact, weight-bearing dancing, along with the promotion of a healthy diet abundant in calcium and vitamin D, provides the best formula for achieving maximal peak bone mass. The recognition by paediatricians of the modifiable factors that influence bone mass in childhood is crucial. As the first line of defence, paediatricians can aid families and dance professionals with evidence-based information regarding how to optimize bone health. Healthy nutritional choices in turn not only enhance performance but also help to protect the skeleton both during and after life on the stage.

References

1. Weeks BK, Young CM, Beck BR. Eight months of regular in-school jumping improves indices of bone strength in adolescent boys and girls: the power PE study. J Bone Miner Res. 2008;23(7):1002–11.
2. Bowerman EA, Whatman C, Harris N, Bradshaw E. A review of the risk factors for lower extremity overuse injuries in young elite female ballet dancers. J Dance Med Sci. 2015; 19(2):51–6.
3. Allen N, Nevill A, Brooks J, Koutedakis Y, Wyon M. Ballet injuries: injury incidence and severity over 1 year. J Orthop Sports Phys Ther. 2012;42(9):781-A1.
4. Leanderson C, Leanderson J, Wykman A, Strender L-E, Johansson S-E, Sundquist K. Musculoskeletal injuries in young ballet dancers. Knee Surg Sports Traumatol Arthrosc. 2011;19(9):1531–5.
5. Steinberg N, Aujla I, Zeev A, Redding E. Injuries among talented young dancers: findings from the UK Centres for Advanced Training. Int J Sports Med. 2014;35(3):238–44.
6. Georgopoulos NA, Markou KB, Theodoropoulou A, Vagenakis GA, Mylonas P, Vagenakis AG. Growth, pubertal development, skeletal maturation and bone mass acquisition in athletes. Hormones (Athens). 2004;3(4):233–43.
7. Davies JH, Evans BAJ, Gregory JW. Bone mass acquisition in healthy children. Arch Dis Child. 2005;90(4):373–8.
8. Prentice A, Schoenmakers I, Laskey MA, de Bono S, Ginty F, Goldberg GR. Nutrition and bone growth and development. Proc Nutr Soc. 2006;65(4):348–60.
9. Karlberg J, Jalil F, Lindblad BS. Longitudinal analysis of infantile growth in an urban area of Lahore, Pakistan. Acta Paediatr Scand. 1988;77(3):392–401.
10. Ekstrand J, Hagglund M, Walden M. Injury incidence and injury patterns in professional football: the UEFA injury study. Br J Sports Med. 2011;45(7):553–8.
11. Shields BJ. Cheerleading-related injuries to children 5 to 18 years of age: United States, 1990–2002. Pediatrics. 2006;117(1):122–9.
12. Roberts KJ, Nelson NG, McKenzie L. Dance-related injuries in children and adolescents treated in US emergency departments in 1991–2007. J Phys Act Health. 2013;10(2):143–50.
13. Jacobs CL, Hincapié CA, Cassidy JD. Musculoskeletal injuries and pain in dancers: a systematic review update. J Dance Med Sci. 2012;16(2):74–84.
14. Russell JA. Preventing dance injuries: current perspectives. Open Access J Sports Med. 2013;4:199–210.
15. Hind K, Burrows M. Weight-bearing exercise and bone mineral accrual in children and adolescents: a review of controlled trials. Bone. 2007;40(1):14–27.
16. Munoz MT, la Piedra de C, Barrios V, Garrido G, Argente J. Changes in bone density and bone markers in rhythmic gymnasts and ballet dancers: implications for puberty and leptin levels. Eur J Endocrinol. 2004;151(4):491–6.
17. Finkelstein JS, Neer RM, Biller BM, Crawford JD, Klibanski A. Osteopenia in men with a history of delayed puberty. N Engl J Med. 1992;326(9):600–4.
18. Pigeon P, Oliver I, Charlet JP, Rochiccioli P. Intensive dance practice: repercussions on growth and puberty. Am J Sports Med. 1997;25(2):243–7.
19. Steinberg N, Siev-Ner I, Peleg S, Dar G, Masharawi Y, Hershkovitz I. Growth and development of female dancers aged 8–16 years. Am J Hum Biol. 2008;20(3):299–307.
20. Bailey DA, Faulkner RA, McKay HA. Growth, physical activity, and bone mineral acquisition. Exerc Sport Sci Rev. 1996;24:233–66.
21. Burckhardt P, Wynn E, Krieg M-A, Bagutti C, Faouzi M. The effects of nutrition, puberty and dancing on bone density in adolescent ballet dancers. J Dance Med Sci. 2011;15(2):51–60.
22. Brown D, Wyon M. The effect of moderate glycemic energy bar consumption on blood glucose and mood in dancers. Med Probl Perform Art. 2014;29(1):27–31.
23. Seeman E. Pathogenesis of bone fragility in women and men. Lancet. 2002;359(9320): 1841–50.

24. Mølgaard C, Thomsen BL, Prentice A, Cole TJ, Michaelsen KF. Whole body bone mineral content in healthy children and adolescents. Arch Dis Child. 1997;76(1):9–15.
25. Amorim T, Wyon M, Maia J, Machado JC, Marques F, Metsios GS, et al. Prevalence of low bone mineral density in female dancers. Sports Med. 2015;45(2):257–68.
26. Chang G, Rajapakse CS, Diamond M, Honig S, Recht MP, Weiss DS, et al. Micro-finite element analysis applied to high-resolution MRI reveals improved bone mechanical competence in the distal femur of female pre-professional dancers. Osteoporos Int. 2012; 24(4):1407–17.
27. Parfitt AM, Travers R, Rauch F, Glorieux FH. Structural and cellular changes during bone growth in healthy children. Bone. 2000;27(4):487–94.
28. Jahreis G, Kauf E, Fröhner G, Schmidt HE. Influence of intensive exercise on insulin-like growth factor I, thyroid and steroid hormones in female gymnasts. Growth Regul. 1991; 1(3):95–9.
29. Turner CH. Three rules for bone adaptation to mechanical stimuli. Bone. 1998;23(5): 399–407.
30. Hoch AZ, Papanek P, Szabo A, Widlansky ME, Schimke JE, Gutterman DD. Association between the female athlete triad and endothelial dysfunction in dancers. Clin J Sport Med. 2011;21(2):119–25.
31. Khan KM, Bennell KL, Hopper JL, Flicker L, Nowson CA, Sherwin AJ, et al. Self-reported ballet classes undertaken at age 10–12 years and hip bone mineral density in later life. Osteoporos Int. 1998;8(2):165–73.
32. Dhillon PS, Currall V, Shannon MN. Traumatic plastic deformation of the tibia: case report and literature review. Ann R Coll Surg Engl. 2012;94(1):e30–2.
33. Weiss DS, Rist RA, Grossman G. When can I start pointe work? Guidelines for initiating pointe training. J Dance Med Sci. 2009;13(3):90–2.
34. Gerrard DF. Overuse injury and growing bones: the young athlete at risk. Br J Sports Med. 1993;27(1):14–8.
35. Stracciolini A, Casciano R, Levey Friedman H, Stein CJ, Meehan WP, Micheli LJ. Pediatric sports injuries: a comparison of males versus females. Am J Sports Med. 2014;42(4):965–72.
36. Tanner JM. Growth and maturation during adolescence. Nutr Rev. 1981;39(2):43–55.
37. Bianchi ML. Osteoporosis in children and adolescents. Bone. 2007;41(4):486–95.
38. Cromer B, Harel Z. Adolescents: at increased risk for osteoporosis? Clin Pediatr (Phila). 2000;39(10):565–74.
39. Brown DD, Challis J. Optimal nutrition for dancers. In: Krasnow D, Wilmerding V, editors. Dancer wellness. Champaign, IL: Human Kinetics Books; 2016. p. 1–20.
40. Rogol AD, Clark PA, Roemmich JN. Growth and pubertal development in children and adolescents: effects of diet and physical activity. Am J Clin Nutr. 2000;72(2 Suppl):521S–8S.
41. Kurz S, van Dyck Z, Dremmel D, Munsch S, Hilbert A. Variants of early-onset restrictive eating disturbances in middle childhood. Int J Eat Disord. 2016;49(1):102–6.
42. Kerstetter JE, O'Brien KO, Caseria DM, Wall DE, Insogna KL. The impact of dietary protein on calcium absorption and kinetic measures of bone turnover in women. J Clin Endocrinol Metab. 2005;90(1):26–31.
43. U.S. Department of Agriculture, U.S. Department of Health and Human Services. Dietary Guidelines for Americans. 7th ed. Washington DC: U.S. Government Printing Office; 2010.
44. Weaver CM, Martin BR, Plawecki KL, Peacock M, Wood OB, Smith DL, et al. Differences in calcium metabolism between adolescent and adult females. Am J Clin Nutr. 1995;61(3): 577–81.
45. Moyer-Mileur LJ, Xie B, Ball SD, Pratt T. Bone mass and density response to a 12-month trial of calcium and vitamin D supplement in preadolescent girls. J Musculoskelet Neuronal Interact. 2003;3(1):63–70.
46. Matkovic V, Heaney RP. Calcium balance during human growth: evidence for threshold behavior. Am J Clin Nutr. 1992;55(5):992–6.
47. Todd JJ, Pourshahidi LK, McSorley EM, Madigan SM, Magee PJ. Vitamin D: recent advances and implications for athletes. Sports Med. 2015;45(2):213–29.

48. Wolman R, Wyon MA, Koutedakis Y, Nevill AM, Eastell R, Allen N. Vitamin D status in professional ballet dancers: winter vs. summer. J Sci Med Sport. 2013;16(5):388–91.
49. Ducher G, Kukuljan S, Hill B, Garnham AP, Nowson CA, Kimlin MG, et al. Vitamin D status and musculoskeletal health in adolescent male ballet dancers a pilot study. J Dance Med Sci. 2011;15(3):99–107.
50. Craig WJ. Health effects of vegan diets. Am J Clin Nutr. 2009;89(5):1627S–33S.
51. Appleby P, Roddam A, Allen N, Key T. Comparative fracture risk in vegetarians and nonvegetarians in EPIC-Oxford. Eur J Clin Nutr. 2007;61(12):1400–6.
52. Lanou AJ, Berkow SE, Barnard ND. Calcium, dairy products, and bone health in children and young adults: a reevaluation of the evidence. Pediatrics. 2005;115(3):736–43.
53. Weaver CM. Should dairy be recommended as part of a healthy vegetarian diet? Point. Am J Clin Nutr. 2009;89(5):1634S–7S.
54. Nkansah N, Nguyen T, Iraninezhad H, Bero L. Randomized trials assessing calcium supplementation in healthy children: relationship between industry sponsorship and study outcomes. Public Health Nutr. 2009;12(10):1931–7.
55. Venkatraman JT, Pendergast DR. Effect of dietary intake on immune function in athletes. Sports Med. 2002;32(5):323–37.
56. Ducher DG, Turner AI, Kukuljan S, Pantano KJ, Carlson JL, Williams NI, et al. Obstacles in the optimization of bone health outcomes in the female athlete triad. Sports Med. 2011;41(7): 587–607.
57. de Vries ALC, McGuire JK, Steensma TD, Wagenaar ECF, Doreleijers TAH, Cohen-Kettenis PT. Young adult psychological outcome after puberty suppression and gender reassignment. Pediatrics. 2014;134(4):696–704.
58. Klink D, Caris M, Heijboer A, van Trotsenburg M, Rotteveel J. Bone mass in young adulthood following gonadotropin-releasing hormone analog treatment and cross-sex hormone treatment in adolescents with gender dysphoria. J Clin Endocrinol Metab. 2015;100(2):E270–5.
59. Couturier J, Pindiprolu B, Findlay S, Johnson N. Anorexia nervosa and gender dysphoria in two adolescents. Int J Eat Disord. 2014;48(1):151–5.
60. Ewan LA, Middleman AB, Feldmann J. Treatment of anorexia nervosa in the context of transsexuality: a case report. Int J Eat Disord. 2014;47(1):112–5.

Chapter 12
Psychological Issues Facing the Injured Adolescent Dancer

Miriam R. Rowan, MS and Katherine L. Wilson, MSW

Pertinent Definitions

Psychopathology: A term describing a mental or behavioral disorder.
Biopsychosocial: A view that explains causes and/or outcomes of disease as occurring through interactions between a variety of biological (e.g., genetic), psychological (e.g., personality), and social (e.g., socioeconomic) factors.
Coping skills: The methods one uses to manage under stressful situations.
Ruminative: Adjective variation on *rumination* (*n.*), which describes a means of coping with negative mood using compulsive and self-focused attention toward symptoms of distress and their causes and consequences, rather than possible solutions.
Cognitive: A term which describes mental actions or processes involved in gaining knowledge or understanding through thought and sensory experience. Cognition includes such faculties as attention, memory (both short- and long-term), judgment, reasoning, computation, problem solving, comprehension, and language production.
Drive for thinness (DT): A construct represented as a subscale on the Eating Disorder Inventory (EDI; a self-report measure of disordered eating attitudes about

M.R. Rowan, MS (✉)
PGSP-Stanford Psy.D. Consortium, 1791 Arastradero Rd., Palo Alto, CA 94304, USA
e-mail: mrowpsyd@stanford.edu

K.L. Wilson, MSW
Boston Ballet School, 19 Clarendon St, Boston, MA 02116, USA
e-mail: kwilson.licsw@gmail.com; katherinewilson@comcast.net

R. Solomon et al. (eds.), *Prevention of Injuries in the Young Dancer*, Contemporary Pediatric and Adolescent Sports Medicine,
DOI 10.1007/978-3-319-55047-3_12

body image, weight, and shape). DT includes perceptual, behavioral, and attitudinal components such as excessive concern with dieting, weight, and the pursuit of thinness.

Compensatory exercise: Unhealthy, excessive, and compulsive exercise engaged in for the primary purpose of purging calories or compensating for eating.

Multiple relationships: A term defined by the APA Ethics Code Standard 3.05 as a relationship that occurs when a psychologist is in a professional role with a person and at the same time is in another role with the same person, at the same time is in a relationship with a person closely associated with or related to the person with whom the psychologist has the professional relationship, or promises to enter into another relationship in the future with the person or a person closely associated with or related to the person, and which presents a variety of possible complications to the quality and integrity of treatment and may cause harm in some circumstances.

Stress-related growth: Positive changes, including a broadened perspective, acquisition of new coping skills, and development of personal and social resources, that may follow stressful life experiences.

Introduction

Martha Graham reminds us: "It takes about ten years to make a mature dancer" [1]. It is of great significance that these training years occur in adolescence, which is a span of time that involves rapid changes across almost every major developmental domain [2]. Developmental events, including increased independence, identity exploration, pubertal changes, cognitive limitations, and risk-taking, exert influence over the elite adolescent dancer's injury experience [2]. Indeed, young dancers who become injured must endure the consequences of this event in the midst of a period that necessitates experimentation, risk-taking, and honest self-evaluation of one's potential relative to one's dreams.

The dancer's elite training experience, which includes high-level competition and early specialization, is of great relevance to his or her response to injury, particularly if a professional career is the primary training goal. This rare achievement is granted to a select few endowed with a distinct talent profile and favorable circumstances. Early dance specialization, which follows a time-urgent path with limited room for error, demands intensive investment and sacrifice. Often, dancers prematurely separate from their caregivers for a boarding environment. The impact of early separation includes both marked advantages (e.g., independence) and weaknesses (e.g., disconnection from family of origin) [3]. Further, with such specialization the balance between life skills and academic schooling may be de-emphasized [4]. In the event of an injury, this combination of cultural and developmental factors can result in amplified psychological duress.

On the one hand, it is no wonder that injuries have been linked to ballet training attrition [5]. On the other hand, as one seasoned dancer interviewed for this chapter noted, "*Injuries are the 'wait' weight room emotionally.*" With support, a break in intensive training due to injury can become less of a setback. Rest can enable the dancer to focus on other priorities, including academic work, family connection, novel life experiences, and interaction with non-dancer peers. Moreover, injuries may present as a potential platform for *stress-related growth* [6]. It is possible that the young dancer will develop adaptive coping skills, increased resilience, improved self-care, and injury prevention strategies that he or she can carry into a fulfilling professional career.

Scope of the Problem

There is a paucity of general research on the mental health needs of adolescent dancers, as well as the specific relationship between injury and psychopathology. To date, literature on this population has focused largely on eating disorders (ED) and the *female athlete triad* [7]. Beyond the prevalence of ED, domains of psychopathology have been insufficiently examined in pre-professional ballet dancers. In lieu of rigorous epidemiological evidence, clinicians working with this population must rely on rates of psychopathology among adolescents in general and the few small studies that have been conducted on dancers.

Among a large sample of male and female adolescents aged 13–18 (National Comorbidity Survey Replication–Adolescent Supplement), there is a lifetime prevalence rate of 49.5% for teens meeting DSM-IV criteria for at least one disorder, with anxiety and mood disorders (including unipolar depression, dysthymia, and bipolar disorder) most commonly represented [8]. Moreover, approximately 40% of teens meeting the criteria for one mental disorder also met criteria for at least one other disorder from another diagnostic class [8]. Given the high prevalence of ED in preprofessional dancers coupled with the prevalence of mood and anxiety disorders in the adolescent general population, we might suspect frequent comorbidity of a mood or anxiety disorder in conjunction with ED symptomatology.

Small experimental and case studies utilizing dancers illustrate some biopsychosocial nuances of the adolescent dancer's injury experience. Such nuances include characteristics of the injury. Specifically, it appears that dancers with chronic or overuse injuries tend to ignore their injuries despite potential consequences ranging from psychological distress to severe physical damage [9].

Pre-existing psychological vulnerabilities may exert influence over the young dancer's reaction to injury, for example, the presence of a pre-existing mental illness (e.g., depression) [10] may impede recovery from injury. Given the prevalence of mental illness in adolescence [8], it follows that injured adolescent dancers may be at least equally vulnerable to the development of mental health issues. It has been suggested, however, that a flexible versus rigid approach to dance activities when injured and engagement in self-motivated injury prevention behaviors are associated with lower rates, duration, and overall suffering from injuries during training [11].

Beyond a dancer's pre-existing vulnerabilities, his or her post-injury behavioral and psychological reactions to injury can also impact the injury experience. Indeed, injuries may threaten one's sense of self [9] and induce ruminative concerns regarding one's self-worth and status in a highly competitive training environment [12]. Such emotional and cognitive reactions can lead certain dancers to deny or hide an injury or return to training prematurely due to his or her drive for success and fear of falling behind classmates and missing opportunities. Implicit efforts to avoid identity disruption and cultural acceptance of pain may additionally exert influence over decisions to train while injured [9]. Notably, most professional dancers do not seek medical attention for their injuries [12], and 28% of professional dancers in one sample reported making a unilateral decision to return to work prematurely [13]. Given inherent adolescent immaturity in foreseeing the consequences of one's behavior, it is possible that pre-professional dancers would also have high rates of premature return to training. Further, among typical adolescents there exists an adolescent *health paradox* [14], which describes marked increases in morbidity and mortality despite peak physical health due to factors such as immature impulse control and decision-making capacities. This paradox can have notable implications for the adolescent dancer's rehabilitation behavior. Factors such as lack of insight into the consequences of dancing injured can further the denial of injury, treatment non-compliance, and a premature return to training.

In addition to the dancer's pre-existing vulnerabilities and post-injury reactions, negative environmental circumstances can also impact the injury experience. Such circumstances have been observed to significantly predict subsequent injuries among ballet dancers [15]. In the midst of negative life events, lack of proper social support appears to further increase vulnerability to injury in young dancers [15].

Diagnoses

These authors have observed a variety of clinical and subclinical presentations of mental suffering accompanying injury in the young dancer. Below, we illustrate diagnostic features of psychopathology and problem behaviors that we have anecdotally observed occurring with dance injury. These include *Adjustment Disorder, Major Depressive Disorder, Anxiety Disorders, Eating Disorders, and Substance Use Disorders.*

A diagnosis of *Adjustment Disorder* is the most conservative diagnosis for many young dancers who initially present with mood and anxiety symptoms following injury. Injury may prompt concerns regarding one's career potential and produce a void in the dancer's activity schedule and social support. Recovery activities take immediate precedent over his or her cohort's regular training schedule. This loss of community at a time when peer relations are developmentally necessary can amplify threats to the adolescent dancer's identity and prompt feelings of isolation. Further, when seeking support from classmates, the injured dancer may experience a paradoxical combination of closeness and competition, which can serve to exacerbate emotional reactions including depression and anxiety. While these depressed and anxious symptoms fall under the diagnostic domain of Adjustment Disorder, a full-blown Major Depressive Episode or Anxiety Disorder may occasionally emerge, as illustrated in the following case:

> Amy[1] is a 17-year-old female pre-professional dancer living in a residential ballet program far from home. Her dance training occurs upward of six hours per day. For the past 6 months she has been struggling with plantar fasciitis. Amy initially managed her pain by skipping classes as needed. Feeling overwhelmed because her pain 'just won't go away', she now presents to her school's on-site psychotherapist. A cascade of tears overcomes her as she describes her intense fear of losing precious time while unable to dance as fully as she wants to and sadness at not being able to be with her family during this difficult time. She additionally reports an inability to concentrate, has been withdrawing from her peers, and feels alone in her struggle.

The emergence of *Major Depressive Disorder (MDD)* has been anecdotally observed in our work with pre-professional dancers. MDD occurs in 4–8% of adolescents [2] and is characterized by frequent crying, irritability, diminished interest or pleasure in regular activities, disrupted sleep and appetite, and social withdrawal [16]. Identification of depressive symptoms in young dancers can be particularly challenging due to their high level of functioning, gritty nature, and active attempts to conceal injury from teachers and treatment providers. Nonetheless, such depressive symptoms may induce significant suffering, interfere with daily functioning, and potentially introduce additional problem behaviors such as self-harm (e.g., cutting and unsafe sex) and substance abuse [2]. Thus, MDD symptoms warrant swift identification and treatment.

Anxiety disorders, including *Generalized Anxiety Disorder, Panic Disorder, Social Anxiety Disorder,* and *Specific Phobia* [16], represent the most common cluster of psychiatric disorders occurring in adolescents, with nearly one in three teens experiencing a lifetime occurrence [8]. Anxiety typically represents a reaction to and subsequent avoidance of a feared event in the future. Given the dancer's goal-directed nature, an injury can precipitate excessive, future-focused worries related to such issues as teacher, classmate, or parental perceptions, compromised career potential, reinjury, or failed recovery.

Eating disorders (ED), which include *anorexia nervosa (AN), bulimia (BN),* and *binge eating disorder*, are characterized by abnormal eating behaviors that drive destructive, potentially life-threatening behaviors [16]. According to the Adolescent Supplement of the National Comorbidity Study, the lifetime prevalence of an ED is 2.7% across genders, with double the occurrence in females (3.8%) versus males

[1] *de-identified.*

(1.5%), and slight increases in prevalence with age [8]. Given the ballet aesthetic (e.g., "anorexic ideal") [4] and the high valuation of body shape and size, it is widely believed that eating disorders occur more readily in dancers versus non-dancers. A recent meta-analysis of studies conducted on male and female professional and pre-professional dancers [17] noted the prevalence rate of ED among female ballet dancers at 16.4% (4% for AN, 2% for BN, and 14.9% for *ED not otherwise specified*, per DSM-IV criteria).

In the context of injury, measures of body dissatisfaction, drive for thinness, bulimic tendencies, and perfectionism have been observed to be significantly higher in injured versus non-injured advanced pre-professional dancers [18]. Indeed, given that injury can impose weeks to years of inactivity and loss of control on a dancer, it is clear that vulnerability to developing disordered eating behaviors and poor body image is heightened post-injury. Further, adolescent dancers and their teachers often perceive typical pubertal changes in weight and shape as a "make-or-break" moment along the professional ballet career path [19]. Coupled with fears of weight gain and loss of technique when injured, it is likely that adolescent dancers may be prone to additionally poor body image when injured [12]. As dancers may tend toward over reliance on external (e.g., teacher) cues [20], students may fear "falling out of favor" with a prized teacher and resort to extreme measures (i.e., disordered eating and dancing with injury) to avoid such threats to their career and identity. The following case illustrates pressures and expressions of ED in the context of injury:

> Patricia[2] is a 16-year-old female advanced pre-professional ballet dancer who reports never feeling her body adhered to her elite program's ideal. Struggling with weight gain following 6 months of weekly episodes of binge eating she sustains a knee injury, which now requires her to cease training for three months. In consultation with her school's psychotherapist regarding her weight problem, Patricia minimizes her binge eating behavior and overemphasizes adherence to a strict diet and an intensive ('as long as it takes to burn it off') exercise regimen of swimming, biking, and physical therapy for injury. Nonetheless, her BN symptoms are evident when recounting an intensive compensatory late-night swimming episode following a bowl of ice cream binge that same evening. Patricia's experience exemplifies a pattern whereby poor body image, forced rest from injury, and compensatory exercise may interact in a destructive ED cycle that will persist if left untreated.

Substance Use and Abuse Disorders, including the use of alcohol, street drugs, and prescription medications, are pervasive among adolescents in the USA, with approximately 6% of adolescents, aged 12–17, having a substance use diagnosis [2]. Adolescence is a time of experimentation, and this often includes experimenting with substances. Young dancers are not immune to this behavioral pattern. For example, Hamilton [10] surveyed 300 dancers and found that 13% of those under the age of 18 self-reported instances of alcohol bingeing (i.e., 3–5 drinks in a row). Experimentation most often begins as and remains a social activity; however,

[2] *de-identified.*

harmful consequences of an adolescent's substance use can occur when he or she uses it to regulate his or her emotions under stress (e.g., parental divorce or academic struggles). Dance injury can indeed function as such a stressor. In one small study with female performers, for example, those who were injured self-reported greater use of alcohol and prescription and street drugs than non-injured performers in the sample [4]. Thus, while limited research exists regarding substance use behavior in injured adolescent dancers, there is a concern that injury-related emotional distress might prompt some adolescent dancers to abuse alcohol and drugs.

Treatment

Dance injuries can occur suddenly, such as breaking a bone, or (far more often) over the course of time, as the result of repetitive microtraumas. The young dancer may experience shock or denial at the onset of injury. At many points along the injury timeline, psychological intervention can be effective in reducing harm to a young dancer's identity, health, and career. When there is denial at onset of injury, psychological intervention can facilitate a dancer's acceptance of injury and prompt him or her to maintain appropriate contact with medical personnel. In the case of immediate injury onset, psychological intervention can be effective in helping a dancer to process psychological adjustment, stress, and grief, increase adherence to prescribed rehabilitation activities, enhance communication with third parties (e.g., medical providers, training program personnel, and parents), and problem solve logistical issues (e.g., decisions to return home to family or remain at the ballet school to observe classes).

Despite the limited number of ballet schools providing in-house psychotherapy support, this chapter's co-author, KW, has the rare opportunity of working on the front lines in treating students at the Boston Ballet School. Such an on-site counseling situation presents both advantages (e.g., accessibility) and disadvantages (e.g., complexities in protecting patient confidentiality). Nonetheless, school counseling is not a new idea and offers convenience and affordability that may be effective and preferable to many students. At the Boston Ballet School KW has taken an integrative approach. She focuses on tailoring empirically supported interventions within a unique and challenging ballet school treatment environment despite limited resources. Indeed, she has found that several such interventions can support the dancer's return to optimal physical and psychological health following injury. We enumerate a few of her most recent treatment approaches below.

Cognitive behavioral therapy (CBT) can be used to help the injured dancer function more effectively by identifying distorted thought patterns and reducing associated negative emotions and problematic behaviors [21]. This structured, concrete, and goal-oriented approach can capitalize on the dancer's signature goal-directed nature. In addition to CBT, *acceptance and commitment therapy (ACT)* can particularly help dancers shift their perspective from denial of injury to acceptance, and thus ACT may temper suffering associated with resistance [22].

Additionally, in the midst of injury-related identity crises, ACT's focus on examining one's values can be used to help the dancer find rewarding, value-congruent activities that support his or her feelings of productivity and purpose despite inability to dance. *Mindfulness-based* approaches can also provide techniques aimed at improving the injured dancer's ability to be present-focused while reducing any tendency that he or she might have to ascribe unhelpful judgments to the self, others, or the situation while en route to recovery [23]. Applicable mindfulness practices may include diaphragmatic breathing, progressive muscle relaxation, guided imagery, brief meditations, connection with nature, and body-centered practices (e.g., yoga). In addition to mindfulness, *hypnosis* techniques can be used to facilitate the dancer's understanding of the mind–body connection and help increase psychophysiological self-regulation skills [24].

The following is an example of an integrated course of treatment for an injured dance student during a 6 month recovery period:

> Celia,[3] an 18-year-old advanced level student, sustained a serious ankle sprain just before her professional audition season. Celia believed her chances of securing a company position would be hampered and she was devastated by her inability to dance at this most crucial moment in her career. Initially she reported a sense of loss regarding her physical limitations and isolation from her healthy peers. Early stages of treatment provided Celia with validation regarding her understandable reactions following injury. Although many of Celia's reactions were appropriate to the pressurized situation, CBT exercises allowed Celia to identify and reframe less helpful appraisals of herself and the situation, such as catastrophic predictions about her future. Specifically, she reinforced new, adaptive ways of thinking about her injury through daily writing assignments. In addition, mindfulness exercises were integrated into Celia's treatment to help her recognize and diffuse ongoing distress regarding loss of training time and improve her ability to exercise self-compassion in her rehabilitation process. Celia engaged in ACT work around accepting her injured circumstance. This allowed her to engage in effective problem solving to develop and embrace her recovery plan, and imbued her with a sense of predictability and control. Problem solving was useful in optimizing Celia's use of time and advocating for support in her new plan. Specifically, after several weeks following her initial recovery plan, which included watching all missed ballet classes, she found herself increasingly depressed and anxious. Observing class served as a poignant reminder that she might be falling behind her classmates. For her the mental health risks of observing all classes outweighed her school's assumed benefits. With the support of her therapist Celia reworked this element of her recovery plan and practiced means of advocating for her needs and communicating her progress to her teachers rather than simply skipping classes and avoiding her teachers entirely. Although Celia indeed missed many auditions she had hoped to attend her injury experience was improved by her active engagement in treatment. Therapy reduced some of the mental suffering she faced at injury onset and fostered her development of new coping skills. Overall, this intervention assisted Celia in achieving significant personal growth in the face of injury, and she returned to dance emotionally fortified. While some dancers may choose to seek treatment off-site to ensure confidentiality of their protected health information, Celia's experience exemplifies the benefits of staffing an on-site ballet school therapist trained in evidence-based, short-term, and dancer-sensitive treatment.

[3]*de-identified.*

Future Directions and Limitations

Several limitations and barriers to accessing necessary mental health care exist for the injured dance student. For example, gaps in knowledge regarding psychopathology among injured dancers present as ripe areas for future research. Little is known, for instance, regarding the intersection between dance injuries and *somatic symptom and related disorders* such as somatic symptom disorder, illness anxiety disorder (hypochondriasis), and factitious disorder (malingering) [16]. Although the assessment of malingering, a disorder motivated by secondary gains, has been considered in other athletic populations [25], it is not clearly understood in dance students. In addition, little is known about possible intersections between abuse of prescription painkillers and dance injuries.

Beyond limited research, clinical practice also has its challenges and limitations. Notably, a trend toward overvaluation of the physical body in ballet training may diminish other aspects of a young dancer's identity [26], in particular the emotional aspects of the dancer's experience and performance. Such undervaluation of emotional experience presents as a barrier to treatment provision among dance schools and treatment seeking among students. Additional barriers to treatment of young dancers include lack of understanding and wariness among dance organizations and their members regarding mental illness. Even in the general population social stigma, reflecting negative attitudes and discrimination based on mental illness [27], prevents individuals from seeking necessary mental health care [28]. As the highly competitive training climate puts dancers under a social microscope and reinforces perfectionistic striving, young dancers may be unwilling to engage in treatment for fear of being "found out". Given their rigorous scheduling, dancers may be unwilling to seek outside help and are often reliant on on-site staff and treatment providers. At the same time, fear of breached confidentiality and social repercussions can deter dancers from approaching the staff psychotherapist regarding issues of mental stress. Thus, it is incumbent upon each dance school and its on-site psychotherapist to develop a clear procedure for protecting dancer confidentiality and managing inherent multiple relationships between the on-site psychotherapist, the student, and the school, including faculty, staff, and management (who often pay for these services). It also behooves schools to consider whether a private space within the school's facilities or a nearby outside location would best suit the on-site psychotherapist's work with the students. Further, there are cases when a dancer's condition warrants outside referral (e.g., psychiatric hospitalization or specialist treatment). It benefits students when dance schools and on-site psychotherapists have an established referral network and procedures detailing involvement in transfer of care.

In addition to the logistics of confidentiality, lack of cultural competence and clinical blind spots among treatment providers can impede dancer-sensitive care. For example, idealization of dancers [29] may bias parents, friends, and clinicians such that they are unable fully to acknowledge, understand, or support the distinct challenges faced by this unique population.

Pre-professional dancers, who are after all minors, may have less insight into and power to act upon their best interests regarding their health care following injury. Informed parents and medical providers can be an essential force for advocacy. Such adult third parties can provide outreach and consultation with dance teachers, directors, and organizations where the benefits of addressing the emotional components of the young dancer are concerned. Given budgetary constraints in the performing arts, limited resources are first allotted to physical therapist and physician services. Mental wellness services are often considered less necessary. These constraints warrant creative, accessible, and affordable means of supporting young dancer's mental health when injured. Augmenting individual counseling services with, for example, preventative educational workshops, faculty and staff training, and new technology (e.g., Web-based interventions; iPhone apps) may broaden the reach of those services.

Summary

Early specialization of the pre-professional ballet dancer occurs during the height of adolescence. Dance injuries occurring during this crucial phase of training can prompt additional mental health challenges. Further, pre-existing psychological vulnerabilities, post-injury reactions, and negative social and environmental circumstances can influence each dancer's injury experience. There is a paucity of research on the specific mental health needs of adolescent dancers and the relationship between dance injury and psychopathology. Nonetheless, some young dancers who experience injury have been anecdotally observed to develop psychopathology and problem behaviors such as Adjustment Disorder, Major Depressive Disorder, Anxiety Disorders, Eating Disorders, and Substance Use Disorders. At many points along the injury timeline, psychological intervention can be effective in reducing harm to a young dancer's identity, health, and career. Drawing on evidence-based psychological therapies a short-term, empirically supported, and dancer-sensitive treatment approach has been used to address the stress and psychopathology emerging from a dancer's injury experience. With psychological support the young dancer may be able to develop adaptive coping skills, increased resilience, improved self-care, and injury prevention strategies that he or she can carry into a fulfilling professional career.

References

1. Graham M. Blood memory: an autobiography. New York: Doubleday; 1991. p. 4.
2. Steiner H, Hall RE. Treating adolescents. Hoboken, NJ: Wiley; 2015. p. 5, 142.
3. Schaverien J. Boarding school syndrome: broken attachments a hidden trauma. Br J Psychother. 2011;27(2):138–55.

4. Hamilton LH. The person behind the mask. Greenwich: Ablex Publishing Corporation; 1997. p. 27–97.
5. Hamilton LH, Hamilton WG, Warren MP, Keller K, Molnar M. Factors contributing to the attrition rate in elite ballet students. J Dance Med Sci. 1997;1(4):131–8.
6. Park CL, Fenster JR. Stress-related growth: predictors of occurrence and correlates with psychological adjustment. J Soc Clin Psychol. 2004;23(2):195–215.
7. Herbrich L, Pfeiffer E, Lehmkuhl U, Schneider N. Anorexia athletica in pre-professional ballet dancers. J Sports Sci. 2011;29(11):1115–23.
8. Merikangas KR, He JP, Burstein M, Swanson SA, Avenevoli S, Cui L, Benjet C, Georgiades K, Swendsen J. Lifetime prevalence of mental disorders in US adolescents: results from the National Comorbidity Survey Replication-Adolescent Supplement (NCS-A). J Am Acad Child Adolesc Psychiatry. 2010;49(10):980–9.
9. Mainwaring LM, Krasnow D, Kerr G. And the dance goes on psychological impact of injury. J Dance Med Sci. 2001;5(4):105–15.
10. Hamilton LH. Advice for dancers: emotional counsel and practical strategies. San Francisco: Jossey-Bass; 1998. p. 76, 134.
11. Rip B, Fortin S, Vallerand RJ. The relationship between passion and injury in dance students. J Dance Med Sci. 2006;10(1–2):14–20.
12. Krasnow D, Kerr G, Mainwaring L. Psychology of dealing with the injured dancer. Med Probl Perform Art. 1994;9(1):7–9.
13. Macchi R, Crossman J. After the fall: reflections of injured classical ballet dancers. J Sport Behav. 1996;19(3):221–34.
14. Dahl RE. Adolescent brain development: a period of vulnerabilities and opportunities. Ann N Y Acad Sci. 2004;1021:1–22.
15. Patterson EL, Smith RE, Everett JJ, Ptacek JT. Psychosocial factors as predictors of ballet injuries: interactive effects of life stress and social support. J Sport Behav. 1998;21(1):101–12.
16. American Psychiatric Association, editors. Diagnostic and statistical manual of mental disorders (DSM-5®). Arlington, VA: American Psychiatric Association Publishing; 2013.
17. Arcelus J, Witcomb GL, Mitchell A. Prevalence of eating disorders amongst dancers: a systemic review and meta-analysis. Eur Eat Disord Rev. 2014;22(2):92–101.
18. Liederbach M, Compagno JM. Psychological aspects of fatigue-related injuries in dancers. J Dance Med Sci. 2001;5(4):116–20.
19. Mitchell SB, Haase AM, Malina RM, Cumming SP. The role of puberty in the making and breaking of young ballet dancers: perspectives of dance teachers. J Adolesc. 2016;47:81–9.
20. van Staden A, Myburgh CP, Poggenpoel M. A psycho-educational model to enhance the self-development and mental health of classical dancers. J Dance Med Sci. 2009;13(1):20–8.
21. Beck JS. Cognitive behavior therapy. New York: Guilford Press; 2011. p. 10.
22. Hayes SC. Get out of your mind and into your life. Oakland: New Harbinger Publications; 2005. p. 2.
23. Pollack SM, Pedulla T, Siegel RD. Sitting together: essential skills for mindfulness-based psychotherapy. New York: Guilford Press; 2014. p. 5.
24. Fromm E, Nash MR. Contemporary hypnosis research. New York: Guilford Press; 1992. p. 307.
25. Rotella RJ, Ogilvie BC, Perrin DH. The malingering athlete: psychological considerations. In: Pargman D, editor. Psychological Bases of sport injuries. 2nd ed. Morgantown: Fitness Information Technologies; 1999. p. 111–22.
26. Wainwright SP, Williams C, Turner BS. Fractured identities: injury and the balletic body. Health. 2005;9(1):49–66.
27. Corrigan PW, Markowitz FE, Watson AC. Structural levels of mental illness stigma and discrimination. Schizophr Bull. 2004;30(3):481–91.
28. Corrigan P. How stigma interferes with mental health care. Am Psychol. 2004;59(7):614–25.
29. Friedler SE, Glazer S. Dancing female: lives and issues of women in contemporary dance. Amsterdam: Harwood Academic Press; 1997. p. 243.

Chapter 13
Preventing Degenerative Hip Injuries from a Dance Technique Perspective

Ruth Solomon Professor Emerita

Pertinent Definitions

Stenosing tenosynovitis: Tenosynovitis refers to a painful inflammatory condition involving the synovial sheath of a tendon. Stenosing tenosynovitis is a specific entity in which a tendon no longer runs smoothly in its sheath, the result of inflammation, swelling, and microtrauma caused by repetitive forceful compression, tensile stress, and resistive flexion.
Iliopsoas tendinitis: *Iliopsoas tendinitis* is an inflammation of the *tendon* or area surrounding the *tendon*. Major causes are acute trauma and overuse resulting from repetitive hip flexion.
Snapping hip: Snapping hip, or coxa saltans, is a general term that describes a snap or click in the hip that occurs with certain movements such as flexion and extension (raising and lowering) of the whole leg or rotation (twisting) of the hip. Tendinitis, or inflammation of the iliopsoas tendon, is a common cause.
Acetabulum: A concave surface of the pelvis. The head of the femur meets the pelvis at the acetabulum, forming the hip joint.
Acetabular labrum: The *acetabular labrum* is a ring of cartilage that surrounds the acetabulum of the hip. It provides an articulating surface for the acetabulum, allowing the head of the femur to articulate with the pelvis. The anterior portion is most vulnerable to labrum tears.
Acetabular dysplasia: Acetabular dysplasia is a condition defined by inadequate development of the acetabulum, which is shallow and dish-shaped rather than cup-shaped.

R. Solomon (✉)
Professor Emerita
Department of Theater Arts, University of California, Santa Cruz, CA 95064, USA
e-mail: ruthsol@ucsc.edu

R. Solomon et al. (eds.), *Prevention of Injuries in the Young Dancer*,
Contemporary Pediatric and Adolescent Sports Medicine,
DOI 10.1007/978-3-319-55047-3_13

Iliofemoral ligament: The iliofemoral ligament is a Y-shaped band of very strong fibers that connects the lower front iliac spine of the coxal bone to a bony line (intertrochanteric line) extending between the greater and lesser trochanters of the femur (thigh bone). The iliofemoral ligament is the strongest ligament in the body.
Pubofemoral ligament: The *pubofemoral* (or pubocapsular) *ligament* is a ligament on the inferior side of the hip joint. It is attached, above, to the obturator crest and the superior ramus of the pubis; below, it blends with the capsule and with the deep surface of the vertical band of the iliofemoral ligament. This ligament prevents hyper-abduction of the hip joint.
Ischiofemoral ligament: Is the only ligament located on the posterior aspect of the hip. It attaches to the posterior surface of the acetabular rim and labrum. This ligament is said to "wind" around the joint and insert on the anterior aspect of the femur. It reinforces the joint capsule posteriorly and guards against excessive extension and internal rotation of the hip joint.
Microinstability: If the femoral head and its center of rotation translate, with or without rotation, the inherent stability of the femoroacetabular articulation may be compromised. Microinstability may be the cause or the effect of several other hip pathologies.
Vacuum sign: It represents a subluxation of the femoral head due to a lever mechanism between the femoral neck and the acetabular rim, and is, therefore, suggestive of a relevant femoroacetabular impingement and hip instability. It is only visible in frog-leg lateral radiographs.
Osteoarthrosis: Osteoarthrosis of the hip is a common non-inflammatory degenerative joint disease characterized by progressive softening and disintegration of articular cartilage with associated new bone formation and capsular fibrosis. In dancers there is considerable loading of the joints, but they also have increased joint laxity. Both factors may contribute to the development of osteoarthrosis.
Rectus femoris tendons: The *rectus femoris* muscle arises by two tendons, one from the anterior inferior iliac spine, the other from a groove above the rim of the acetabulum. The rectus femoris, sartorius, and iliopsoas are the flexors of the thigh at the hip.
Sartorius: A long, flat, narrow muscle extending obliquely from the front of the hip to the inner side of the tibia, assisting in bending the hip or knee joint and in rotating the thigh outward. It is the longest muscle in humans.
Arabesque: A movement in which the body weight is supported by one leg. The supporting leg may be straight or half-bent, while the gesturing leg is straight and extended to the rear.
Attitude: A position in which the body weight is supported by one leg. The supporting leg may be straight or bent, with the arm on the same side opened front, side, or back. The other leg is extended to the back and bent 90° at the knee.
Développé: A movement whereby the dancer's working leg is drawn up to the knee of the supporting leg and extended to an open position. The unfolding movement can be performed in numerous directions—to the front, side, the back, and in parallel position.

Rond de jambe: A circular action of the gesturing leg. It moves from first position through fourth front, second, and fourth back, and then passes through first position again. It can be performed with the toe of the gesturing leg in contact with the floor (rond de jambe à terre) or in the air (rond de jambe en l'air).

Introduction

One assumes, given the amount of attention it has received in the dance medicine and science literature, that there are few teachers of dance (especially ballet) out there who do not know by now that to require their students to achieve 180° of turnout of the feet is to ask of them something that is not only beyond the capability of virtually all of them, but is also potentially injurious. I begin with this observation because it is the best known example of the fact that a misconceived approach to the teaching of dance technique can, over time, do serious damage to the generally ever anxious to please but anatomically naïve young student of dance. The unfortunate truth of the matter is that there are innumerable other things that teachers traditionally ask of their students, and students find for themselves to do, that are equally injurious. This chapter will utilize two under-researched pathologies of the hip to expand the knowledge of medical personnel who deal with young dancers, the parents of those dancers, and the dancers themselves regarding how biomechanically unsound practices acquired in the earliest years of training can lead, through the mechanism of "overuse," to unwanted medical consequences later on.

Before moving on to specifics I offer several global qualifications. First, virtually all of the other chapters in this book are authored by either MDs or PTs, i.e., people who have spent all of their professional lives in the practice of medicine, although several of them have had some training in dance along the way. Hence, those chapters deal with dance injuries to the anatomical region in question in their entirety, and for that perspective I happily refer you to those sources. Mine has been the opposite experience; since the age of seven onward my life has been devoted to the practice of dance, and my medical experience is limited to a 36-year apprenticeship under the mentorship of Dr. Lyle Micheli. It is appropriate, therefore, that in this chapter I limit my perspective to the etiology of dance injuries, drawing largely on what I have experienced and seen over many years in dance studios, rehearsal halls, and on stage.

Second, etiology is a surprisingly complex subject, complicated by the well-established fact that the vast majority of dance injuries are attributable to the aforementioned overuse. The problem with this is that the specifics of overuse have seldom been spelled out; all too often the term is blithely used and passed over as simply referring to the fact that the development of dance technique inevitably requires endless repetition of the same movements, class after class, and that leaves moot the question of why most of the students in those classes experience few if any ill effects, while others break down and ultimately require medical attention. My own explanation of that phenomenon was described long ago: Overuse injuries in dancers occur at the point where the stress of training, rehearsals, and performance intersects with weakness in the individual dancer's anatomy. So how are the persons who oversee the development of young dancers' careers to identify those who are especially susceptible to injury? The answer to that question is multi-faceted but clear: (1) through being willing and able to see in each individual not only how well the material presented is being performed, but also how it is being executed in biomechanical, or anatomical terms; and (2) by making use of the increasingly widespread process of screening (discussed in Chaps. 2 and 3 of this book).

Lastly, it is by no means always possible to visualize the etiology of an injury in an unadulterated straight line. As dancers become increasingly committed to the art form they inevitably spend more and more of their time in practicing it. However, they also continue to participate in activities unrelated to dance, some of which may be the actual cause of, or at least a contributing factor to, an injury that is slowly becoming manifest over time. Thus, the eight-year-old who both takes dance class and plays soccer into her adolescence, at which time she develops pain in her hip, may require the services of a medical practitioner specifically trained in dance medicine to determine the actual cause of the injury, and this problem may be extended even into her twenties by dancers' traditional unwillingness to seek appropriate medical assistance for their pain. Indeed, it is not unusual for a dancer to reach the end of a career that has been marred by "dancing through pain" without ever fully understanding its cause(s).

The bottom line of this introduction is that to a greater extent than any of the previous chapters this one is based on subjective or "anecdotal" observation, supported by some of the research in the field that will be referenced where appropriate for substantiation. Nonetheless, I am hopeful that the dancer's perspective represented here will be found to add something of value to the book as a whole.

It all begins in early ballet classes, where the joy of dance and play intermingle, and motor learning skills are taught (Fig. 13.1). As the child becomes more seriously interested in dance, she (for the sake of convenience the female pronoun is used throughout this chapter) moves progressively through the hierarchy of classes and the demands become more strict and codified. If she seeks to pursue a career she will eventually need to audition for a professionally oriented school and be assessed by ballet teachers as to whether her body might accommodate to those demands. Unhappily, most youngsters "fail the test" because their potential for acquiring the requisite combination of strength and flexibility appears limited. At this point it is important to recognize that from an anatomical point of view young people develop uniquely and can grow to be effective and efficient dancers at decidedly different stages in their development. Emphatically, teachers of dance must be aware of the need not to impose a traditionally derived image onto a body that is not yet ready to assimilate it. Also, there is the humane imperative to avoid "breaking a heart" by way of a precipitous rejection.

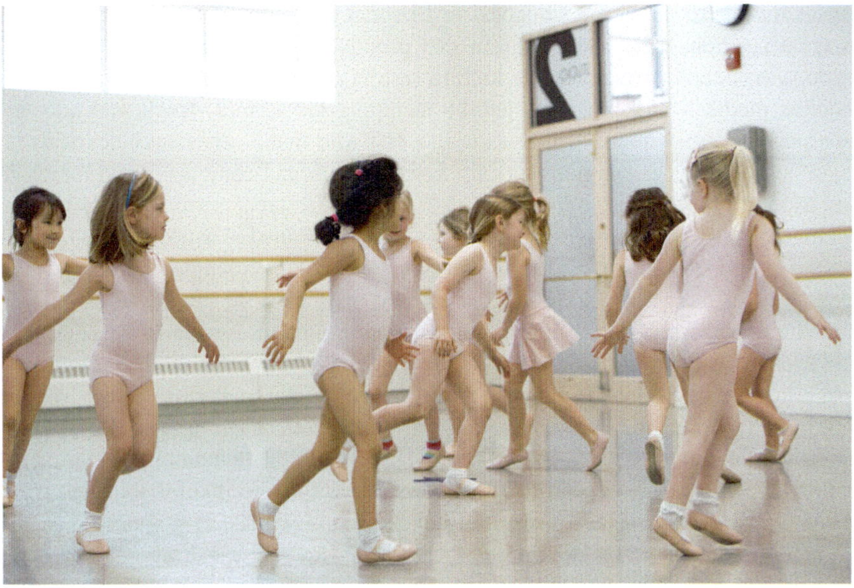

Fig. 13.1 Where the joy of dance and play intermingle. *Photo* by Igor Burlak, Courtesy of Boston Ballet School

Here I would like to emphasize that it is up to the individual dancer, especially as she progresses into adolescence, to be as informed as possible about her own anatomic and biomechanical status during all phases of training, in order to resist doing damage that may not appear until years later, or could inhibit healthy progress through a long dance career. The basic take-away message from this chapter is that one really can dance from beginning to end of a career and *beyond* without causing hip pathology.

Snapping Hip

Although it is frequently mentioned in the literature of dance pedagogy, the widespread condition known as "snapping hip" is seldom taken seriously enough to be subjected to in-depth study. Nor does it tend to receive anywhere near its proper due in the dance studio. As this syndrome is intimately associated with several highly debilitating injuries in dancers, most notably iliopsoas tendinitis and acetabular labrum tears, it seems vitally important to raise awareness of its true significance among dancers and their teachers.

Clicking and popping about the hip in athletes and dancers is a common phenomenon, and generally remains asymptomatic. In certain circumstances, however, especially where the hip is subjected to frequent and extreme hyperextension and external rotation, the same condition that produces these sounds (the "snapping" tendon) may cause pain severe enough to restrict or prohibit activity, and therefore requires medical attention. This painful snapping hip is most frequently encountered in dancers, gymnasts, and soccer players, who make very heavy demands on the iliopsoas muscle-tendinous unit for both strength and endurance, and therefore are especially prone to hypertrophy of these structures, setting the stage for derangement of the iliopsoas mechanism at the anteromedial aspect of the hip [1].

Early reports of snapping hip treated the condition as a single entity involving movement of the tensor fascia lata or iliotibial band over the greater trochanter on the lateral aspect of the hip [2–6]. With Moreira [7] and especially Nunziata [8], however, a distinction came to be made between this variety and an "internal" snapping hip experienced in the groin area on the anterior aspect of the hip. Initially, some observers suggested that this medial snapping was due to a tear of the labrum, and in some instances surgical exploration of these hips was carried out [9]. However, subsequent investigative studies, spearheaded by Schaberg et al. [10, 11], demonstrated that it results from the iliopsoas tendon snapping over the neck of the femur. This finding was subsequently replicated by several other investigators [12–14]. Deslandes et al. found that the hip movement that generates the snapping consists of bringing the hip from flexion-abduction-external rotation back to the neutral position. According to these authors the snapping is provoked by the sudden flipping of the iliopsoas tendon over the iliac muscle, allowing abrupt contact of the tendon against the pubic bone and producing an audible snap [15].

Internal snapping hip poses a greater problem for the population at risk than the external variety, as the pain associated with it tends to be more intense and therefore more debilitating. The doctors with whom I work in the Sports Medicine Division of Children's Hospital in Boston, headed by Dr. Lyle Micheli, were apparently the first to propose that this pain is the result of a stenosing tenosynovitis of the iliopsoas tendon near its insertion on the femur—essentially, an iliopsoas tendinitis [16]. Others implicate the iliopsoas bursa, which lies between the iliopsoas tendon and the anterior hip capsule [17, 18]. Whether the injury we are attempting to manage is strictly defined as a tendinitis, a bursitis, or damage done by a simple anatomical malfunction, the preferred initial treatment involves: "relative" rest; the use of anti-inflammatory medication and therapeutic modalities such as deep heat or ultrasound; anti-lordotic exercises; and peripelvic stretching and strengthening exercises, particularly of the iliopsoas, both for immediate relief and to correct the biomechanical conditions that caused the problem in the first place [1]. To this we have recently added ultrasound-guided injection, either intra-articular or into the psoas bursa (see Chap. 10 for a more complete discussion of these procedures). Ultrasound is a convenient and low-risk tool that can be used to aid in the diagnosis of common injuries seen in the adolescent dancer and as imaging guidance for diagnostic and therapeutic injections.

These "conservative" measures have generally been found to be quite efficacious [19–25], particularly if diagnosis is made early and intervention begun immediately thereafter. Unfortunately, many dancers and their teachers tend to dismiss snapping hip in its early stages as a minor mechanical problem. In other cases, ineffectual treatment which simply approaches it as an inflammatory condition, without attempting to correct the excessive tightness and muscle imbalances about the hip that precipitated it, can result in persistence of this condition to the point where chronic inflammation of the tendon sheath and bursa occurs [1]. Once this point is reached medical interventions up to and including surgery, all of which portend at the very least a prolonged rehabilitation and potentially even the end of a dance career, may appropriately be considered.

As an aside, it should be mentioned that when discussing snapping and pain about the hip one must consider the possible differential diagnosis of a labral tear, a condition that can mimic, or even exist simultaneously with, iliopsoas tendinitis [9]. Labral tears of the hip are associated with painful and unpredictable catching sensations in the groin, especially with internal rotation at 90° of hip flexion and abduction. Anderson posits that labral tears may be related to subluxations (which I discuss below in the section on microinstability) and underlying acetabular dysplasia [26]. No one has actually witnessed the emergence of a labral tear; hence, our understanding of the etiology of this injury remains somewhat theoretical [9]. On the other hand, anyone who has ever danced (especially ballet), or witnessed dance with an anatomically critical eye, will have no problem conceptualizing the mechanism of injury. Simply to stand in first or second position, with the feet "turned out" to 180°, rotates the head of the femur in the acetabulum to an extent that most people seldom experience in their daily lives. When the dancer elevates the leg through développé into the various extensions front, side, and to the rear that are an essential component of all choreography, this rotation is carried to truly unique extremes. As the dancer performs these maneuvers hundreds (perhaps thousands) of times over the course of a typical work week, it is not surprising that the labrum occasionally tears.

In medical circles there is a belief that one etiology for labral tears involves an underlying structural abnormality in the hip. While it is no doubt true that such abnormalities are often contributing factors in the development of labral tears, it is our belief that these factors are secondary to what is widely understood to be the basic mechanism of most dance injuries in general: The labral tear is just another overuse injury that results from the interplay between the dancer's unique anatomy and the extreme demands of the art form. Dancers who develop this condition are simply among those relative few whose hips could not stand up to the rigors of the daily routine, or, alternatively, whose faulty dance technique exacerbated the effect of the routine on the anatomy.

Fully fifty percent of the dancer-patients seen at our clinic over the past three years have presented for assessment and treatment of hip pain. The most frequently diagnosed injuries were labral tears, "snapping hip" syndrome (iliopsoas tendinitis), muscle-tendon strains, stress fractures, and joint disease (e.g., chondral defect, or degenerative joint disease). Labral tears were the most common, accounting for forty percent of the total hip injuries and twenty percent of injuries generally in this population [9]. In his summary of these findings, Dr. Kocher states that dancers and their teachers should be educated on reliable strategies for avoiding hip injuries. A focused rehabilitation program of peripelvic conditioning and biomechanically sound dance technique may obviate the need for operative treatment. Prevention, he says, is clearly preferable to surgery [9].

In the context of complications associated with labral tears and chondral flaps, some mention should be made of degenerative joint disease (DJD). DJD may contribute to the initial onset of labral injury in the hip. Of even greater concern is the risk to any hip in which labral damage has occurred of developing long-term DJD after the original injury has been treated. Any dancer who undergoes arthroscopic hip surgery should be aware that the relief produced thereby may be temporary; resulting DJD could cause recurrent problems at some future date [9].

As indicated previously, in its early stages medial snapping hip is usually painless, and therefore seemingly benign. It is only with repetition over time that the tendon becomes irritated and inflamed enough to stick in its sheath and sustain the tearing and scarring that characterize tendinitis. This no doubt explains in part why many dance teachers advise that snapping hip is really nothing to worry about unless it is painful. Such advice may also mask an ignorance of how to correct dance technique to eliminate the snapping. At any rate, it is widely known that dancers are prone to snapping hip, and one might well wonder why *more* of them do not progress to iliopsoas tendinitis.

Our theory is that when many dancers say their hips snap/click/pop they mean *occasionally*; that this is something they have experienced and taught themselves to avoid by subtly altering their technique when performing hip abducting movements (many dancers can intentionally snap their hips; hence, it is to some extent a controllable phenomenon). The unfortunate few who come to us with full blown iliopsoas tendinitis are those who have taken too much to heart the ill-informed injunction not to worry about the snapping until there is pain.

It should be obvious by now that in this author's view responsible dance teachers must be alert to evidence of snapping hip in their students and learn how properly to respond to it. In fact, the appropriate response is a fairly simple matter. First, take the situation seriously yourself and see to it that the student involved does the same. Second, reach a mutual agreement with that student that it will be all right for her to work at less than 180° of turnout (no matter what the other students in class are doing) until you both feel that she is ready to "go for it." Third, make a permanent part of your teaching repertory exercises that are intended to aid the student in identifying her proper placement in turnout, and provide the wherewithal to increase the height of her extension within that range. This includes specific mechanisms for extending range of motion and developing the strength (particularly of the iliopsoas muscle complex) required to achieve whatever turnout and extension are possible given the individual student's anatomical limitations. (For an extensive demonstration of such exercises see this author's video, "Anatomy as a Master Image in Training Dancers.") [27].

It is anticipated that this information will "trickle down" to those teachers and students everywhere who still do not have a handle on how to address the problems connected with snapping hip in a technique class, and have therefore chosen to ignore them in hopes that they will magically disappear. As this almost never happens, such communication should help to ward off numerous unnecessary injuries in dancers [28].

Microinstability of the Hip

Before addressing microinstability of the hip per se we need to discuss some anatomy. There are three longitudinal ligaments of the hip joint that form a helical spiral structure around the proximal femur: the iliofemoral ligament, the pubofemoral ligament, and the ischiofemoral ligament. All three ligaments help to stabilize the hip joint. In dance training these fibers sequentially twist and unwind in movements such as arabesque, attitude, développé, and rond de jambe. The iliopsoas group, if strong enough, also provides stability and assists in resisting anterior translation of the femur in the acetabulum during these movements.

Kalisvaart and Safran published a significant article in 2015 regarding the importance of recognizing the phenomenon of microinstability of the hip [29]. These authors state that this pathology has not received much attention in the past as it has a "less dramatic clinical presentation" than numerous other potential sources of hip pain. "It recently has emerged as a significant cause of pain and disability in younger patients and athletes," to which we, from clinical experience, add dancers. Microinstability begins with subtle anatomic abnormalities combined with repetitive hip joint rotation [29]. Causes may be ligamentous laxity or weakness of the musculature surrounding the hip joint, which in the case of dancers can often be exacerbated by the use of exteme stretching techniques in attempting to increase turnout. This allows for excessive range of movement of the head of the femur in the acetabulum, which can eventually lead to damage of the labrum and surrounding structures as the dancer continues to demand extreme external rotation of the joint. Once joint laxity exists, it places the dancer at greater risk for instability and potential injury. If the suction effect of an intact labrum is compromised by a labral tear or degeneration, 60% less force is required to distract the hip joint, leading to instability [30, 31]. This microinstability may result in damage to the bony and chondral surfaces, causing early degenerative changes of the hip joint [29].

Dancers are given detailed instruction on technique and asked to achieve certain "requirements" that their bodies might not be prepared to handle. However, they dutifully follow these instructions and in addition work on their own to gain flexibility and range of motion. Some of their choices may not be carefully considered. The most glaring current example is the demand by those directing "dance teams" and competitions to do "tricks" such as splits or over-splits. Young bodies are stretched into extreme ranges, particularly at the hip joint, in an effort to achieve these requirements. Another example from our clinic: A mother described a technique used in her daughter's dance class by a teacher who sat her students on the floor in a front split position and then placed a book under each foot, then another, and another, raising the legs into what is now commonly termed an over-split. One needs to ask, is there a masochistic psyche that subjects itself to this kind of training (or a sadistic one on the part of the teacher) without a thought of the outcome. Needless to say the dancer in question presented in clinic with hip pain.

In January 2016 Harris, Gerrie, et al. published an article discussing the case of a dancer presenting with deep groin pain suggestive of microinstability. The authors took plain radiographs of the dancer in a front split position, which revealed lateral femoral head translation and a vacuum sign. In this case study the dancer had pain in the split position, hip flexion, and extension with external rotation. There were clear impingement signs. They describe the imaging technique used on a bed or table and the positioning of the pelvis and femurs to achieve the best views of the hip joint. This radiographic technique may illustrate trochanteric-pelvic impingement and similar subsequent effects of subluxation. According to Harris, in addition to the musculature surrounding the hip the iliopsoas musculotendinous unit may provide stability to resist anterior femoral head translation [32].

Charbonnier, Kolo, and Duthon published a series of studies related to this subject [33–35]. Their article in 2013 involved imaging of 59 ballet dancers and demonstrated that while in the splits position all hips subluxated, and the ballet dancers had significantly more acetabular cartilage lesions and labral tears than the controls. It also showed that in certain ballet movements the mean translation of the femur in the acetabulum was as high as 4.6 mm. These authors questioned whether this microinstability would lead to early osteoarthrosis in the future [33].

(As an aside: Splits are not a necessary part of a dancer's vocabulary. They represent "tricks" that are often incorporated into competitions for whatever reason, do not contribute to the aesthetics or serious choreographic intent of what is being presented, and may indeed, as demonstrated by enough research at this juncture, prove to be injurious at least in the long run.)

There is a widespread clinical impression that dancers are more prone to hip pathologies as their careers progress, and may even have significantly increased degeneration leading ultimately to the need for hip replacement. As yet there is no study addressing this concern, but clearly one is needed. The difficulty is in tracking mature dancers once they leave the ranks of a company or professional dance in general.

The question of how to avoid arriving at this kind of condition and level of pain is what concerns us. The well-prepared teacher must help each dancer to find the optimum placement of the femur to achieve her highest développé and maximal external rotation. This is a place where the femur moves freely into extension (which is actually flexion in medical terminology) and no impingement or pain is experienced. It is probably not at 90° of external rotation for the gesturing leg, but somewhere closer to 75–80°. Once the femur flexes in abduction above 90° if the placement is correct the dancer will be able to release the rectus femoris, sartorius, and iliopsoas tendons. If the placement is not biomechanically correct for that individual those tendons will remain contracted, and snapping and popping will occur (see Fig. 13.2). Strengthening of the psoas and musculature surrounding the hip should be an essential component of training [36, 37] (Figs. 13.2 and 13.3).

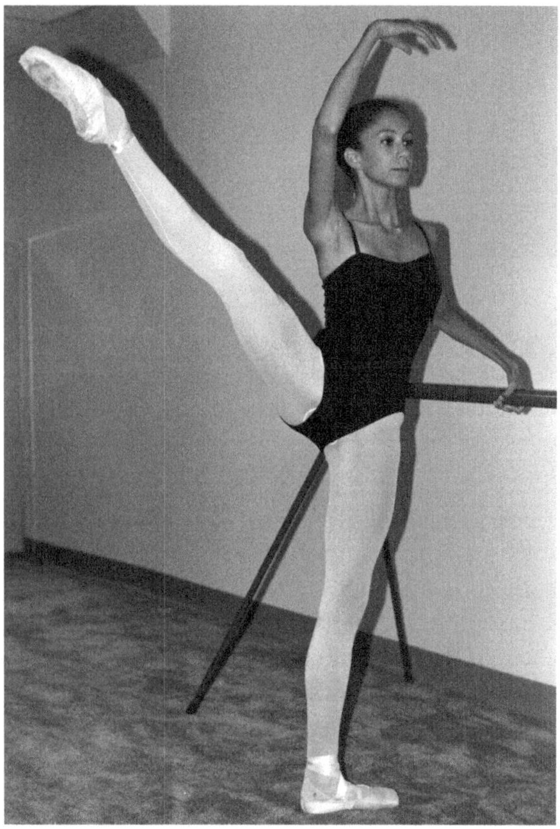

Fig. 13.2 Développé à la seconde with relatively correct placement of the gesturing leg. *Photo* courtesy of Karen Clippinger. *Model* Maurya Kerr

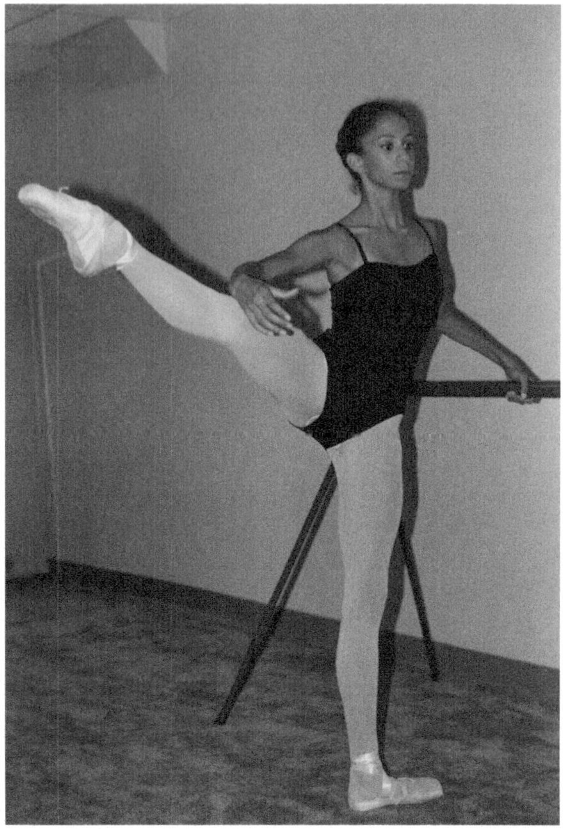

Fig. 13.3 Incorrect placement of développé à la seconde with the hip lifted and quadriceps contracted. *Photo* courtesy of Karen Clippinger. *Model* Maurya Kerr

Summary

This chapter deals with two seemingly marginal medical issues, "snapping hip" and "microinstability" of the hip, that are commonly found in dancers. The intention in doing so is to provide examples of why it is necessary to take conditions of this sort seriously and do what is necessary to correct them before they give rise to major problems. In my view those most specifically charged with assuming this responsibility are dance teachers, as they are in frequent contact with their students in situations that are under their control. This means getting beyond the traditional practice of unthinkingly teaching what one was taught, reading as much as possible of the exponentially expanding literature of dance medicine and science, and being willing to put into practice the new information that is available there. In closing, I would like to reiterate, however, that it is also up to the individual dancer to be as informed as possible about her own anatomic and biomechanical limitations during all phases of training (especially as she progresses into adolescence), in order to resist doing damage that may not appear until years later, or could inhibit healthy progress through a long dance career.

References

1. Micheli LJ, Solomon R. Treatment of recalcitrant iliopsoas tendinitis in athletes and dancers with corticosteroid injection under fluoroscopy. J Dance Med Sci. 1997;1(1):7–11.
2. Binne JF. Snapping hip (hanche a ressort; Schnellend Hefte). Ann Surg. 1913;58:59–66.
3. Mayer L. Snapping hip. Surg Gynecol Obstet. 1919;29:425–8.
4. Jones FW. The anatomy of snapping hip. J Orthop Surg. 1920;1–3.
5. Dickinson AM. Case reports by Dr. Arthur M. Dickinson. Bilateral snapping hip. Am J Surg. 1929;6:97–101.
6. Parsons EB. The snapping hip. Texas State Med J. 1930;26:361–2.
7. Moreira FEG. Anca a scatto (snapping hip). J Bone Joint Surg. 1940;22A:506.
8. Nunziata A, Blumenfeld I. Cadeva a resorte. A proposito de una variedad. Prensa Med Argentina. 1951;38:1997–2001.
9. Kocher MS, Solomon R, Lee BM, Micheli LJ, Solomon J, Stubbs A. Arthroscopic debridement of hip labral tears in dancers. J Dance Med Sci. 2006;10(3&4):99–105.
10. Schaberg JE, Harper MC, Allen WC. The snapping hip syndrome. Am J Sports Med. 1984;12:361–5.
11. Schaberg JE, Harper MC, Allen WC. Snapping hip syndrome. Adv Ortho Surg. 1985;12:340–2.
12. Harper MC, Schaberg JE, Allen WC. Primary iliopsoas bursography in the diagnosis of disorders of the hip. Clin Orthop Rel Res. 1987;221:238–41.
13. Staple TW, Jung D, Mork A. Snapping tendon syndrome: hip tenography with fluoroscopic monitoring. Radiology. 1988;166:873–4.
14. Silver SF, Connell DG, Duncan CP. Case report 550. Skeletal Radiol. 1989;18:327–8.
15. Deslandes M, Guillin R, Cardinal E, Hobden R, Bureau NJ. The snapping iliopsoas tendon: new mechanisms using dynamic sonography. AJR Am J Roentgenol. 2008;190(3):576–81.
16. Micheli LJ. Overuse injuries in children's sports: the growth factor. Orthop Clin North Am. 1983;14:337–60.
17. Staple TW. Arthrographic demonstration of iliopsoas bursa extension of the hip joint. Diag Radiol. 1972;102:515–6.
18. Lyons JC, Peterson LFA. The snapping iliopsoas tendon. Mayo Clin Proc. 1984;59:327–9.
19. Quirk R. Ballet injuries: the Australian experience. Clin Sports Med. 1983;2:507–14.
20. Sammarco GJ. The dancer's hip. Clin Sports Med. 1983;2:485–98.
21. Sammarco GJ. The hip in dancers. Med Prob Perf Artists. 1987;2:5–14.
22. Micheli LJ. Dance injuries: the back, hip, and pelvis. In: Clarkson PM, Skrinar M, editors. Science of dance training. Champaign, IL: Human Kinetics Books; 1988. p. 193–207.
23. Reid DC. Prevention of hip and knee injuries in ballet dancers. Sports Med. 1988;6:295–307.
24. Taunton JE, McKenzie DC, Clement DB. The role of biomechanics in the epidemiology of injuries. Sports Med. 1988;6:107–20.
25. Paletta GA, Andrish JT. Injuries about the hip and pelvis in the young athlete. Clin Sports Med. 1995;14:591–628.
26. Anderson K, Strickland SM, Warren R. Hip and groin injuries in athletes. Am J Sports Med. 2001;29(4):521–33.
27. Solomon R. Anatomy as a master image in training dancers. [DVD]. Santa Cruz, CA: University of California, Santa Cruz; 1988.

28. Solomon R. Addressing the 'snapping hip' in technique class. In: Solomon R, Solomon J, editors. Proceedings of the 17th annual meeting of the international association for dance medicine & science, Canberra, Australia, 2007. International Association for Dance Medicine & Science; 2007. p. 162–6.
29. Kalisvaart MM, Safran MR. Microinstability of the hip—it does exist: etiology, diagnosis and treatment. J Hip Preserv Surg. 2015;2(2):123–35.
30. Ferguson SJ, Bryant JT, Ganz R, Ito K. An in vitro investigation of the acetabular labral seal in hip joint mechanics. J Biomech. 2003;36(2):171–8.
31. Crawford MJ, Dy CJ, Alexander JW, Thompson M, Schroder SJ, Vega CE, et al. The 2007 Frank Stinchfield Award. The biomechanics of the hip labrum and the stability of the hip. Clin Orthop Relat Res. 2007;465:16–22.
32. Harris JD, Gerrie BJ, Lintner DM, Varner KE, McCulloch PC, Harris JD, et al. Microinstability of the hip and the splits radiograph. Orthopedics. 2016;39(1):e169–75.
33. Charbonnier C, Kolo FC, Duthon VB, Magnenat-Thalmann N, Becker CD, Hoffmeyer P, et al. Assessment of congruence and impingement of the hip joint in professional ballet dancers: a motion capture study. Am J Sports Med. 2011;39(3):557–66.
34. Kolo FC, Charbonnier C, Pfirrmann CW, Duc SR, Lubbeke A, Duthon VB, et al. Extreme hip motion in professional ballet dancers: dynamic and morphologic evaluation based on magnetic resonance imaging. Skeletal Radiol. 2013;42(5):689–98.
35. Duthon VB, Charbonnier C, Kolo FC, Magnenat-Thalmann N, Becker CD, Bouvet C, et al. Correlation of clinical and magnetic resonance imaging findings in hips of elite female ballet dancers. Arthroscopy. 2013;29(3):411–9.
36. Solomon R. An efficient warm-up based on anatomical principles. In: Solomon R, Solomon J, Minton SC, editors. Preventing dance injuries. 2nd ed. Champaign, IL: Human Kinetics; 2005. p. 113–4.
37. Micheli LJ, Solomon R. Training the young dancer. In: Ryan AJ, Stephens RE, editors. Dance medicine: a comprehensive guide. Chicago, IL: Pluribus Press, Inc.; 1987. p. 58–65.

Index

Note: Page numbers followed by *f* and *t* indicate figures and tables, respectively

R. Solomon et al. (eds.), *Prevention of Injuries in the Young Dancer*,
Contemporary Pediatric and Adolescent Sports Medicine,
DOI 10.1007/978-3-319-55047-3

The manufacturer's authorised representative in the EU is Springer Nature Customer Service Centre GmbH, Europaplatz 3, 69115 Heidelberg, Germany. If you have any concerns regarding our products, please contact ProductSafety@springernature.com

Printed and bound by CPI Group (UK) Ltd, Croydon, CR0 4YY
28/07/2026
02179159-0004